Cancer Modeling

STATISTICS: Textbooks and Monographs

A Series Edited by

D. B. Owen, Coordinating Editor
Department of Statistics
Southern Methodist University
Dallas, Texas

R. G. Cornell, Associate Editor
for Biostatistics
University of Michigan

W. J. Kennedy, Associate Editor
for Statistical Computing
Iowa State University

A. M. Kshirsagar, Associate Editor
for Multivariate Analysis and
Experimental Design
University of Michigan

E. G. Schilling, Associate Editor
for Statistical Quality Control
Rochester Institute of Technology

ADDITIONAL VOLUMES IN PREPARATION

Cancer Modeling

edited by

James R. Thompson

Department of Statistics
Rice University
Houston, Texas

Barry W. Brown

Department of Biomathematics
University of Texas
System Cancer Center
M.D. Anderson Hospital
and Tumor Institute
Houston, Texas

Marcel Dekker, Inc.   New York and Basel

Library of Congress Cataloging-in-Publication

Cancer modeling.

(Statistics, textbooks and monographs ; v. 83)
Includes index.
1. Cancer--Mathematical models. 2. Cancer--Research--
Statistical methods. I. Thompson, James R. (James
Robert). II. Brown, Barry W. III. Series.
[DNLM: 1. Models, Biological. 2. Neoplasm--
etiology. 3. Research--methods. QZ 206 C2146]
RC262.C29116 1987   616.99'4'00724   87-15516
ISBN 0-8247-7773-5

MARCEL DEKKER, INC.
270 Madison Avenue, New York, New York   10016

Current printing (last digit):
10 9 8 7 6 5 4 3 2 1

PRINTED IN THE UNITED STATES OF AMERICA

To my wife, Ewa, and to my mother, Mary H. Thompson

James R. Thompson

To the four women in my life: Diane, Sheryl, Marion, and Lisa,
and my parents, George and Lucille Brown

Barry W. Brown

Preface

In the "war on cancer" the primary function of biometry has been more confirmatory than innovative. So it is that statisticians have spent more time in testing whether one mode of treatment was better than another than in actually designing therapy. In this testing role, the primary response variables examined have been response rates or survival times of patients. Relatively little energy has been expended in innovative examinations of possible mechanisms of tumor origination and progression of tumors and the consequences of these mechanisms for prevention or therapy.

The role of statisticians in designing and analyzing clinical trials is essential to oncology. However, in and of itself, confirmatory statistics provides no new directions, and so has been secondary in importance to the contributions of, say, biochemistry or radiotherapy.

In a sense, biometricians have been the most conservative force in oncology. We have been the great debunkers of "quack" cures and quick fixes. Our testing protocols fulfill an almost sacerdotal role in cancer. Like a medieval *censor librorum* the oncological statistician does not engage in "theology." Rather he applies fairly standard and lengthy tests to the work of those who do.

We wonder whether biomathematics might not have a great deal more to contribute to the war on cancer. Perhaps we ought to get involved more in conjecture and speculation—even at the risk of making mistakes leading, on occasion, to heresy.

At one level, statistics is simply an orderly implementation of the scientific method itself. Someone makes a claim, and the statistician checks it for empirical plausibility. At this level, there is little necessity for the statistician to become much involved in the scientific field in which the claim is made.

But at a deeper level, the oncological biometrician can, if he is so disposed, examine the very mechanisms involved in the neoplastic process: he can attempt to model bits and pieces of that process and try to use the insights gained from his models to suggest improved means of treatment and prevention. Many will regard such a role as inappropriate, possibly presumptuous. After all, a clinical oncologist has undertaken years of biomedical training generally not experienced by the statistician or mathematician.

It might be noted in this regard that quantitative and modeling methods have been in widespread use for decades in some areas of basic sciences directly concerned with cancer, particularly in the areas of cellular kinetics and radiobiology. Many of the workers in these areas initially had training in a quantitative discipline, particularly physics. Most of these researchers learned the appropriate biological laboratory methods so that they could produce experimental results as well as the theory relating to them.

Our view is that one can indeed grasp the essentials of many biological situations without engaging in years of laboratory work in the area. On the other hand, the process of model building requires a fair amount of mathematical maturation. Experience indicates that it is easier for a biometrician to get involved in modeling than for a physician, although certainly both routes are possible, since both individuals trained in statistics and mathematics and those trained in medicine are included among the authors of the papers in this volume.

The statistician who does modeling is handicapped in that he cannot perform the experiments or collect the clinical data that will elucidate aspects of the theory. Moreover, unless he makes a reasonably major effort to acquaint himself with the current ideas of the field, he may produce models that are hopelessly naive.

The clinician or experimental scientist who does not avail himself of modeling techniques takes the risk of missing important gaps in knowledge which might be filled were he cognizant of them. He may not be able to decide between hypotheses which are easily discriminable when stated quantitatively, although very difficult to choose between using purely qualitative arguments. Also, he may draw conclusions which, when examined quantitatively, are absurd.

The obvious solution of extensive training in both biometry and a clinical or experimental discipline is not likely to be generally feasible due to the large investment of time and money required. Perhaps the best work will result from collaborations between biometricians and clinical and experimental scientists.

One of the main problems confronting the oncological modeler is the paucity of data recorded by most clinicians. Simply noting the survival times of cancer patients gives very little insight into the kinetics of cancer progression. The fault here is with the failure of biometricians to propose models which would require, say, the volumes of primary and secondary tumors. Data is collected in the light of models. A primary obligation of the biomathematician is to propose models for whch supporting data are currently unavailable or parti al but which with some effort could be obtained. The challange to biometricians to engage in speculative modeling is one which many will reject, yet it must be made. Over the last fifty years oncological biometry has mainly contented itself with ad hoc linear models using survival times and various prognostic factors. Considering the efforts expended, the results of such an approach have been poor. If biometry is to make a positive and significant impact in the war on cancer, then biometricians must break out of purely confirmatory data analysis and extend themselves to exploratory data analysis (EDA). Beyond that, they must go further into the murky depths of speculative data analysis (SDA).

This volume represents a collection of chapters dealing with a number of aspects of the oncological modeling process. Each chapter is expository and self-contained, so that a reader interested in a particular topic may proceed to it immediately. The variety of the aspects of the modeling process go from EDA to SDA to supporting algorithms. Many of the models considered will no doubt subsequently be found to be wrong. All will be found to be incomplete. That is simply the way things are in real-world science. But those who wish to begin the study of oncological modeling will find that this book presents a number of inviting paths into the subject.

The editors wish to extend their thanks to Dr. Maurits Dekker, Chairman of the Board of Marcel Dekker, Inc., who proposed that the present project be undertaken, Vickie Kearn, Executive Editor, and Brian Black, Production Editor, who facilitated its progress. We wish to thank the United States Army Research Office (Durham), the National Cancer Institute and the Office of Naval Research, who supported our work, in part, under DAAG-29-85-K-0212, CA11430, and N00014-85-K-0100, respectively. The contributors to the volume are all due our thanks for their contributions and for following deadlines and predetermined composition guidelines.

James R. Thompson

Barry W. Brown

Contributors

E. Neely Atkinson, Assistant Professor, Department of Biomathematics, University of Texas System Cancer Center, M.D. Anderson Hospital and Tumor Institute, Houston, Texas

Robert Bartoszyński, Ph.D. Professor, Department of Statistics, Ohio State University, Columbus, Ohio

Barry W. Brown, Ph.D. Larry and Pat McNeil Professor of Cancer Research, Department of Biomathematics, University of Texas System Cancer Center, M.D. Anderson Hospital and Tumor Institute, Houston, Texas

Andrew J. Coldman, Ph.D. Head of Biometry, Divisions of Epidemiology Biometry, and Occupational Oncology, Cancer Control Agency of British Columbia, Vancouver, British Columbia, Canada

Kenny S. Crump, Ph.D.* Executive Vice President, K. S. Crump/ Clement, Inc., Ruston, Louisiana

Roger S. Day, Sc.D.† Research Fellow, Department of Biostatistics, Harvard School of Public Health, Boston, Massachusetts

---

Current affiliation:
*Executive Vice President, Clement Associates, Inc., Ruston, Louisiana.
†Assistant Professor, Department of Biostatistics, University of Pittsburgh Graduate School of Public Health and Associate Member, Pittsburgh Cancer Institute, Pittsburgh, Pennsylvania.

James H. Goldie, M.D. Head, Division of Medical Oncology, Cancer Control Agency of British Columbia, Vancouver, British Columbia, Canada

Birger Jansson, Ph.D. Professor, Department of Biomathematics, University of Texas System Cancer Center, M.D. Anderson Hospital and Tumor Institute, Houston, Texas

Marek Kimmel, Ph.D. Visiting Investigator, Investigative Cytology Laboratory, Memorial Sloan-Kettering Cancer Center, New York, New York

Daniel R. Krewski, Ph.D. Chief, Biostatistics and Computer Applications, Environmental Health Directorate, Health and Welfare Canada, Ottawa, Ontario, Canada

Duncan J. Murdoch, B. Math., M. Sc. Statistical Analyst, Environmental Health Directorate, Health and Welfare Canada, Ottawa, Ontario, Canada

George W. Swan, B.Sc., Ph.D. Consultant, Biomedicine and Bioengineering, Edmonds, Washington

Howard D. Thames, Jr., Ph.D. Professor, Department of Biomathematics, University of Texas System Cancer Center, M.D. Anderson Hospital and Tumor Institute, Houston, Texas

James R. Thompson, Ph.D. Professor and Chairman, Department of Statistics, Rice University, Houston, Texas

Susan L. Tucker, Ph.D. Assistant Professor, Department of Biomathematics, University of Texas System Cancer Center, M.D. Anderson Hospital and Tumor Institute, Houston, Texas

Contents

Cancer Modeling

1
Intracellular Electrolytes and their Role in Cancer Etiology

BIRGER JANSSON *University of Texas System Cancer Center,*
M.D. Anderson Hospital and Tumor Institute, Houston, Texas

I. INTRODUCTION

Scientific work generally proceeds along similar avenues. It starts
with observations generated by the researcher or obtained from the
literature. Regularities noticed in the observations lead to the formulation of hypotheses. The validity of these hypotheses can be tested
either by experiments designed directly for that purpose or by results
obtained from further and more extensive literature search. If we
assume that a hypothesis is true, some of its consequences can be
deduced and used for further testing (similarly to corollaries deduced
rigorously from theorems). In an inductive way the hypotheses may
also lead to formulations of other possible and probable consequences
(in the same way as, from known mathematical relations, we can
inductively guess that other relations might be true and ready for
testing). Confirmatory tests increase our beliefs in the hypotheses;
refutory results force us to modify our hypotheses or maybe even to
abandon them. Our knowledge increases, and the hypotheses converge
toward a refined hypothesis, which might evolve into a theory, by
this switching between confirmations and refutations. From a practical
point of view the philosophical discussion of what is most important—
"verifications" or "refutations," a discussion introduced by Popper
[1,2] and, for epidemiological theory building, commented on by
Maclure [3]—is of little interest even if one must admit that refutations
are more important because by limiting and modifying they make the

hypotheses more specific. It often happens not least within biology and medicine that a hypothesis has been found to be almost unrefutable, and still the mechanisms behind it are not understood. It may take a long time before the final step is taken and the explanation reached.

We thus find that the scientific procedure includes

1. Observations
2. Formulations of hypotheses
3. Testing
4. Improvements of the hypotheses in an iterative process involving tests and modifications
5. Explanations of the mechanisms

All observations and results of the different steps in the procedure shall be reported, even if they are negative, and the different phases documented until eventually the explanatory report is published and accepted. This is well expressed by Shimkin [4]: "Research should begin and end in a library."

Most often, different researchers are involved in the different steps. As an example, let me remind you of the development of our knowledge of the laws of planetary motion. The Danish astronomer Tycho Brahe painstakingly observed and recorded the positions of the planets as functions of time. This was almost his lifelong work. Later, his student Kepler entered. He plotted the paths of the planets and inductively found, formulated, and tested the laws of the planetary movements, which are now named after him. Kepler, however, could not explain the laws. The explanation had to wait for more than half a century, when Newton, using his gravitational theories, could show why Kepler's laws describe planetary motions. In biology the development of the Mendelian laws in genetics follows the same pattern. After making his own experiments and interpreting the observed results Mendel could formulate his laws. They were published in 1865 but were forgotten and then discovered by other researchers in 1900. A first explanation was presented by Sutton in 1903, based on the knowledge of chromosomes, which had evolved since Mendel's time. A final (?) explanation, however, was not possible until Watson and Crick in 1953 published their model of the DNA molecule. We conclude that a model or a theory can be "true" and usable long before it is fully understood. If we know that moving a lever down always moves another lever up and that moving the first lever up always moves the second one down, the mechanism hidden in the black box between the two levers does not need to be known in order to use this apparatus. Human nature and curiosity will, however, sooner or later produce the explanation.

Biological and medical problems are often vast and comprehensive, seemingly more so today than yesterday. Understanding cancer is a typical example. Knowledge is needed in a number of areas to attack

such problems. Therefore myriads of specialists are working on different parts of problems and publishing their results in myriads of
articles. To build bridges between the high narrow peaks on which
these specialists are sitting, another type of researcher is needed. Let
us call this type a generalist. The tasks of a generalist are to find the
common denominators among the specialized results and bring them
together into comprehensive hypotheses, models, or theories. Generalists often have to filter the specialized information to retain only the
parts most relevant for the comprehensive model. They also have to
find and retrieve information from a number of different subjects
sometimes seemingly unrelated to the main problem. Mathematicians or
mathematically oriented persons are often most suitable for such gener-
alistic approaches. They are, by education and traits, used to finding
relations among observed data sets and to formulating hypotheses.
Their roles in scientific teams are thus, above all, to use observed
data to construct hypotheses and to suggest experiments for testing
the hypotheses. Burkitt [5] has compared epidemiological work with
trying to assemble a giant jigsaw puzzle. This is a good picture,
which shows the specialists as producers of the puzzle pieces and the
generalists as the ones who try to assemble the puzzle. They are
equally important. Without the pieces the puzzle can never be assembled,
and without anyone to take the scattered pieces and assemble them
into a complete picture the puzzle will remain unsolved. A further
complication is that some pieces may not have been produced. The
generalists can in such cases point out for the specialists where the
puzzle has holes that must be filled before the final solution is reached.
And now comes the time for the specialists to enter again and to
finally give the biological explanation to the relations found by the
generalists. All the team members play important roles in solving the
problem. The persons who give the final explanation undoubtedly are
the ones most honored. Newton's explanation of the mechanics behind
Kepler's laws must be considered superior to Kepler's inductively
found formulations, which in turn shine brighter than Tycho Brahe's
collection of data. Likewise more honor falls on Watson, Crick, and
Sutton, who explained the biological mechanisms behind Mendel's laws,
than on Mendel himself, who merely observed the data and formulated
the laws. But again all three types of members of the scientific team—
the data producers, the hypotheses formulators, the explanators—are
necessary to attain the final solution.

Many pieces are known in the cancer puzzle. Some are

Some chemical compounds cause cancer in animals.
Dietary fats increase the risk of cancer.
Smoking increases the risk of cancer.
Alcohol intake increases the risk of cancer and acts synergistically
    with smoking.

Salt-cured meat increases the risk of cancer.
Salt increases the risk of gastric cancer.
Sunlight increases the risk of skin cancer.
Obesity increases the risk of cancer.
Aging increases the risk of cancer.
Patients with some diseases are at higher risk of cancer.
Patients with some other diseases are at lower risk of cancer.
Dietary intake of vegetables reduces the risk of cancer.
Dietary intake of fruit reduces the risk of cancer.
The trace element selenium (Se) reduces the risk of cancer.
Dietary intakes of vitamins A and C reduce the risk of cancer.
Dietary intake of fiber reduces the risk of cancer.

Can all these disparate pieces be brought together into one comprehensive picture?

This chapter describes the development of a hypothesis that combines all these pieces and acts as a common denominator for all these observations. This hypothesis states the following:

Intracellular sodium (Na) is positively associated with cancer.
Intracellular potassium (K) is negatively associated with cancer.
The ratio intracellular K/intracellular Na is negatively associated
    with cancer and, in this respect, more important than each
    of the elements.

This hypothesis arose from studying the geographic distribution of colorectal cancer and finding a region unexpectedly low in this cancer. The geochemical uniqueness of the water in the region hinted at the importance of the Na and K concentrations. The geographical findings were confirmed in other regions and led to studies of these two elements in our diet. When the dietary results were also confirmatory, other areas were included, such as gerontology, changes due to differences in oxygen pressure (altitude dependencies), hyper- and hypokalemic diseases, electrolyte differences between healthy cells and the corresponding cancer cells, results from animal experiments, etc. The work, which started in 1974, will be described mainly chronologically, however, some more recent results will be discussed in the contexts where they logically belong. The development of the hypothesis will be reported more or less as I subjectively saw it evolve.

As already pointed out, explanations of the mechanisms behind the results belong to other specialities than the one concerned with the formulation of hypotheses. Some possible mechanisms will, however, be briefly discussed. Intracellular ions influence condensation of the chromatin, transcription rate from DNA to RNA, membrane fluxes, and maybe even off/on switches of oncogenes. These explanations or others may be behind the obtained results.

II. GEOPATHOLOGY: THE FIRST LEADS

When President Nixon, in 1971, signed the National Cancer Act, an intensified war against cancer was declared under the motto, "Cancer will be wiped out in our lifetime." The increased funds for cancer research were among other projects used for the creation, in 1973, of three organ site projects for studies of large bowel cancer, bladder cancer, and prostate cancer. These three projects were later increased by a project for pancreatic cancer.

The Headquarters for the National Large Bowel Cancer Project was located at the M. D. Anderson Hospital and Tumor Institute in Houston, Texas, under the guidance of the late Dr. Murray M. Copeland, who became its project director. A biomathematical unit was included in the headquarters from the very beginning. Besides automation of the project's administrative routines, and participation in the review processes of grant applications, the unit became engaged in epidemiological studies. This occurred partly because grant applications in carcinogenesis were dominant and partly because of a feeling that the epidemiology of large bowel cancer could lead to an increased knowledge of the etiology of the disease and then to possible preventive actions. In 1974 research on the identification of possible carcinogens strongly outweighed research on prevention, and we felt that prevention ought to take a much larger part of this type of study. Also contributing to our decision to concentrate on preventive epidemiology was the 1973 Department of Health, Education and Welfare (HEW) *U.S. Cancer Mortality by County, 1950—1969* [6], which was one of the tools we needed. From my monthly report for August 1974 I quote:

> We have decided to make a survey of epidemiological data concerning incidence rates and mortality rates in different parts of the world and above all in different parts of the United States. These rates will be compared to and correlated with geographic and cultural data such as soil differences, water pollution differences, etc. Preliminary results based on the above-mentioned HEW publication indicate some interesting possibilities.

Looking back at our first efforts, we see that they are characterized by a searching for suitable tracks along which the problems could be explored. We studied clusters of high- and low-rate areas for stomach, colon, and rectum cancers, both nationally and internationally, as well as statistical distributions for cancer rates over a number of regions, sex differences of cancer rates, etc. The results mainly confirmed already known results, but it gave us a platform to start from. The most important result of these first fumbling efforts was that it led to an invitation to take part in and present our results at a National Academy of Sciences workshop "Relations between Geochemistry and Diseases," held on Captiva Island off Florida's west coast in October 1974. The workshop was organized by the Subcommittee on Geochemical Environment Related to Health and Disease. The motto of the workshop coincided completely with my own ideas on how inter-disciplinary epidemiological work should be performed, and there is no doubt that this workshop played a fundamental role for our future work. A quote from the objectives of the workshop clearly points out the research direction to follow:

> How can we improve the way we select appropriate data scattered among many disciplines, governmental agencies, etc., bring them together and evaluate their reliability, make them miscible for automatic processing, determine the appropriate computer mani-pulation and the most effective form of output? With respect to output we will emphasize maps as an effective way to display information, also as a *research tool* that provides unique oppor-tunities for pattern comparison and cluster analysis in a time/place framework.

At this workshop I met for the first time Dr. Raymond Shamberger of the Cleveland Clinic, who informed me of his and others' successful experiments to reduce chemically induced cancers by administering Se compounds. For years to come Se became our greatest interest as an anticarcinogen.

Inspired by the motto from the Captiva Island workshop, we initiated a county by county mapping of colon, rectum, stomach, and breast cancers in the United States, dividing the rates roughly in quintiles. The known positive associations between colon, rectum, and breast cancers were confirmed through the great similarities of their geographic distributions. That stomach cancer had a different geo-graphic distribution was also evident. The distribution maps were presented in 1975 in our first publication in cancer epidemiology [7]. Besides showing the known high rates in the northeast corner of the United States, the colon and rectum cancer maps demonstrated that the Ohio River to the south and the Mississippi River to the west constituted rather sharp borders between high and low colorectal cancer rate areas, and we concluded that this strongly indicated that geochemical and geophysical properties must play bigger roles in car-cinogenesis than was generally believed. The dominating idea at the time was that the agents that caused colorectal cancer were found in the diet. That the rates were very different on the two sides of the rivers, even though the diets must be considered to be mainly the same, told us that factors other than diet strongly contributed to the differences in cancer rates. This was further emphasized by a study of the coefficients of variation over the states for cancers of different organs (Fig. 1). It was obvious that environmentally exposed organs

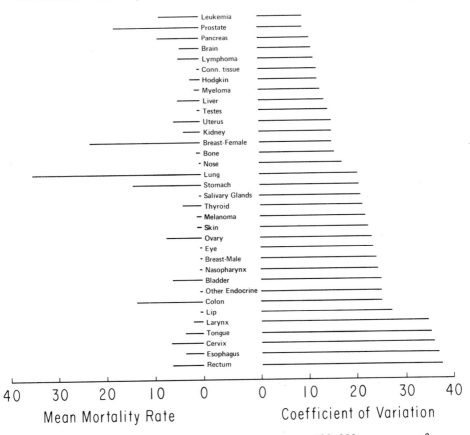

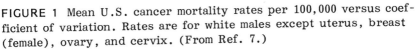

FIGURE 1 Mean U.S. cancer mortality rates per 100,000 versus coefficient of variation. Rates are for white males except uterus, breast (female), ovary, and cervix. (From Ref. 7.)

like the rectum, esophagus, tongue, larynx, lip, and colon have more geographic dependence than less exposed organs [7]. In November 1974 I wrote in my diary: "It is not the diet but a geochemical factor, which is the foremost cause of colorectal cancer."

When our maps were presented in June 1975 at a conference entitled "Trace Substances in Environmental Health," it was pointed out that the high colorectal cancer rate area north of the Ohio River and west of the Mississippi River coincided very well with the extension of the glacier at the last glaciation period about 20,000 years ago. We considered it possible that the sand, which was brought with the ice and remained when the ice melted, buried and covered some essential elements, thereby giving rise to nutritional deficiencies that

caused the increased cancer rates. Most interesting in this context
was the trace element Se. The geographic distribution of Se-deficient
areas was shown to be almost identical to the high colon, rectum, and
breast cancer ares. Since Shamberger [8] had shown that Se could
reduce chemically induced skin cancer rates and Schrauzer and
Ishmael [9], in 1974, reported that spontaneous mammary cancer in
mice could be almost eliminated by Se added to the drinking water, we
suggested that a similar study should be done with intestinal cancer.
Maryce Jacobs, a biochemist at M. D. Anderson and later a member
of the scientific cadre of the National Large Bowel Cancer Project,
challenged rats with dimethylhydrazine (DMH), a specific intestinal
carcinogen, and was able to demonstrate that Se in the drinking water
significantly reduced the cancer incidence rates [10].

Our efforts the first year were severely handicapped because the
cancer mortality data by county were available to us only as a printed
table. Not until May 1975 did we obtain from the National Cancer
Institute (NCI) a magnetic tape with the data necessary to initiate
more comprehensive studies.

The statistical fluctuations of the rates in the counties are big.
In counties with small populations, one cancer case more or less may
change the rate considerably. It is thus clear that mainly large trends
can be considered in the crude maps of cancer distributions. To combine rates from different organ sites was considered unsuitable because that would give too high a weight to an organ with a high cancer
rate. We therefore decided that rankings of the counties in rate order
from the county with the highest rate (rank 1) to the county with the
lowest rate (rank 3055) would give a better base for comparisons.
Since colon and rectum cancers for males and for females were considered to have almost identical geographic distributions, we could
reduce the statistical fluctuations by ranking the counties within each
of the four categories (male colon cancer, male rectum cancer, female
colon cancer, female rectum cancer), adding the four ranks for each
county, and then rerank the sum of ranks from the county with the
highest ranksum to the one with the lowest ranksum. This procedure
cuts the statistical deviations in half. Refined maps were constructed,
using the reranked ranksums, and the results were striking. Almost
all the 600 counties highest in colorectal cancer were located north of
the Ohio River and east of the Mississippi River. The borders were
now much more sharply defined than in the crude rate maps. The low
colorectal cancer area consisted of a broad band over the southeast
United States and the Rocky Mountain area. Mapping the 100 counties
highest in colorectal cancer revealed that most of them formed a band
along the New England coast from the Maine—Canada border down to
and including New Jersey. This concentration along the Atlantic coast
in the northeast United States has not been explained. The band con-

sists of highly industrialized counties in the South and nonindustri-
alized counties in the North. These maps, which were already constructed in early 1976, were not published until 1985 [11].

The same ranking procedure was used to compare colorectal
cancer rates for males and females. The results confirmed that the two
sexes have the same geographic distribution of colorectal cancer. Likewise colon cancer for males and females was compared to rectum cancer
for males and females. The geographic distributions were found to be
almost identical, with a possible tendency for rectum cancer to take a
greater proportion of the sum of these two cancers in coastal areas
than inland.

Another very important discovery, was that in Seneca County,
New York, the colorectal cancer rates were surprisingly low. Comparing
the ranks for the 3055 U.S. counties, we noted that there was a difference of more than 1000 ranks between Seneca and its neighboring
counties. This finding became the basis for our coming interest in
intracellular K and Na ions and their roles in cancer etiology. I will
return to a detailed description of the Seneca findings in the next
section.

Let me conclude this section by briefly describing a spin-off
result. Working with maps and observing possible clusters in maps are
sources of possible mistakes. For example, mark on a map the quartile
of counties that have the highest rates of some disease, it may be difficult to distinguish between real clusters and spurious ones. This
problem was solved by using a Monte Carlo technique. Clusters were
defined as connected areas of counties. Two statistics were analyzed:

1. The statistical distribution of the largest observed clusters
   in a map
2. The statistical distribution of the number of observed
   clusters in a map

The results are presented as graphs in which p-values can be read
for the number of assigned regions (e.g., number of counties with
rates higher than a given rate) and the observed size of the largest
cluster or the observed number of clusters. Such graphs were published
for the states and for Texas counties [12]. The graphs are reproduced
here as Fig. 2—5.

III. SENECA COUNTY: KEY PIECE IN THE PUZZLE

When we discovered in the early spring of 1976 that Seneca County,
New York, had exceptionally low colorectal cancer rates for males and
females, we first suspected that it could be a randomly caused artefact.
This led us to the study of other cancers in Seneca, and we then found

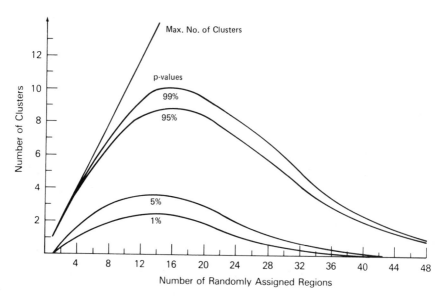

FIGURE 2 U.S. states, p-values for obtaining as many clusters or more than an observed number. (From Ref. 12.)

that, with very few exceptions, all cancers had low rates compared to other counties in New York. This is illustrated in Fig. 6 for colon, rectum, and breast cancers and for all malignancies combined.

That random orderings of the rates gives a ranksum at most equal to an observed value can be tested in the following way. Assume that we have n categories (such as colon cancer for males, colon cancer for females, etc.) and k ranks within each category (such as the number of counties in a state). Then the coefficient c_s in

$$(x + x^2 + \ldots + x^k)^n = \sum_{s=n}^{nk} c_s x_s$$

gives the number of combinations for which the ranksum is equal to s. The probability of randomly obtaining a ranksum s is then c_s/k^n, and the probability p_i that the ranksum is i or less is

$$p_i = \sum_{s=n}^{i} \frac{c_s}{k^n}$$

Since

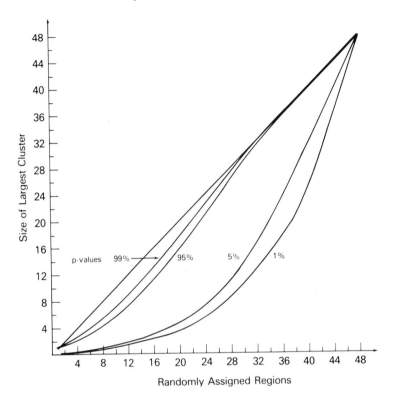

FIGURE 3 U.S. states. p-values for obtaining a largest cluster as large as or larger than the observed one. (From Ref. 12.)

$$(x + x^2 + \cdots + x^k)^n = \frac{x^n (x^k - 1)^n}{(x - 1)^n}$$

a long division can be used to determine the value of c_s. We get

$$c_s = \sum_{j=0}^{\infty} (-1)^j \binom{n}{j} \binom{s-1-jk}{s-n-jk}$$

where the summation is extended over all terms for which $s-n-jk \geqslant 0$. By symmetry, $c_{n+m} = c_{nk-m}$, showing that we can let Rank = 1 be either the highest rate or the lowest one. The double sum in the expression for p_i can be simplified. Changing the order of the summations and applying the relation

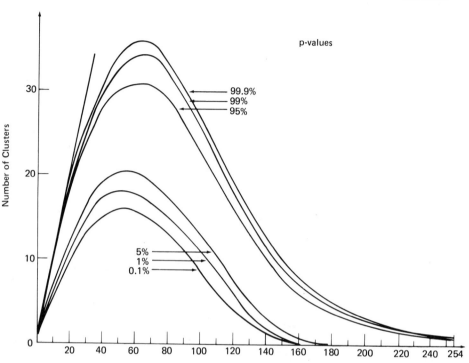

Number of Subregions (counties)

FIGURE 4 Texas counties. p-values for obtaining as many clusters
or more than an observed number. (From Ref. 12.)

$$\binom{n-1}{0} + \binom{n}{1} + \binom{n+1}{2} + \cdots + \binom{i-2}{i-n-1} + \binom{i-1}{i-n} = \binom{i}{n}$$

gives

$$p_i = \frac{1}{k^n} \left\{ \binom{n}{0}\binom{i}{n} - \binom{n}{1}\binom{i-k}{n} + \binom{n}{2}\binom{i-2k}{n} - \binom{n}{3}\binom{i-3k}{n} + \cdots \right\} \tag{1}$$

where the summation continues as long as $i - jk \geqslant n$.

For our case with colon and rectum cancers for males and females
($n = 4$) over the 58 counties in New York ($k = 58$), Fig. 6 shows that
the ranksum for Seneca is $2.5 + 1.5 + 1 + 2.5 = 7.5$, where rank $= 1$
refers to the county with the lowest rate. For $i = 8$ formula (1) gives
$p_8 = \binom{4}{0}\binom{8}{4}/58^4 = 0.000006$, and we conclude that the low colorectal
cancer rate in Seneca is not a random event.

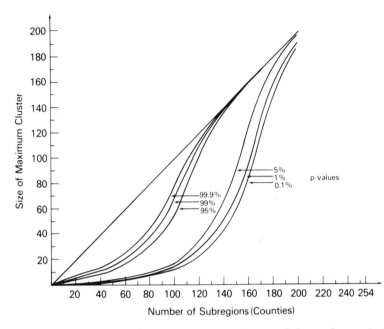

FIGURE 5 Texas counties. p-values for obtaining a largest cluster as large as or larger than the observed one. (From Ref. 12.)

In September 1983 NCI updated the cancer mortality rates by county [13]. This makes it suitable to abandon the chronological development and now discuss the updated data for Seneca County. The mortality rates are given in the new tables by decade for the 1950s, 1960s, and 1970s. The number of counties in New York is increased to 62 (k = 62) because the boroughs in New York City, which were combined in the old tables are now included as separate units. The ranks, the ranksums, and the p-values to get a ranksum as high as or lower than the observed one are presented in Table 1. This update, which has never been published, confirms and considerably strengthens the previous results. Especially significant are the low ranksums for all malignancies, rectum cancer, and breast cancer for whites. It is also remarkable that the ranksum for all malignancies of nonwhites, although there are only about 400 nonwhites in Seneca, is very low (a p-value of 0.001). For the 12 categories (2 races × 2 sexes × 3 decades) the ranksum is 55, for which the p-value is

$$p_{55} = \binom{55}{12}/62^{12} = 0.0000000001$$

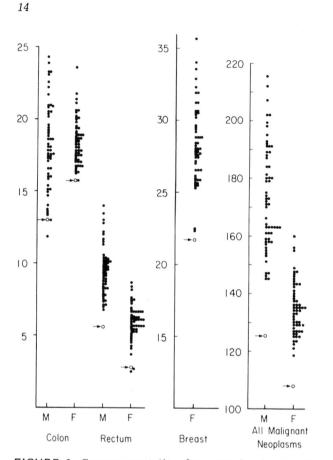

FIGURE 6 Cancer mortality for counties in New York State. ○ Seneca County. ● other counties, M = Males, F = Females. (From Ref. 16.)

The low cancer rates in Seneca were puzzling and forced us to search for an explanation. We learned that Seneca is a small rural county in the Finger Lakes region in northern New York. The population, which is declining, is about 30,000—35,000. Industries are few and small. The north-south water divider cuts over Seneca, contributing to a low pollution situation. The county is enclosed between two deep glacial lakes, Lake Seneca to the west and Lake Cayuga to the east.

Since at this phase of our study Se was highest on our list of anticarcinogenic elements, we contacted the New York State Department of Health and the United States Geological Survey to get information on the prevalence of this trace element in Seneca. The result was very promising. The Se concentration in the water in Seneca is, we

Table 1   Ranks of Seneca County among 62 Counties in New York State.[a]

	Males			Females				
	1950s	1960s	1970s	1950s	1960s	1970s	Ranksum	p-Value
All malignancies White	1	1	4	1	4	1	12	0.00000002
Colon cancer White	3	17	6	2	27	5	60	0.0009
Rectum cancer White	2	6	2	2	3	2	17	0.0000002
Breast cancer White	-	-	-	3	2	1	6	0.00008
All malignancies Nonwhite	15	12	4	1	8	3	43	0.0001

[a]Lowest rate has Rank = 1.

were told, twice as high as in New York State in general, and, very important, the soil in Seneca is alkaline, whereas it is acid almost everywhere else in the state. Alkaline soil facilitates the uptake of selenium by plants. It seemed quite possible that Se could be the explanation of the low cancer rates. A study of cancer rates in the northeast corner of the United States and their relation to selenium concentrations, however, changed our opinion on Se from being the *anticarcinogen* to being just one contributing anticarcinogen among many, and probably not the most important one. Since we knew that the colorectal cancer rates were highest in the country along the northern part of the Atlantic coast and then decreased steadily as a function of the distance from the coast, we expected that the Se concentration should be lowest at the coast and increase inland. To study this, we divided New England into four 130-mile-wide strips parallel to the coastline and estimated the average colorectal cancer mortality rate and the average Se concentration in water in each of the four strips. We had expected a negative association between these two sets of averages, but to our surprise the result was the opposite. The Se concentration was highest in the coastal strip, and then it decreased, as did the cancer rates, as the distance from the coast increased [14]. This made us conclude that even if Se contributed to the low cancer rates in Seneca, it was not a dominating factor.

The Seneca riddle remained in our minds asking for a solution.
Many attempts were made and discarded. One of these has an anecdotal
interest and may be worth mentioning. The Mormons are reported to
have low cancer rates, which is believed to be caused by their life-
style and their dietary restrictions. The state of Utah, where 75% of
the population are Mormons, has the lowest cancer rates in the United
States. This made me interested in the Mormon Church, its rules and
regulations, and its history. To my astonishment, I learned that
Joseph Smith, the founder of the Mormon Church, was born in Wayne
County just north of Seneca County. In Wayne he met the angel who
gave him the golden tablets on which the Book of Mormon is written.
Smith then moved to Seneca County, where he and his followers
interpreted the text of the tablets. When the Mormons were persecuted,
they moved from Seneca and ended up in Utah. Could it be that the
people in Seneca still followed the Mormon rules and thereby reduced
their cancer risks? To follow this possible lead, I contacted both the
Mormon headquarters in Salt Lake City and the president of the Seneca
branch of the Church. The answers were similar. Few Mormons remain
in Seneca, and the non-Mormons "do not at all live as the Mormons
do," as I was told by the head of the local branch of the Church. It
is thus only a coincidence that Seneca, where the Mormon movement
was born, and Utah, where so many Mormons live, both are outstanding
by their low cancer rates.

The contacts with the Mormon Church in Seneca, however, gave
us information on Seneca that we otherwise would not have found. A
table of the age structure in 1970 in Seneca reveals that despite an
out-migration of retired people, the people in Seneca are older than
the people in New York State, in general. Only 10% of the persons
in New York State in 1970 were over 60 years of age but the corresponding figure for Seneca was 15%. The difference in cumulative age
distributions between Seneca and New York State is very significant.
It indicates that persons in Seneca have lower mortality rates and
longer lifespans than persons in New York State, in general.

In early 1979 we again took up the Seneca problem. Reading
literature on the industries in Seneca and on saline intrusions into
the Seneca lake led us to a reference describing the limnology in North
America. One chapter in this book discussed the Middle Atlantic
states [15]. This reading became a turning point in our Seneca studies.
The author describes the Finger Lakes, and from his description the
geochemical uniqueness of the land between Seneca and Cayuga lakes
became evident. Some observations are especially important:

Seneca Lake and Cayuga Lake are deeper than the other Finger
lakes.

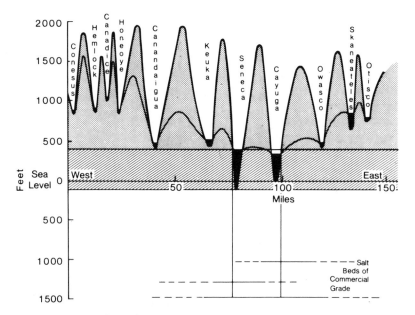

FIGURE 7 Profile of the lakes in the Finger Lakes region and of the land between the lakes. The thin line represents the land profile at the north ends of the lakes and the thick line that at the south ends (Modified from Ref. 15). (From Ref. 16.).

These two lakes are situated at the lowest elevation of the Finger Lakes region.

There are salt strata below the lakes. Salt has been mined from the shores of Seneca and Cayuga lakes (see Fig. 7).

In the Seneca and Cayuga lakes the Na + K and the Cl concentrations are 10 to 20 times higher than in the other lakes (see Fig. 8).

The low elevation of Seneca and Cayuga lakes combined with their greater depths make these two lakes penetrate soil strata that the other lakes do not reach [16].

In September 1976 the European Institute of Ecology and Cancer held a meeting in Cremona, Italy. I did not participate in the meeting, but I submitted a paper on colorectal cancer distribution in the United States [17]. In April 1979, when the geochemical uniqueness of Seneca had just been discovered, the proceedings from the Cremona conference appeared. Glancing through the different contributions, I stumbled on a paper by Valsé Pantellini "Hydrogen (H) bonds and their salifi-

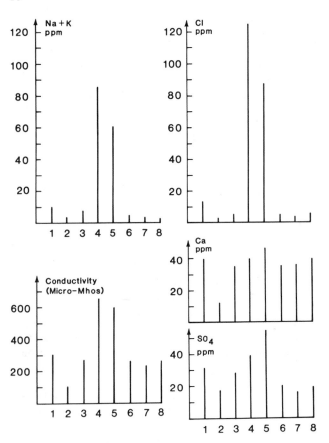

FIGURE 8 The conductivity and the concentration of some chemical ions from west to east in (1) Conesus, (2) Canadice, (3) Canandaigua, (4) Seneca, (5) Cayuga, (6) Owasco, (7) Skaneateles, and (8) Otisco Lakes. (From Ref. 16.).

cation by potassium (K) in the structure of living matter" [18]. Pantellini formulates four postulates:

All basic living structures are made up of H bonds.
The H bonds are formed by the K cation.
The equilibrium between H bonds and salifying K cations is constant for every structure but differs from structure to structure.
The lack of salification of the H bonds by the K cation linked to them in their natural structuring leads to modification of the structures due to opening of valencies of the bases and to distortion of the genetic information.

The author concludes that loss of intracellular potassium and its substitution by Na causes the opening of valence bonds and the altering
of the genetic information apparatus leading to the beginning of the
formation of neoplasms. He states, "In the process, concomitant factors
may intervene such as viruses, toxins, stress, toxic elements, radiations and energy variations of a chemical, physical and biological
nature." What Pantellini postulates is thus a general theory for the
formation of neoplasms.

Our findings of high K concentrations in Seneca, supported by
Pantellini's postulates on the importance of intracellular K for pro-
tection against neoplasms, were the pieces of information needed to
formulate a working hypothesis. This could be further specified by
Pantellini's belief that when Na replaces K in the cells the probability
for formation of neoplasms increases.

We thus formulated the following hypothesis:

Intracellular and dietary K protects against cancer.
Intracellular and dietary Na increases the risk of cancer.

This hypothesis had to be confirmed or refuted by further studies.

IV. CANCER RATES IN OTHER POTASSIUM-RICH AREAS

Seneca County seems to be unique in the country by having exceptionally low cancer rates compared to other counties in the same state. A
complete study of this has not yet been done. A preliminary study of
nine states has been performed, and the results are presented in
Table 2. The counties with the lowest ranksums in their states are
ordered by increasing p-values. Seneca has an outstanding low ranksum, and we do not expect to find other counties in the country with
similar geochemical uniqueness. However, a few lakes have been reported to have very high concentrations of K cations. Examples are
Mono and Modoc counties in California and Grant County in Washington
state. We find that Mono and Modoc have, respectively, the second
and the third lowest ranksum in California for all malignancies combined,
and Grant has the fourth lowest in Washington. (For white women
in Mono County the rate in the 1960s for a number of rare cancer sites
combined has been excluded. This is so high that it must be suspected
to be an error.)

In 1981 Bopp and Biggs [19] reported on the minerals found in
the sediments in Delaware Bay. They observed that the K concentrations was high and the Na concentration low outside Kent County,
Delaware, located in the middle of the Bay. The high K concentration
in the sediment was interpreted as being eroded from land, indicating

Tabe 2 States for Which the Ranksums Have Been Calculated for Every County for Three Decades and for Both Sexes (n = 6)[a]

State	County with lowest ranksum	Number of counties	Ranksum	Ranksum	
				Number of counties	p-Value
New York	Seneca	62	12	0.19	0.00000002
Texas	Jeff Davis	254	128	0.50	0.000020
Massachusetts	Hampshire	14	10	0.71	0.000028
Washington	Skamania	39	30	0.76	0.00026
Montana	Judith Basin	56	47	0.84	0.00035
California	Trinity	58	50	0.86	0.00042
Arizona	Mohave	14	19	1.36	0.0036
North Dakota	Stutsman	53	68	1.28	0.0049
Rhode Island	Bristol, Kent	5	12	2.40	0.056

[a]Counties with lowest ranksums in their states are listed and ordered after increasing p-values.

high K concentration in the soil and water in Kent. They found sediments further out in the bay originating from the continental shelf with reduced K concentrations and increased Na concentrations. In the innermost parts of the bay both K and Na concentrations were low. The sediments in these parts were dominated by metals associated with upstream pollution. The six counties along the coast of the Delaware Bay are Newcastle, Kent, and Sussex in Delaware and Salem, Cumberland, and Cape May in New Jersey. If our hypothesis on low cancer rates in areas with high K and low Na concentrations is correct, we expect Kent County to have the lowest cancer rates of these six counties. With 12 categories (3 decades, 2 sexes, 2 races; n = 12) and six counties (k = 6), Table 3 gives the ranksums for all malignancies combined. As expected, Kent has a significantly low ranksum. Using formula (1), we find that p_{21} = 0.00013 to get a ranksum of 21 or lower. This result thus supports our hypothesis. Cumberland County on the New Jersey side opposite Kent has the second lowest cancer rates of the six counties in the bay. It is reported to have high to moderate K concentration and low to moderate Na concentration. The counties around the mouth of the bay, Sussex and Cap May, where the Na concentration is high and the K concentration is low, have higher ranksums corresponding to higher cancer rates. We conclude that the data from the Delaware Bay confirm our hypothesis.

A report from the Texas Water Development Board [20] gave us information on salinity and depths of the saline ground water in the Texas Counties. We used this information to study cancer rates in relation to the salinity of the ground water. The texas counties were grouped as follows:

1. One group (56 counties) in which the Cl ion concentration in the ground water was above 300 ppm and at the same time depth to the saline water was less than 300 feet.
2. The remaining 199 counties.

It was found that in the first group, 49% of the counties had cancer rates (colon + rectum + breast) belonging to the lowest 10% in the United States. The corresponding figure for the other group was 18%. The difference is very significant. A χ^2-test gives a p-value of 0.00001. We conclude that there is a very significant negative association between ground water salinity and cancer rates. The study has the weakness that Cl ions were used for indicating salinity since information on the K concentration was not available. It is quite possible that some of the saline counties have high Na concentrations. If a further grouping in high and low K concentrations had been possible, the 48% low cancer rate counties could have been still higher in the high K group.

Table 3   Counties around Delaware Bay.[a]

State	County	Ranksum	p-Value
	Newcastle	59	0.0021
Delaware	Kent	21	0.00013
	Sussex	36	0.18
	Salem	55	0.017
New Jersey	Cumberland	33	0.073
	Cape May	43	0.47

[a]Six Counties (k = 6), 3 decades × 2 races × 2 sexes (n = 12), ranksums and p-values to get these ranksums or lower.

The studies reported in this section—the counties with K-rich lakes, Delaware Bay with outflow from Kent County of K-rich sediments, and the ground water salinity in Texas—may not by themselves give much weight to the support of our hypothesis. They are, however, all supportive and contribute to the combined confirmation. One conclusion seems evident. The intake of local water is either directly or indirectly (through plants and animals) associated with cancer rates. This is an almost unstudied subject.

V.   ALTITUDE, ACID-BASE BALANCE, INTRACELLULAR ELECTROLYTES

After we concluded that high K concentrations in soil and water are associated with low cancer rates, the logical next step would be to find other areas where intracellular concentrations of K and Na differ from "normal." That diet influences these concentrations is most likely. We further see from reading physiological literature that hormones, such as aldosterone, insulin, and epinephrine take part in the regulation of the K/Na balance extracellularly and intracellularly. From geriatric literature we learn that aging changes the electrolytic concentrations, and from pathology we see that patients with some diseases are hypokalemic and patients with some other diseases are hyperkalemic. From knowledge on how such phenomena act on the intracellular K/Na balance, our hypothesis can be used to predict expected cancer rates. By comparing it with actually observed cancer rates, we obtain confirmations or refutals of our hypothesis. This is

in analogy with inductive conclusions in mathematics and their testing
for proof or disproof. All the aforementioned areas will be discussed
in this chapter. Here we discuss another phenomenon, which is related
to geopathology.

Burton [21] has commented on the change of blood pH as a
function of altitude. When we move from a low altitude to higher
altitudes, the pH of the blood rises. This changes the acid-base
balance toward the basic side. It has been shown [22] that when the
extracellular pH rises, K enters the cells and Na leaves the cells.
Consequently the intracellular K/Na ratio is higher at high altitudes
than at low altitudes. If our hypothesis is true, we expect that people
living at high altitudes have lower cancer rates than people living at
low altitudes. This can be studied. The results confirm the hypothesis,
as the following examples show.

From the cancer mortality data by states [6], we extracted the
cancer mortality rates for all organ sites, for organs directly exposed
to the oxygen pressure (lip, salivary glands, nasopharynx, tongue,
esophagus, larynx, lung) and, by subtraction, for all remaining
organs. The state geographic mean elevations were determined as
population elevations by calculating the weighted mean elevations for
the largest cities in the states, using the population sizes of the cities
as weights. (For Arizona, California, and Nevada the mean population
elevation has been estimated.) The correlation coefficients were as
follows: between elevation and cancer of all organ sites, -0.55 (p =
0.0001), between elevation and cancers of lip + . . . + lung, -0.62
(p < 0.0001), and between elevation and cancer of the remaining organ
sites, -0.44 (p = 0.002). In this example there are very significant
negative associations between altitude and these three groups of
cancers. The correlation is especially strong for the organs directly
exposed to the oxygen pressure. This is illustrated in Fig. 9, where
the correlation coefficients are presented for a number of organ sites
and where the significance levels are included. In further examples
we will see that this organ site specificity for the relation between
altitude and cancer is a rule. Figure 10 illustrates the relation between
cancer rates of all organ sites for white males and the elevation of
the states. Note that the relation is exponential or hyperbolic rather
than linear!

In some other studies we defined and used a coefficient (R) for
describing the relation between a cancer rate at low altitude and the
corresponding cancer rate at high altitude. R was then defined as
the mean rate at low altitude divided by the mean rate at high altitude.
For organ sites with higher rates at low altitudes than at high altitudes,
R > 1. Table 4 gives R-values. Data have been taken from the following
sources:

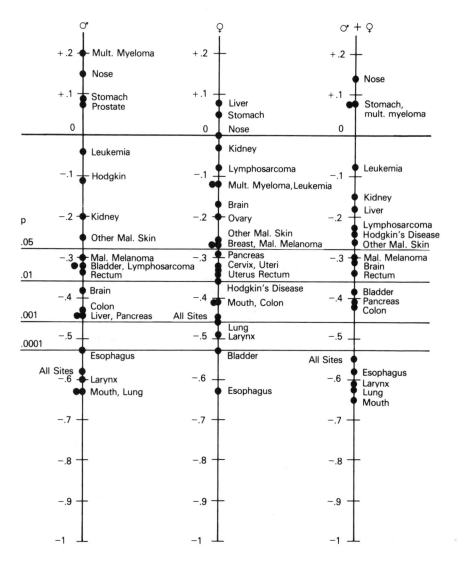

FIGURE 9 Correlations between altitudes of the United States and cancer mortality. p value levels for the estimation of significance are included. (From Ref. 24.)

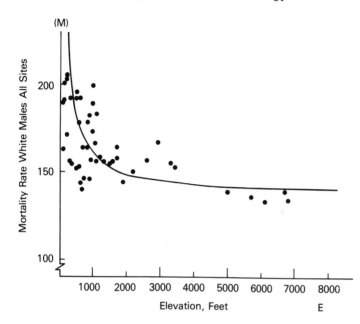

FIGURE 10 Relation between cancer mortality of all sites for white males and average elevations for the United States: $M = 138 + 22,600/E$. (From Ref. 24.)

1. *The Third National Cancer Survey* (TNCS) [23]. Of the nine regions in this survey Colorado is the only high-altitude one. The rate in Colorado is thus divided by the mean rate over the other eight regions.
2. The mean rate in the four lowest states (Delaware, Florida, Louisiana, Mississippi) as well as the District of Columbia is divided by the mean rate in the five highest states (Colorado, Montana, New Mexico, Utah, Wyoming) [24].
3. During a visit to Sydney, Australia, I met with Dr. Leicester Atkinson. While discussing completely different subjects, he gave me a book on cancer rates in Papua, New Guinea (PNG), and told me that he was one of the founders of the cancer registry in this country. At that time I had no use for the book, but when my interest in relationships between altitude and cancer awoke, the PNG data turned out to be useful. This stresses how important it is to always be alert to obtain data from all possible—and impossible—sources and to know where to retrieve the data when needed. Without

Table 4 Ratios (R) between Cancer Rates for Low- and High-Altitude Regions

Organ sites	TNCS[a]		Five lowest contra five highest states		PNG, lowland contra highland[b]		Average of normalized Rs	
	Males	Females	Males	Females	Males	Females	Males	Females
All sites	1.14	1.10	1.27	1.10	2.49	1.96	1.00	1.00
Mouth	1.47	1.31	2.34	1.49	14.54	7.84	2.99	2.18
Esophagus	1.43	2.04	1.95	1.66	2.25	7.00	1.23	2.31
Stomach	1.12	1.26	0.81	0.81	1.86	1.51	0.79	0.88
Colon	1.37	1.15	1.36	1.21	0.74	1.02	0.86	0.89
Rectum	1.39	1.49	1.29	1.18	1.17	1.22	0.90	1.02
Pancreas	1.06	0.97	1.16	1.10	1.07	.075	0.75	0.75
Larynx	1.18	1.17	2.25	1.87	5.09	∞	2.03	∞
Lung	1.38	1.34	1.68	1.41	4.52	∞	1.45	∞

Mal. melanoma	0.91	0.93	1.44	1.32	1.28	0.56	0.82	0.78
Breast	—	1.04	—	1.08	—	1.09	—	0.83
Cervix uteri	—	1.32	—	1.19	—	2.26	—	1.14
Corpus uteri	—	1.13	—	1.02	—	1.16	—	0.85
Ovary	—	0.98	—	1.02	—	1.08	—	0.79
Prostate	0.86	—	0.95	—	0.79	—	0.61	—
Bladder	0.91	0.96	1.32	1.39	0.83	0.25	0.72	0.75
Kidney	1.02	1.13	1.06	1.00	0.90	2.75	0.70	1.11
Brain	1.27	1.16	1.23	1.09	2.61	1.15	1.04	0.88
Lymphomas	1.25	1.14	1.11	1.00	4.09	3.29	1.20	1.21
Leukemias	1.16	0.90	1.07	1.05	0.91	1.18	0.74	0.79

[a]TCNS = Third National Cancer Survey.
[b]PNG = Papua New Guinea.
Source: Ref. 24.

my brief encounter with Dr. Atkinson, the PNG data would never have been known to me. Papua, New Guinea, is divided into a lowland region and a highland region, and the ratio between the mean cancer rates in these two regions was used in the R-calculations.

Finally, averages of the R-values from these three sources have been calculated after normalization by dividing each value in the table by the R-value of each site in the top of the corresponding column. Table 4 shows that cancers of the mouth, esophagus, larynx, and lung have the highest R-values—i.e., the organs most exposed to the differences in oxygen pressure have the greatest differences in cancer rates between low altitude and high altitude.

A number of articles from the literature confirm these results. Amsel et al. [25] compared cancer rates in high-altitude and low-altitude counties and included only counties with populations between 50,000 and 100,000. They found significantly lower rates in the high-altitude counties for cancers of the tongue, mouth, esophagus, larynx, and lung, and for melanoma. By stratification these authors showed that neither industrialization nor urbanization nor the number of Spanish-speaking people influenced the difference in cancer rates at different altitudes. Similar results have been reported from South America [26], the Soviet Union [27], and Italy [28].

The organ site specificity of the altitude dependence is interesting. One would expect that permanent living at high altitudes would lead to an equilibrium resulting in the same acid-base balance in all parts of the body. By comparing the oxygen pressure in different parts of the body for people living at sea level and people living at a 4500-meter altitude, Hurtado [29] showed that the difference in oxygen pressure gets smaller and smaller from the tracheal air to the alveolar air to the arterial blood and capillary blood until it has almost disappeared in the venous blood (see Table 5). The organ specificity is thus to be expected.

The discussion in this section leads us to believe that persons spending considerable time under above normal oxygen pressure can be expected to have increased cancer rates in the mouth, esophagus, and respiratory organs. This has not been studied. Good candidates for such studies would be, for example, miners, who sometimes work 1 km or more below sea level. It is known that such workers have high lung cancer rates. This is believed to be caused by the dust in the mines or by radiation from radon daughters. It is quite possible, however, that the increased oxygen pressure to which these workers are exposed contributes significantly to their increased rates of cancer in respiratory organs. The problem is also very suitable for animal experiments.

Table 5 Differences between Partial Oxygen Pressures (mmHg, mean ± SE) in Different Parts of the Body at Sea Level and at High Altitude

	Lima, Peru (sea level)	Morococha, Peru (4540 m)	Difference
Tracheal air	147.2 ± 0.09	83.4 ± 0.09	63.8
Alveolar air	96.2 ± 0.55	46.7 ± 0.36	49.5
Arterial blood	87.3 ± 1.58	45.2 ± 0.73	42.1
Mean capillary blood	57.2 ± 0.46	38.3 ± 0.52	18.9
Mixed venous blood	42.1 ± 0.53	34.8 ± 0.54	7.3

Adapted from Hurtado.
Source: Ref. 24.

VI. POTASSIUM AND SODIUM IN THE DIET AND THEIR RELATIONS TO CANCER RATES

In the discussion on salts in water and soil in Seneca County and in other regions we have tacitly assumed that what we eat and drink affects our cancer risks. The diet is certainly a very important, perhaps the most important, factor in our intracellular K/Na balance.

Let us set the stage for the discussion by briefly reviewing the difference that has occurred in our intake of K and Na over a dozen or so millenia. Before the agricultural revolution about 10,000 years ago, humans were gatherers of plants, roots, berries, fruits, etc. and hunters of mainly small animals. They did not preserve their food and, like other mammals, they did not use salt. The K and Na they consumed were natural ingredients in their food. Eaton and Konner [30] recently estimated the K and Na intakes in the Paleolithic era and concluded that the dietary K/Na ratio at that time was about 16. They pointed out that some primitive tribes today that still live in hunter-gatherer societies also have dietary K/Na ratios of this order. As a comparison the Na intake today in most developed countries is greater than the K intake and the dietary K/Na is reported to be 0.2 to 1. We thus find that this ratio over 10,000 years has been reduced by a factor of 20 or more. This great change is almost completely caused by the use of Na in preservation, preparation, and eating of food. Human evolution is slow, and it is not unreasonable to believe that we have not yet adapted to this dietary change. Since reproduction most often occurs before the onset of cancers, the evolutionary pressure to adapt to the new dietary situation must, moreover, be expected to be less successful.

Shah and Belonje [31], in a Canadian study, showed that the processing of food from raw natural ingredients to a ready-to-eat product changes the K/Na from about 10 in the unprocessed form to about 1 as processed. Since their study did not take salting at the table into account, which further increases the Na intake, the changes of K/Na caused by preparing food for eating will result in a 10- to 20-fold reduction, which agrees well with the Eaton-Konner estimate. A striking illustration of the same effect of food processing has been presented by Henningsen et al. [32]. These authors found that the K/Na ratio in a raw potato is 104. When the potato was peeled and boiled in 1% salt water, the ratio was reduced to 0.7, 140 times lower than before processing. As a comparison, a steamed and unsalted potato still kept a K/Na ratio of 100, which is almost unchanged from the one in the raw form. We conclude that our great use of sodium in food processing and eating has changed the dietary K/Na dramatically, for which we seemingly have to pay a price in the form of increased risks of a number of diseases, among them cardiovascular diseases and cancer. The relation between cancer and dietary K/Na will be demonstrated by several examples.

Researchers interested in the roles of K and Na in hypertension and other cardiovascular diseases have published reports in which the dietary intakes of these minerals have been estimated for white males and females as well as for black males and females. Three of these reports are especially important since all kinds of salting are included—i.e., salt used in cooking and at eating. That makes these studies unique and most valuable. Grim et al. [33] were interested in the high blood pressures of black males in Evans County, Georgia; they used a 24-hr duplicate dietary collection to estimate the K and Na intakes. Frank and his co-workers [34] during an eight-day observation period used stool samples, urine samples, and a food inventory program for the same determinations. Their study was performed in New Orleans, Louisiana. Finally, Voors et al. [35] similarly estimated the K and Na intakes among young persons in Bogalosa and Franklinton, Washington County, Louisiana. For cancer comparisons we used cancer rates for all organ sites and for digestive organs (esophagus, stomach, colon, rectum, liver, pancreas), and we used subtraction for nondigestive organs. The cancer data were obtained from the tables of cancer mortality by county [13]. The rates were averaged over the three decades given in the tables. The results are presented in Table 6 and, for cancer of the digestive tract, in Fig. 11. The negative associations between dietary K/Na and cancer are evident in all three sets. The relations seem to be hyperbolic rather than linear, in analogy with what was seen in the relation between altitude and cancer (Fig. 10). The two sets from Louisiana fit together well; the Georgia set is shifted to the left, compared to these two. Georgia has, in general, lower cancer rates than Louisiana, indicating that factors

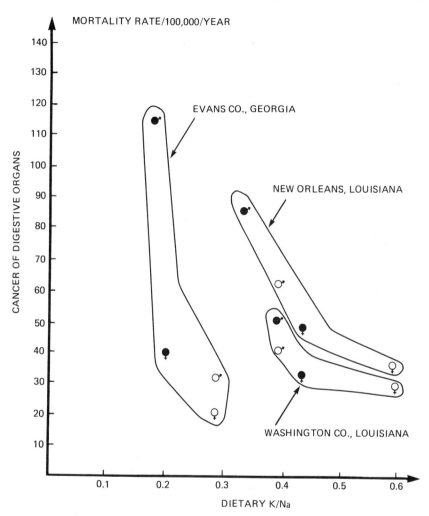

FIGURE 11 The mortality rate for cancer of the digestive organs as a function of the dietary K/Na. Three different samples. ♂ black males, ♀ black females, ♂ white males, ♀ white females.

Table 6   Cancer Mortality Rates for All Organ Sites, Digestive Organs, and Nondigestive Organs in Relation to Dietary K/Na[a]

	Whites		Blacks		Location of study
	Males	Females	Males	Females	Source
All sites	200	122	201	120	Washington Co., La.
Digestive	41	34	51	35	Voors et al. (35)
Nondigestive	159	88	150	85	
K/Na	0.39	0.60	0.39	0.43	
All sites	244	139	271	169	New Orleans, La.
Digestive	63	38	86	48	Frank et al. (34)
Nondigestive	181	101	185	121	
K/Na	0.39	0.59	0.33	0.43	
All sites	178	109	260	108	Evans Co., Ga.
Digestive	34	22	116	40	Grim et al. (33)
Nondigestive	144	87	144	68	
K/Na	0.29	0.29	0.17	0.20	

[a]Data from three different studies.

other than diet contribute to the differences. To compare the three sets we ranked the cancer rates and the K/Na values within each set. The points (K/Na rank, rate rank) were then plotted for each sex, race, and set combination ($2 \times 2 \times 3 = 12$ points) for digestive tract cancer [Fig. 12(a)] and for nondigestive tract cancer [Fig. 12(b)]. The lesson from this figure is that the digestive organs are more sensitive to changes in the dietary K/Na values than are the non-digestive organs. This parallels the organ specificity results from the altitude study in the previous section, where it was found that organs most exposed to reduced oxygen pressure were the most protected against cancer.

We conclude this section with two international examples. The first one uses data published by the Organization for Economic Co-operation and Development (OECD), and the second one uses data from the studies of esophageal cancer in Iran. In both examples the K and Na contents of the food has been estimated by using tables

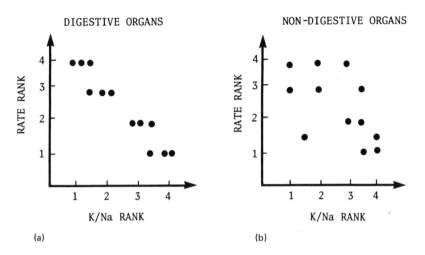

FIGURE 12 Relation between the dietary K/Na rank and (a) the rate rank of cancer of digestive organs and (b) the rate rank of cancer of the nondigestive organs.

prepared by the U.S. Department of Agriculture [36] together with information on per capita consumption of different food commodities. Because information was not available on salting at food preparation and at the table the Na content of the food is underestimated, probably by a factor of 10 or more in the OECD case.

The OECD [37] annually obtains data on the per capita consumption of about 100 commodities from their 20-member counties (17 European countries, United States, Canada, and Japan). In this study these commodities were arranged in 11 groups: grains and cereals, sugars, potatoes, pulses, vegetables, fruits, meats, eggs, milk and cheese, fish, and fats. For each group the K, Na, and Ca contents were estimated and summed to total consumptions. For correlation calculations cancer mortality rates were obtained from the American Cancer Society [38]. The resulting correlations between food intake and different cancers are presented in Table 7. The Ca part of the table will be discussed in the next section; here we concentrate on K and Na. The positive correlation between Na and cancer, the lack of correlations between K and cancer, and the strong negative correlation between the K/Na ratio and cancer is evident. An exception is stomach cancer for which the signs of the correlations are reversed. For the food groups we note negative correlations above all for grains and cereals, pulses, vegetables, fruits, and fish, and positive correlations for sugars, potatoes, meats, eggs, and fats. The positive correlation

Table 7 Correlations between Cancer and Calcium, Sodium, Potassium, and Different Food Groups[a].

	All sites		Colorectal		Lung		Breast	Stomach	
	Males	Females	Males	Females	Males	Females	Females	Males	Females
Ca	0.34	0.42	0.34	0.39	0.49	0.29	0.50	-0.35	-0.34
Na	0.41	0.66	0.58	0.64	0.49	0.21	0.68	-0.42	-0.43
K	0.19	-0.15	0.00	-0.01	-0.02	-0.05	-0.10	-0.05	0.01
Ca/Na	-0.52	-0.71	-0.76	-0.79	-0.46	-0.19	-0.77	0.47	0.48
K/Ca	-0.35	-0.54	-0.48	-0.49	-0.55	-0.37	-0.66	0.50	0.53
K/Na	-0.53	-0.69	-0.73	-0.74	-0.59	-0.30	-0.82	0.58	0.60
Grains + cereals	-0.43	-0.66	-0.72	-0.76	-0.40	-0.27	-0.75	0.45	0.46
Sugar	0.44	0.73	0.73	0.78	0.56	0.56	0.88	-0.53	-0.54
Potatoes	0.33	0.42	0.44	0.52	0.23	0.05	0.34	-0.13	-0.08
Pulses	-0.40	-0.52	-0.62	-0.63	-0.46	-0.14	-0.75	0.69	0.69
Vegetables	-0.11	-0.42	-0.30	-0.35	-0.32	-0.20	-0.35	0.11	0.12
Fruits	0.02	-0.13	-0.05	-0.16	-0.06	-0.38	0.00	-0.19	-0.18
Meats	0.54	0.56	0.82	0.79	0.54	0.54	0.79	-0.65	-.066
Eggs	0.51	0.62	0.76	0.77	0.55	0.66	0.72	-0.46	-0.46
Milk + cheese	0.36	0.47	0.40	0.45	0.50	0.30	0.55	-0.37	-0.36
Fish	-0.52	-0.37	-0.41	-0.33	-0.64	-0.36	-0.47	0.32	-0.35
Fats	0.35	0.65	0.52	0.57	0.42	0.08	0.60	-0.32	-0.34

aData from OECD (37). $p < 0.001$ for $0.68 < |r|$, $0.001 < p < 0.01$ for $0.56 < |r| < 0.68$, $0.01 < p < 0.02$ for $0.52 < |r| < 0.56$, $0.02 < p < 0.05$ for $0.44 < |r| < 0.52$.

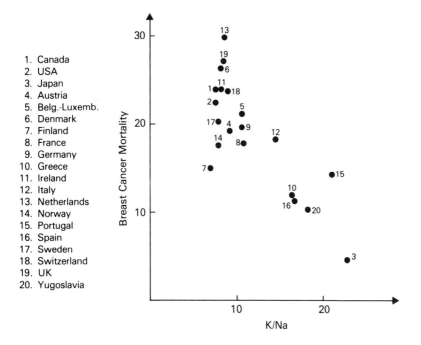

1. Canada
2. USA
3. Japan
4. Austria
5. Belg.-Luxemb.
6. Denmark
7. Finland
8. France
9. Germany
10. Greece
11. Ireland
12. Italy
13. Netherlands
14. Norway
15. Portugal
16. Spain
17. Sweden
18. Switzerland
19. UK
20. Yugoslavia

FIGURE 13 Relation between breast cancer mortality/100,000/year and dietary K/Na ratios in 20 OECD countries ($r = - .80$, $t_{18} = 5.6$, $p < .0001$). Salting in preservation, preparation, and eating is not included. (From Ref. 24.)

between potatoes and cancer is probably due to boiling the potatoes in salt water, which, as noted earlier, reduces the K/Na ratio by a factor of 140, or salting them (french fries). The correlation between dietary K/Na and breast cancer is illustrated in Fig. 13, where the negative association is clear. Some comments are necessary to explain this figure. The K/Na values are too high because salting during food preparation and eating is not included. Japan, where deliberate salting at the table is very high, has the lowest K/Na value of the 20 countries involved. In these correlation calculations the K and Na concentrations in the food ingredients have been used. A very high intake of grains (rice) and pulses gives Japan its high K/Na ratio. Japan has low cancer rates in almost all cancers. The exception is stomach cancer, where the rate is among the highest in the world. It is quite possible that the NaCl added at the table directly damages the gastric mucosa and thereby increases the cancer risk, as recently suggested by Charnley and Tannenbaum [39]: "NaCl increases the gastric cancer risk through the mitogenesis which results from the damage caused to the mucosa by this agent." Sodium as a natural ingredient in the food and used as a condiment seems to play different roles in cancer etiology.

The esophageal cancer rates are among the highest in the world along the Caspian littoral in Iran. The diets and the habits of people living there have been thoroughly investigated by the Joint Iran– International Agency for Research on Cancer Study Group. We use their data [40] on the esophageal cancer rates and food intakes in each of 14 regions. The intakes of bread and rice dominate the total intakes, and we observe that the sum of these two foods is about 700 g/day in all regions. This is illustrated in Fig. 14(a) where the data points have been fitted by

$$B = 610 - 0.78R \tag{2}$$

where B and R are, respectively, the daily bread and rice intakes in grams. The relation between the esophageal cancer incidence rate (I) and the bread intake is shown in Fig. 14(b). It is fitted by the hyperbola

$$B = 580 - \frac{11,000}{I} \tag{3}$$

From a food table [36] we estimate that 1 g of bread has 5 mg Na and 1 mg K, and 1 g of rice has 0.1 mg Na and 2 mg K. The daily Na and K intakes from bread and rice consumptions can then, from (2), be expressed in terms of daily bread intake:

$$Na = 5B + \frac{0.1(610 - B)}{0.78} = 5B + 78$$

$$K = B + \frac{2(610 - B)}{0.78} = 1,600 - 1.6B$$

which, combined with (3), gives relations between the esophageal cancer rates and the intakes of Na, K, and the K/Na ratio. Thus

$$Na = 2900 - \frac{55,000}{I} \qquad K = 670 + \frac{18,000}{I} \qquad \frac{K}{Na} = 0.23$$

$$+ \frac{11}{I - 19} \tag{4}$$

The derived relations (4) are displayed in Fig. 14(c)–(e) together with the corresponding observed data points. The positive correlation

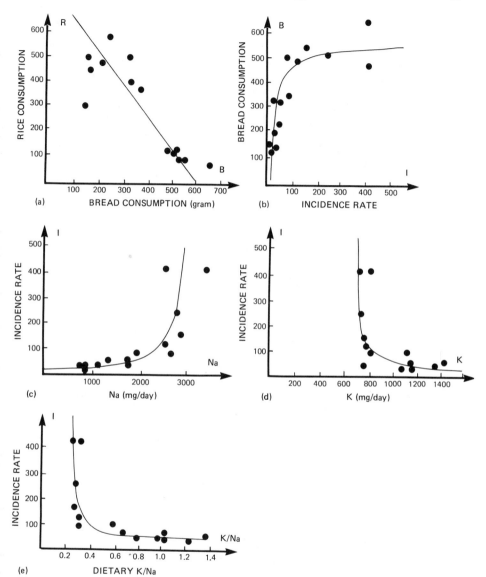

FIGURE 14 Esophageal cancer in Iran. (a) Relation between bread consumption and rice consumption in 14 regions. (b) Relation between esophageal cancer incidence rate and the consumption of bread. (c) Relation between esophageal cancer rate and the intake of Na. (d) Relation between esophageal cancer rate and the intake of K. (e) Relation between esophageal cancer rate and the dietary K/Na ratio.

between cancer rate and Na intake and the negative correlations
between cancer rate and K intake and between cancer and the K/Na
ratio are clearly illustrated. The nonlinearity is obvious also in this
example. As in the examples from New Orleans and Georgia (Fig. 11),
we again find that when K/Na < 0.5 the cancer rates strongly increase.

Vegetarians have lower cancer rates than meat eaters. Ophir et
al. [41], in a study of low blood pressure in vegetarians, determined
the urinary excretion of Na and K for vegetarians and for a control
group of nonvegetarians. The average urinary K/Na ratios were
found to be 0.94 for vegetarians and 0.65 for nonvegetarians. Since
the urinary K/Na ratio is assumed to be equal to the dietary K/Na
ratio, the higher value of this ratio for vegetarians may explain their
reduced cancer rates.

Some animal experiments and some human epidemiological studies
have shown that an increased intake of table salt (NaCl) increases
the risk of stomach cancer. At least one experiment was performed in
which K was given to animals to study its preventive effect. Jacobs
[42] added KCl to the drinking water of rats and showed that the
incidence of intestinal cancer, induced by DMH, was reduced. More
comprehensive animal experiments are being conducted.

Let us return to the Burkitt analogy solving the cancer riddle
and assembling a jigsaw puzzle. The Seneca findings were the piece
of the puzzle that gave a first vague idea of the picture in the
assembled puzzle. If the idea was right, we expected the existence
of an "altitude piece" and a "diet piece" that should fit into the
puzzle. These pieces were found, and it was shown that they fitted
the puzzle excellently. The picture in the puzzle thereby began to
take a more precise form.

VII. DIETARY CALCIUM AND ITS RELATION
TO POTASSIUM AND SODIUM

This chapter concentrates on the dietary and intracellular concentrations of K and Na. The other important elements in the cancer context
are Mg and Ca. Magnesium has not been discussed much regarding its
effects on cancer etiology. It is, however, mentioned as an element
with anticarcinogenic properties [43]. Newmark, Lipkin, and their co-
workers have recently suggested that Ca prevents colorectal cancer.
We therefore include a brief discussion on Ca and its relation to intracellular K and Na.

Newmark et al. [44] note that dietary Ca prevents colon cancer
by forming almost insoluble Ca soaps with fatty acids and bile acids.
This will eliminate the carcinogenic effects caused by intake of fats
according to these authors. The suggestion has been followed up by
Lipkin and Newmark [45], who showed that adding Ca to the diet of

persons with high risk of familial colon cancer changes the proliferation of the epithelial cells in the colonic crypts from a high-risk pattern to a low-risk pattern.

Independently Garland et al. [46] based a study of colorectal cancer and Ca intake on the assumption that people living in areas with low amounts of natural sunlight have low vitamin D production and low Ca absorption. In a case control study (49 cases, 1095 controls) they compared the intakes of vitamin D and Ca for colorectal cancer patients and controls. They found that these intakes were lower for cases than for controls. The differences were weakly significant (p < 0.05).

Repeating Garland's study, Heilbrun et al. [47], with a sample of 100 colon and 59 rectum cancer cases, could not confirm Garland's results. In a later study the same group of authors [48], using 99 colon cancer patients and 378 cancer-free controls, again could not repeat the Garland results and thus could not confirm the Newmark hypothesis that dietary Ca is negatively associated with colon cancer. A low Ca, high fat diet did not considerably increase the risk of colon cancer. In the two Heilbrun studies a 24-hr diet recall was used.

In the OECD study described in the previous section, Ca intake was included, and we see from Table 7 that there is a positive correlation between Ca and colorectal cancer. Hormozdiari et al. [49], using data from the esophageal cancer study in Iran, determined the Ca intake in the 14 regions involved. Correlating their data with the esophageal cancer rates, we again obtain a weak positive correlation. The correlations between cancer and dietary intakes of Ca, K, Na, K/Ca, K/Na, and Ca/Na for the OECD and the Iran data are presented in Table 8, where male and female cancers are combined. With both organ sites Na has a strong positive correlation and Ca a weak positive correlation. Potassium has a negative correlation with esophageal cancer and no correlation with colorectal cancer. Of greatest interest are the ratios between these elements and their correlations with the cancers.

Table 8 Correlation Coefficients between Colorectal and Esophageal Cancer and Calcium, Sodium, and Potassium and Their Ratios

	Ca	Na	K	Ca/Na	K/Ca	K/Na
OECD Colorectal cancer	0.36	0.61	0.00	-0.78	-0.48	-0.74
Iran−IARC Esophageal cancer	0.19	0.75	-0.58	-0.76	-0.48	-0.68

Both Ca and K are able to eliminate or reduce the increased cancer risks caused by a high Na intake. Furthermore, K reduces the increased cancer risks caused by a too high Ca intake. It is a great Na intake that causes the greatest increases in cancer risks.

Milk and other dairy products are the foods that have the highest Ca concentrations. We see from Table 7 that milk and cheese are, in general, positively correlated to cancer. The exception is stomach cancer, where the correlations are negative. Similar results were obtained by Bjelke [50, Table II.3]. In his data from 27 countries the milk consumption was positively and significantly correlated to colorectal cancer and breast cancer. For all the different food groups included in Table 7, Bjelke's results from 27 countries and ours from the 20 OECD countries are almost identical.

A few reports describe relations between Ca, Na, and K. Kino et al. [51], working on vascular smooth muscle cells, showed that extracellular Ca plays a role in the intracellular K and Na concentrations: "Removal of Ca from the extracellular medium has been shown to result in a net gain of cellular Na and a net loss of cellular K." Edelman et al. [52] showed that the intracellular K activity increased significantly when metatarsal hypertrophic cells were incubated with the vitamin D metabolite $1,25(OH)_2D_3$. It is thus very likely that dietary Ca is negatively associated with intracellular Na, positively associated with intracellular K, and, consequently, positively associated with the intracellular K/Na ratio. This is in good agreement with the correlations obtained between cancer and the Ca/Na and K/Ca ratios.

These results indicate that we need H a high K intake, a moderate Ca intake, and, most importantly, a low Na intake to reduce the risk of cancer.

VIII. SPECIFIC CARCINOGENIC AND ANTI-CARCINOGENIC AGENTS AND THEIR INFLUENCE ON INTRACELLULAR POTASSIUM AND SODIUM

We have so far mainly discussed direct relations between cancer rates and K, Na, and the K/Na ratio. Differences in diets or in oxygen pressure were found to be related to changes in concentrations of the alkali metals, which were in turn associated with changes in cancer rates. This section discusses indirect relations between carcinogenic or anticarcinogenic agents and the intracellular electrolytes. It will be shown that the carcinogenic agents reduce the intracellular K/Na ratio, whereas the anticarcinogenic agents increase this ratio. Information regarding the influence of these agents on the cellular electrolytes is often taken from noncancer sources. This is similar to looking for puzzle pieces in boxes belonging to other puzzles but with some pieces fitting into more than one of the puzzles.

A. Intake of Fat

Dietary intake of fat is believed to be associated with increased risks of cancer, especially of the breast and the large bowel. Although primarily all fats were suspected, later results have shown that, above all, the unsaturated and polyunsaturated fatty acids are positively correlated with cancer. Data from an animal experiment reported by Carroll [53] illustrates this point. Rats in his experiment were challenged with DMBA, an agent inducing mammary tumors. Nine groups of rats were fed semisynthetic diets, which contained 20% by weight of fats, with different degrees of saturation. From tables of the composition of various fats, I estimated the average number of double bonds for the nine fats and correlated these averages with the total number of tumors per 30 rats as given by Carroll. The results are shown in Fig. 15. The correlation is +0.90, which differs very significantly from 0 ($p = 0.0002$). That polyunsaturated fats

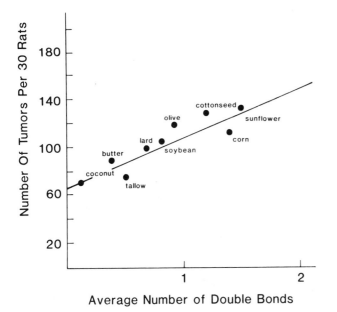

FIGURE 15 Number of tumors per 30 rats (Ref. 53) as a function of the degree of saturation of different types of dietary fats.

enhance the formation of mammary tumors and large bowel tumors
more than saturated fats do is discussed in other articles.

Zidek et al. [54] have shown that the composition of dietary fats
affects the intracellular electrolytes. These authors report that
during a two-week-long diet containing mainly saturated fats the
cellular Na activity was reduced by 13%, whereas during a diet with
mainly polyunsaturated fats this activity increased by 8%. Potassium
activity was not measured, but it can be expected to vary in an
opposite direction. We thus conclude that polyunsaturated fat diets
decrease the intracellular K/Na ratio and increase the risks of breast
cancer and intestinal cancers.

B. Obesity

Obesity has been linked to increased cancer risks. Zidek et al. [55]
report that during a two-week weight reduction period the ratio of
active K ions to active Na ions in the cells increased by 30%. Decreased
obesity is thus related to an increased cellular K/Na ratio.

C. Cholesterol

Dietary cholesterol has been shown to increase the risk of colon
cancer. Kutscherskij et al. [56] showed that the intracellular K/Na
ratio is significantly lower after intake of cholesterol rich diets than
after control diets.

D. Alcohol

Alcohol is believed to increase the risk of cancer. Studying humans as
well as animals, Pierson et al. [57] showed that intake of alcohol decreased the ratio of total body K to total body Na, and they concluded
that this reflected an increase in intracellular Na and a decrease in
intracellular K and, thus, a reduced K/Na ratio.

E. Licorice

There are no reports on direct relations between licorice and cancer.
Licorice is, however, a well-known K depleter. There are reports
that licorice consumption or chewing tobacco has caused hypokalemia,
which led to severe myopathy. Licorice is used in manufacturing
tobacco—90% of the U.S. licorice consumption is used for this purpose.
It is thus a possibility that licorice enhances the cancer risks caused
by smoking or chewing tobacco products. Licorice is also used as a
foaming agent in beer manufacturing. Beer is suspected to cause
rectal cancer.

F. Dimethylhydrazine

DMH is a carcinogen that specifically induces intestinal tumors. It is frequently used in animal models to study such tumors. Cameron [44] reports on the change in K/Na during a period of DMH administration to rats. The intracellular K/Na was 2.1 before the administration of DMH, after eight weeks it was 1.8, and after 16 weeks 1.4. In adenocarcinoma cells the ratio had dropped to 0.95 after 16 weeks of DMH administration. Over the treatment period Na increased more than K decreased, but both elements showed considerable changes. Similar changes were reported by Zs.-Nagy et al. [58] from studies on human material. They found that the intracellular K/Na ratio was four to five times lower in a cancer cell than in the corresponding healthy cell and that Na was the element that varied most.

G. Radiation

Radiation of cells and tissues is, besides smoking, the best-recognized cancer-inducing activity. Radiation causes an outflow of K from the cells and an inflow or Na, thereby reducing the intracellular K/Na ratio.

H. Scarification and Surgical Wounds

Increased cancer risks have been reported in scars and surgical wounds [59]. Cellular K and Na changes may be involved. Kimura et al. [60] studied the intracellular K and Na activities after the healing of myocardial infarctions in cats. They found that the scar cells in the infarct zone and cells in the normal zone had a K/Na activity ratio between 8 and 9. In a border area around the infarct zone, however, the K/Na was less than 4. These changes were reported to be persistent. Since similar changes may occur in all scar formations, they may be associated with an increased cancer risk around the scars.

All the carcinogenic activities just described have as a common property a reduced intracellular K/Na ratio. Let us now turn the coin around and look at activities known to be anticarcinogenic.

I. Vitamin A

In animal and human epidemiological studies, vitamin A has been found to have anticarcinogenic properties. During a 10-day period, Ferrini and Gambaro [61] administered 10,000 IU/day of vitamin A to rats. They found that the intracellular K/Na ratio increased by a factor of 5 from 9.8 before to 50.9 after the experiment period. Although K concentration was almost unchanged, the Na concentration decreased by a factor of 5. The anticarcinogen vitamin A thus increased the intracellular K/Na ratio, thereby supporting our hypothesis.

J. Vitamin C

Linus Pauling is the foremost proponent for the use of vitamin C as a preventor of a number of diseases, among those cancer. Hanck [62] reports that an intake of 1000 mg of vitamin C per day did not change the urinary excretion of K and Na. In a review part of his paper, however, he mentions that in scurvy, a vitamin C deficiency disease, the intracellular Na concentration increases by more than 50%. He also reports that in guinea pigs on a vitamin C deficient diet the intracellular Na concentration goes up while the K concentration goes down. The cellular K/Na ratio is thus negatively associated with vitamin C intake, as our hypothesis predicts.

K. Selenium

A large number of animal studies have shown that Se reduces cancer incidence rates. Similar conclusions have been reached from human epidemiological studies. No articles have been found that directly discuss relations between Se intake and intracellular K and Na concentrations. There are, however, indications that Se is negatively correlated to Na and positively correlated to K and, thus, to the K/Na ratio. Intake of Se has been reported to lower blood pressure, which indicates higher K and lower Na concentrations. Selenium has also been shown to be an antagonist to Cd, which is known to cause retention of Na. It is thus quite possible that Se acts as an anticarcinogen by increasing the intracellular K/Na ratio.

L. Fiber

Burkitt has forcefully advocated that dietary fiber is protective against various diseases of the digestive tract, including cancer. How does this relate to K and Na? Demigné and Rémésy [63] fed rats a very high fiber diet and studied the absorption of Na, K, and other ions in the cecum. They observed a moderate absorption of Na and a contrastingly high absorption of K. Similar results have been reported by Schwartz et al. [64], studying the flux of the Na in the jejunum of rats. A fiber intake is shown to increase the volume of the stool. Says Vaamonde [65]: "Generally, however, as a stool volume increases so does its sodium concentration, while potassium concentration diminishes." A fiber diet thus changes the K/Na ratio in the intestines toward higher values, thereby, if our hypothesis is correct, reducing the risk of cancer.

M. Indomethacin

Pollard and Luckert [66] showed that the drug indomethacin reduced the incidence of DMH-induced intestinal tumors in rats. Similarly,

Lynch and Salomon [67] reported that indomethacin reduced the growth of fibrosarcomas grafted in mice and, in some of the mice, even caused rejection of the tumors. It is known that indomethacin can cause hyperkalemia in patients [68, 69] with or without changing the blood K [70]. This indicates an increase in intracellular K caused by the indomethacin. Since indomethacin did not only reduce the incidence of tumors but also decreased the growth rate of the tumors or completely rejected the grafted tumors, a preventive as well as a curative effect was observed. How Na is affected by indomethacin has not been reported. It is, however, most likely that the drug reduces the intracellular concentration of Na and consequently increases the intracellular K/Na ratio.

We have found that activities known to be carcinogenic cause the intracellular K/Na ratio to decrease, and that activities known to be anticarcinogenic cause the ratio to increase. The assumption that Se and indomethacin are positively associated to the intracellular K/Na ratio remains to be confirmed. Other known carcinogenic and anticarcinogenic activities must be investigated to determine if they behave, as those mentioned in this section, by decreasing or increasing the intracellular K/Na ratio.

Let me finish by mentioning a case control study performed by Marquart-Moulin and her co-workers [71]. She compared the diets of 251 colorectal cancer patients with the diets of as many matched controls regarding the amounts of different nutrients in the diets and their influence on the cancer rates. The conclusion of the study was that, among all the nutrients involved, K was the one that especially had to be taken into account as negatively related to the risk of cancer of colon and rectum.

IX. AGING, POTASSIUM, SODIUM, AND CANCER

When we get older, we lose total body K and gain total body Na. There is an outflow of K from our cells and an inflow of Na. Said Cox and Shalaby [72]: " . . . the change of potassium content of the body seems to be related to a gradual leak of the potassium by the aged cells. . . . The leak of potassium by the cells might be, in actual fact, one of the contributory factors of cell aging."

If our K-Na-cancer hypothesis is true, cancer rates must be expected to increase with age, which is a well-known fact. Figure 16 illustrates the relation between the total body K/total body Na ratio and the incidence rate of cancer for white females and for all malignancies. Cancer data for six different age intervals are taken from Ref. [23] and matched with K/Na values taken from Macgillivray et al. [73]. The nonlinear negative association is very obvious.

Pierson and his co-workers [74] estimated the intracellular concentrations of K and Na for different ages and fitted the obtained data

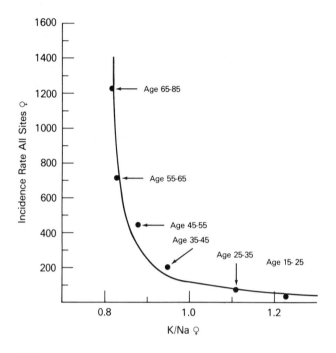

FIGURE 16 Relation between female incidence rate of cancer of all sites and total body K/total body Na ratio at six age intervals. • observed, — expected. I = 22.2/(K/Na − .80). (From Ref. 24.)

with linear expressions. From these expressions we derive the hyperbolic relations

$$\frac{K}{Na} = \frac{560}{A + 58} - 0.76 \quad \text{for males}$$

$$\frac{K}{Na} = \frac{1102}{A + 161} - 1.73 \quad \text{for females}$$

where A is the age in years. Combining these expressions with cancer incidence rates for all sites gives the relations in Fig. 17. The non-linearity is still stronger in the intracellular case than what we observed in the total body case. There seems to be a threshold somewhere around 5; when K/Na < 5, cancer rates increase dramatically.

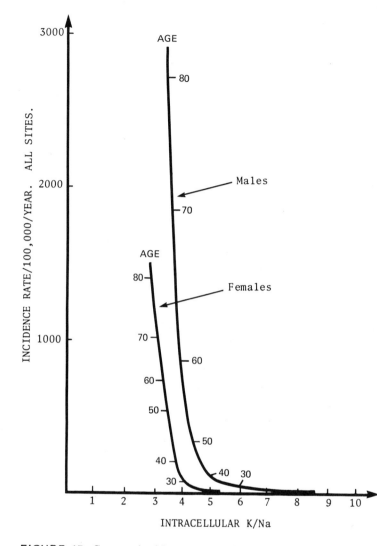

FIGURE 17 Cancer incidence rates for all organ sites combined as a function of the intracellular K/Na ratio.

X. CANCER RATES FOR PATIENTS WITH HYPO-
OR HYPERKALEMIC DISEASES

Ninety-seven percent of the K in the human body is contained within
the cells. The distribution of Na is the opposite, with about 90% being
extracellular. Hypo- and hyperkalemia are defined as less or more
than normal amounts of K in the blood plasma. It has been shown that
there is no obvious or significant correlation between the concentrations
of K within the cells and outside the cells. It follows that the total
body potassium (TBK) gives a better estimate of the intracellular K
than the blood values. We are above all interested in the intracellular
K concentrations, and therefore in this section we define less than
normal values of TBK as hypokalemia and more than normal values as
hyperkalemia. Delwaide [75] and Ellis et al. [76] have determined TBK
for patients with different diseases and compared it with the values
for healthy persons. For this, Ellis developed a formula by which TBK
for healthy persons can be determined as a function of age, sex, body
weight, and height. Examples of diseases with low TBK are alcoholism,
osteoporosis, Cushing's syndrome, diabetes, cirrhosis, obesity,
Crohn's disease, epilepsy, and renal diseases. Some examples of
diseases with high TBK are Parkinson's disease, Addison's disease,
acromegaly, and schizophrenia. We expect that patients with hypokalemic diseases are at increased risk of cancer and that patients
with hyperkalemic diseases are at reduced cancer risks. This section
discusses these topics.

A. Hypokalemic diseases

1. Alcoholism. We have already said that alcohol intake decreases
K and increases Na concentrations. Alcoholism is believed to increase
cancer risks.
2. Cushing's Syndrome. Cushing's syndrome is associated
with cancers of the lung, pancreas, thymus, ovary, and thyroid as
well as with tumors of the pituitary and adrenal glands.
3. Crohn's Disease. Crohn's disease is associated with increased
risks of intestinal cancers. That patients with Crohn's disease have
reduced concentrations of intracellular K was recently reported [77].
4. Cirrhosis and Epilepsy. Both cirrhosis and epilepsy have
been reported to be associated with increased cancer risks.
5. Diabetes. Diabetics have, according to Delwaide [75], 10–20%
lower TBK than nondiabetics. Kessler [78], among others, has reported that the risk of pancreatic cancer is greatest for patients with
diabetes. One function of the hormone insulin, which is deficient in
diabetics, is to take part in the regulation of intracellular K concentrations. An increased secretion of insulin forces K to flow into
the cells; lack of insulin causes an outflow of K from the cells. It is

thus quite possible that untreated diabetics are at increased cancer risk, whereas patients to whom insulin is adminstered are at a normal risk.

6. Stress. The stress hormone aldosterone behaves oppositely to insulin. Increased aldosterone levels will cause decreased intracellular K levels. We thus expect higher caner risks for persons living under stress. It has been reported that during periods of depression intracellular Na goes up and K goes down and that this is reversed after the depression period [79].

7. Muscular Dystrophy. Boys with the inherited Duchenne type of muscular dystrophy have progressively lower and lower total body K, as reported by Edmonds et al. [80]. At 16 years of age their TBK is less than half the normal value. One would thus expect an increased cancer risk among these patients. Since they rarely survive until 20 years of age, it is difficult to determine if they are at an increased cancer risk.

B. Hyperkalemic Diseases

1. Addison's Disease. Patients with Addison's disease are hyponatremic and hyperkalemic, and we thus expect them to be at reduced cancer risks. Nerup [81] reported that of 108 patients with Addison's disease none had developed a cancer.

2. Schizophrenia. Schizophrenic patients have low Na and high K intracellular concentrations [82]. Several investigators have reported low cancer rates among such patients [83, 84].

3. Multiple Sclerosis. Low cancer rates among patients with multiple sclerosis was reported by Palo et al. [85]. Values of total body K and Na or of the intracellular concentrations of these elements have, however, not been found in a literature search. This gap in the puzzle is waiting to be filled in.

4. Parkinson's Disease. In 1954 Doshay [86] wrote that "for reasons as yet unclear, cancer is phenomenally rare in paralysis agitans (parkinsonism), despite the fact that the patients are in the age group 45 to 75, when the expectancy of cancer in the general population is high." This statement has been tested in several studies, with varying results. Having access to the charts for patients with Parkinson's disease at Baylor College of Medicine in Houston, Texas, we determined the number of cancers among 406 patients and compared it with the expected number. This study is described in Jansson and Jankovic [87].

The expected values were determined as follows: Assume that

p_i is the probability of a person's getting cancer when i years old.

q_{ij} is the probability that a person who develops a cancer at age i is still alive j years later (i.e., at age i + j).

The probability of not having developed cancer at age N is then

$$A_N = (1 - p_1)(1 - p_2) \cdots (1 - p_N)$$

and the probability of having developed cancer at age i and still be living at age N is

$$B_N = p_1 q_{1,N} + (1 - p_1)p_2 q_{2,N-1} + (1 - p_1)(1 - p_2)p_3 q_{3,N-2}$$
$$+ \cdots + (1 - p_1)(1 - p_2) \cdots (1 - p_{N-1})p_N q_{N,1}$$

The probability that a person who is alive at age N has developed a cancer some time before that age is then $B_N/(A_N + B_N)$. Summing over all patients in the sampel gives the wanted expected value. The p_i's for all malignancies combined (except nonmelanoma skin cancer) were obtained from the Third National Cancer Survey [23] and these for nonmelanoma skin cancer from Scotto et al. [88]. The q_{ij}'s were calculated as the products of the general survival rate, obtained from life tables, and the relative survival rate, obtained from Ref. 89. The result of the study was that there were only 18 Parkinson patients with cancer (all malignancies) when 41.9 were expected (p < 0.0001), and only 10 with nonmelanoma skin cancer when 49.9 were expected (p < 0.0001). The risk of cancer increased but still remained low during treatment with levodopa. The results of a couple of studies can explain this. Granerus et al. [90] and Sundstrom et al. [91] showed that levodopa increases K excretion.
We have thus confirmed our expectations that patients with hypokalemic diseases are at an increased cancer risk, whereas patients with hyperkalemic diseases are at a decreased cancer risk. Thereby still another puzzle piece could be put in its place.

XI. CONCLUSIONS

From the initial key observation of the low cancer rates in Seneca County and its possible relation to concentrations of K and Na, a hypothesis was formulated regarding a negative relation between cancer rates and intracellular, total body, or dietary K/Na ratios. The hypothesis was tested in two different ways: Either phenomena known to change the K/Na ratio were tested regarding influence on cancer or phenomena known to change cancer rates were tested regarding influence on the K/Na ratio.

To the first group belong diet, change in oxygen pressure, hypo- and hyperkalemic diseases, aging, etc. To the other group belong nutrients and carcinogenic agents such as vitamins, Se, fiber, alcohol, obesity, DMH, etc. Aging could be also included in this group, because we know that aging increases the risk of cancer and that it decreases the total body K. All tests confirmed the hypothesis, and it seems safe to say that even if K/Na is not the causative agent in cancer etiology it is certainly an important marker. The model that was developed combines observations from a number of different specialities and shows how the K/Na ratio, as a common denominator in all these studies, increases when the cancer rates decrease and decreases when the cancer rates increase.

As in all modeling many gaps need to be filled. Here are some:

How does Se change the intracellular K/Na ratio?
Does hyperbaric oxygen pressure increase the cancer rates?
Do patients with multiple sclerosis have a higher than normal
  total body or intracellular K/Na ratio?
Does the tobacco additive licorice play a role in the high cancer
  risks caused by smoking?

Two general findings of this study were

1. *Organ site specificity*: when oxygen pressure was increased, the respiratory organs were afflicted, and when the dietary K/Na was reduced, the digestive organs were afflicted.
2. *Nonlinearity between K/Na and cancer rates*: Even if K/Na decreases as a linear function of the concentration of some agent, the cancer rates increase faster than linearly. This also explains that two carcinogenic agents, even if they are independent of each other, act in a synergistic, not an additive way.

As noted in the introduction, the role of the epidemiologist or the mathematical modeler is to reveal and point out possible relations between observed phenomena. Other specialists, such as biochemists, physiologists, molecular biologists, are needed to explain why these relations exist and to find the mechanisms behind them. A few specu- lations on possible explanations as to how the intracellular K/Na ratio affects cancer rates may nevertheless be permitted:

A high ionic strength within the cells increases the condensation of the chromatin, which in turn might protect against car- cinogens. Potassium contributes more to the intracellular ionic strength than Na does.
The transcription rate from DNA to RNA is faster in a high K concentration in the cells than in a low one.

Cellular oncogenes may belong to the on/off switch system in differentiation and embryogenesis [92]. The intracellular K/Na ratio could be a branching signal in the system. When the ratio is above some value, the oncogene switch may be off; when the ratio drops below this value, the switch goes on. Low K/Na, necessary in the early stages of embryogenesis, may, after differentiation, be replaced by a higher K/Na. When, due to wrong diet, high age, etc., K/Na later falls below the threshold, the switch turns on again and an unwanted return to a more primitive and immature cell type occurs.

Some other explanation of the mechanisms may eventually be shown to be right. That a relation between K/Na concentrations and cancer rates exists seems to be convincingly shown by the results of this study.

Quantitatively this study indicates that the dietary K/Na and the total body K/Na should be above 1, whereas the intracellular K/Na ratio ought to be above 5 or 6. A recommendation for a good diet would thus be to avoids salting in preservation, preparation, and eating of our food, avoid too much fat, and too many calories, in the diet and increases the intake of fruits and vegetables and of other foods rich in vitamins.

REFERENCES

1. Popper K. R. *Objective Knowledge: An Evolutionary Approach,* Clarendon Press, Oxford, (1972).

2. Popper, K. R., *The Logic of Scientific Discovery,* Harper & Row, New York, (1968).

3. Maclure, M. Popperian refutation in epidemiology. *Am. J. Epidemiology 121*:343 (1985).

4. Shimkin, M. B., *Contrary to Nature . . . Cancer,* DHEW Publ. No. (NIH) 76–720, (1977).

5. Burkitt, D. P. Large-bowel cancer: An Epidemiologic jigsaw puzzle, *JNCI, 54*:137 (1975).

6. Mason, T. J. and McKay, F. S., *U.S. Cancer Mortaility by County, 1950–1969,* DHEW Publ. No (NIH) 75–165, (1974).

7. Jansson, B., Seibert, G. B., and Speer, J. F. Gastrointestinal cancer. Its geographic distribution and correlation to breast cancer. *Cancer, 36*:2373 (1975).

8. Shamberger, R. J. Relationship of selenium to cancer, I. Inhibiting effect of selenium on carcinogenesis. *JNCI, 44*:931 (1970).

9. Schrauzer G. N. and Ishmael, D. Effects of selenium and arsenic on the genesis of spontaneous mammary tumors in inbred C$_3$H mice. *Ann. Clin. Lab. Sci.*, *4*:411 (1974).

10. Jacobs, M. M., Jansson, B., and Griffin, A. C. Inhibitory effects of selenium on 1,2-dimethylhydrazine and methylazoxymethanol acetate induction of colon tumors. *Cancer Lett.*, *2*:133 (1977).

11. Jansson, B. Geographic mappings of colorectal cancer rates: A retrospect of studies, 1974—1984. *Cancer Detection and Prevention*, *8*:341 (1985).

12. Jansson, B. Statistical significance of geographical clusters. *Med. Biol. Environ.*, *10*:1 (1983).

13. Riggan, W. B., van Bruggen, J., and Mason, T. J., *U.S. Cancer Mortality Rates and Trends, 1950—1979*, EPA-600/1-83-015a, NCI, (1983).

14. Jansson, B., Jacobs, M. M., and Griggins, A. C. Gastrointestinal cancer: Epidemiology and experimental studies, in *Inorganic and Nutritional Aspects of Cancer* (G. N. Schrauzer, ed.), Plenum Press, New York, p. 305, (1978).

15. Berg, C. O., Middle Atlantic states, in *Limnology in North America* (D. G. Frey, ed.), Univ. Wisconsin Press, Madison, p. 191, (1963).

16. Jansson, B. Seneca County, New York: An area with low cancer mortality rates. *Cancer*, *48*:2542 (1981).

17. Jansson, B. The geographical distribution of colorectal cancer in the United States. *Med. Biol. Environ.*, *4*:119 (1976).

18. Pantellini, G. V. Hydrogen (H) bonds and their salification by potassium (K) in the structuring of living matter. *Med. Biol. Environ.*, *4*:467 (1976).

19. Bopp, F. and Biggs, R. B. Metals in estaurine sediments: Factor analysis and its environmental significance. *Science*, *214*:441 (1981).

20. Texas Water Development Board, *Chemical Analysis of Saline Water. A Survey of the Subsurface Saline Water in Texas*, Report 157, Austin, (1978).

21. Burton, A. C. Cancer and altitude. Does intracellular pH regulate cell division. *Europ. J. Cancer*, *11*:365 (1975).

22. Sterns, R. H., Cox, M., Feig, P. U., and Singer, I. Internal potassium balance and the control of the plasma potassium concentration. *Medicine*, *60*:339 (1981).

23. S. J. Cutler, J. L. Young, Jr., eds., *Third National Cancer Survey:Incidence data*, DHEW Publ. No (NIH) 75–787, (1975).

24. Jansson, B. Geographic cancer risk and intracellular potassium/sodium ratios. *Cancer Detection and Prevention, 9*:171 (1986).

25. Amsel, J., Waterbor, J. W., Oler, J., Rosenwaike, I., and Marshall, K. Relationship of site-specific cancer mortality rates to altitude. *Carcinogenesis, 3*:461 (1982).

26. Rios-Dalenz, J., Correa, P., and Haenzel, W. Morbidity from cancer in La Paz, Bolivia. *Int. J. Cancer, 28*:307 (1981).

27. Akhtiamov, M. G. and Kairakbaev, M. K. Incidence of esophageal cancer on the plains and in the mountainous regions of Kazakh, SSR. *Vopr. Onkl. 29*:49 (1983).

28. Mastrandera, V., LaRosa, F., Pannelli, F., and Cresci, A. Malignant neoplasm mortality in different zones of a central Italian region: The moutains, hills and coast of the Marches. *Zbl. Bakt. Hyg. I. Abt. Orig. B., 165*:269 (1977).

29. Hurtado, H., Animals in high altitudes: Resident man. Adaptation to the environment, (D. B. Dill, E. F. Adolph, and C. G. Wilber, eds.), *Am. Physiological Soc.*, Washington D. C. p. 834, (1964).

30. Eaton, S. B. and Konner, M. Paleolithic nutrition, A consideration of its nature and current implications, *N. Engl. J. Med., 312*:283 (1985).

31. Shah, B. G. and Belonje, B. Calculated sodium and potassium in the Canadian diet if comprised of unprocessed ingredients. *Nutr. Res., 3*:629 (1983).

32. Henningsen, N. C., Larsson, L., and Nelson, D. Hypertension, potassium, and the kitchen. *Lancet. Jan. 15*, p. 133 (1983).

33. Grim, C. E., Luft, F. C., Miller, J. Z., Meneely, G. R., Battarbee, H. D. Hamer, C. G., and Dahl, L. K. Racial differences in blood pressure in Evans County, Georgia: Relationship to sodium and potassium intake and plasma renin activity. *J. Chronic. Dis., 33*:87 (1980).

34. Frank, G. C., Nicolich, J., Voors, A. W., Webber, L. S., and Berenson, G. S. A simplified inventory method for quantitating dietary sodium, potassium, and energy. *Am. J. Clin. Nutr., 38*:474 (1983).

35. Voors, A. W., Daferes, E. R., Frank, G. C., Aristimuno, G. G., and Berenson, G. S. Relation between ingested potassium and sodium balance in young blacks and whites. *Am. J. Clin. Nutr., 37*:583 (1983).

36. Watt, B. K. and Merrill, A. L. *Composition of Foods—Raws, Processed, Prepared.* Agriculture Handbook No. 8, U.S. Department of Agriculture, Washington D.C., (1963).

37. Organization for Economic Cooperation and Development, *Food Consumption Statistics 1960—1968*, Paris, (1970).

38. American Cancer Society, Inc., *American Cancer Society. Cancer Facts and Figures 1979*, (1978).

39. Charnly, G. and Tannenbaum, S. R. Flow cytometric analysis of the effect of sodium chloride on gastric cancer risk in the rat. *Cancer Research*, 45:5608 (1985).

40. Joint Iran—IARC Cancer Study Group. Esophageal cancer studies in the Caspian littoral of Iran: Results of population studies—a prodrome. *JNCI*. 59:1127 (1977).

41. Ophir, O., Peer, G., Gilad, J., Blum, M., and Aviram, A. Low blood pressure in vegetarians: the possible role of potassium. *Am. J. Clin. Nutr.*, 37:755 (1983).

42. Jacobs, M. M. Trace element inhibition of carcinogenesis and angiogenesis. *Biol. Trace Element Res.*, 5:375 (1983).

43. Blondell, J. M. The anticarcinogenic effect of magnesium. *Medical Hypothesis*, 6:863 (1980).

44. Newmark, H. L., Wargovich, M. J., Bruce, W. R., Boynton, A. L., Kleine, L. P., Whitfield, J. F., Jansson, B., and Cameron, I. L., Ions and neoplastic development, in *Large Bowel Cancer, Clinical and Basic Science Research*, (A. J. Mastromarino, and M. G. Brattain, eds.), Praeger, New York, p. 102, (1985).

45. Lipkin, M. and Newmark, H. Effect of added dietary calcium on colonic epithelial-cell proliferation in subjects at high risk for familial colonic cancer. *N. Engl. J. Med.*, 313:1381 (1985).

46. Garland, C., Shekelle, R. B., Barrett-Connor, E., Criqui, M. H., Rossof, A. H., and Paul, O. Dietary vitamin D and calcium and risk of colorectal cancer: A 19-year prospective study in men. *Lancet. Feb 9*:307 (1985).

47. Heilbrun, L. K., Nomura, A., Hankin, J. H., and Stemmermann, G. N. Dietary vitamin D and calcium and risk of colorectal cancer. *Lancet, April 20*:925 (1985).

48. Heilbrun, L. K., Nomura, A., Hankin, J. H., and Stemmermann, G. N. Colon cancer and dietary fat, phosphorus, and calcium in Hawaiian-Japanese men. *Am. J. Clin. Nutr.*, 43:306 (1986).

49. Hormozdiari, H., Day, N. E., Aramesh, B., and Mahboubi, E. Dietary factors and esophageal cancer in the Caspian littoral of Iran. *Cancer Res.*, *35*:3493 (1975).

50. Bjelke, E., *Epidemiological Studies of Cancer of the Stomach, Colon, and Rectum, with Special Emphasis on the Risk of Diet*, Ph.D. Thesis, Univ. of Minnesota, (1973).

51. Kino, M., Tokushigo, A., Tamura, H., Hopp, L., Searle, B. M., Khalil, F., and Aviv, A. Cultured rat vascular smooth muscle cells: extracellular calcium and Na^+-K^+ regulation. *Am. J. Physiol.*, *248*:C436 (1985).

52. Edelman, A., Thil, C.-L., Garabedian, M., Plachot, J.-J., Guillozo, H., Fritsch, J., Tomas, S. R., and Balsan, S. Vitamin D metabolite effects on membrane potential and potassium intracellular activity in rabbit cartilage. *Mineral Electrolyte Metab.*, *11*:97 (1985).

53. Carroll, K. K. Experimental evidence of dietary factors and hormone-dependent cancers. *Cancer Res.*, *35*:3374 (1975).

54. Zidek, W., Karoff, C. H., Losse, H., and Vetter, H. Intracellulaere Elektrolyte und Serumlipide in Abhaengigkeit von der diaetetischen Fettsaurezufuhr. *Schweiz. Med. Wschr.*, *112*:1787 (1982).

55. Zidek, W., Karoff, C., Losse, H., and Vetter, H. Intracellular electrolytes and hormonal parameters during weight reduction. *Ann. Nutr. Metab.*, *28*:65 (1984).

56. Kutscherskij, E., Gunther, J., and Mehley, E. K-p-nitrophenyl-phosphatase activity, Na and K content, Na permeability and membrane lipid composition in rabbit myocardium after cholesterol rich diet. *Experientia*, *40*:812 (1984).

57. Pierson, R. N., Wang, J., Frank, W., Allen, G., and Rayyes, A., Alcohol affects intracellular potassium, sodium, and water distribution in rats and man, *Currents in Alcoholism* (F. A. Seixas, ed.), Grune & Stratton, New York, p. 161, (1977).

58. Zs.-Nagy, I., Lustyik, G., Zs.-Nagy, V., Zarandi, B., and Bertoni-Freddari, C. Intracellular Na^+: K^+ ratios in human cancer cells as revealed by energy dispersive x-ray micro-analysis, *J. Cell. Biol.*, *90*:769 (1981).

59. Matthias, J. Q. Trauma—clinical aspects, in *The Prevention of Cancer* (R. W. Raven and F. J. C. Roe, eds), Butterworths, London, p. 47, (1967).

60. Kimura, S., Bassett, A. L., Gaide, M. S., Kozlovskis, P. L., and Myerburg, R. J. Regional changes in intracellular potassium and sodium activity after healing of experimental myocardial infarction in cats. *Circ. Res.*, *58*:202 (1986).

61. Ferrini, O. and Gambaro, G. C. Studi sull'equilibro idro-salino plasmatico-tissurale. Contenuto in aqua e sali del plasma e del tessuti di ratti trattati con vitamina. A. *Archivio E. Maragliano di patologia e clinica*, *9*:1091 (1954).

62. Hanck, A. B. Der Einfluss von 1,000 mg Vitamin C pro Tag und das renale Ausscheidungsverhalten einiger Elektrolyte im Harn des gesunden Menschen. *Int. J. Vit. Nutr. Res.*, *43*:34 (1973).

63. Demigné, C. and Rémésy, Stimulation of absorption of volatile fatty acids and minerals in the cecum of rats adapted to a very high fiber diet. *J. Nutr.*, *115*:53 (1985).

64. Schwartz, S. E., Levine, G. D., and Starr, C. M. Effects of dietary fiber on intestinal ion fluxes in rats. *Am. J. Clin. Nutr.*, *36*:1102 (1982).

65. Vaamonde, C. A. Sodium depletion, in *Sodium: Its Biological Significance* (S. Papper, ed.), CRC Press, Boca Raton, p. 207, (1982).

66. Pollard, M. and Luckert, P. H. Prolonged antitumor effect of indomethacin on autochthonous intestinal tumors in rats. *JNCI*, *70*:1103 (1983).

67. Lynch, N. R. and Salomon, J.-C. Tumor growth inhibition and potentiation of immunotherapy by indomethacin in mice. *JNCI*, *62*:117 (1979).

68. Galler, M., Folkert, V. W., and Schlondorff, D. Reversible acute renal insufficiency and hyperkalemia. *JAMA*, *246*:154 (1981).

69. Findling, J. W., Beckstrom, D., Rawsthorne, L., Kozin, F., and Itskovitz, H. Indomethacin-induced hyperkalemia in three patients with gouty arthritis. *JAMA*, *244*:1127 (1980).

70. M. N. G. Dukes, Ed., *Side Effects of Drugs*, Annual 6. A worldwide yearly survey of new data and trends, Excerpta Medica, Oxford, p. 93, (1982).

71. Marquart-Moulin, G., Durbec, J. P., Cornée, J., Berthezène, P., and Southgate, D. A. T. Alimentation et cancer recto-colique. *Gastroenterologie Clinique et Biologique*, *7*:277 (1983).

72. Cox, J. R. and Shalaby, W. A. Potassium changes with age. *Gerontology*, *27*:340 (1981).

73. Macgillivray, I., Buchanan, T. J., and Billewicz, W. Z., Values of total exchangeable sodium and potassium in normal females based on weight, height and age. *Clin. Sci., 19*:17 (1960).

74. Pierson, Jr., R. N., Wang, J., Colt, E. W., and Neuman, P. Body composition measurements in normal man: The potassium, sodium, sulfate and tritium spaces in 58 adults. *J. Chron. Dis., 35*:419 (1982).

75. Delwaide, P. A. Body potassium measurements by whole-body counting: Screening of patient populations. *J. Nucl. Med., 14*:40 (1973).

76. Ellis, K. J., Shukla, K. K., Cohn, S. H., and Pierson, R. N. A predictor for total body potassium in man based on height, weight, sex, and age: Applications in metabolic disorders. *J. Lab. Clin. Med., 83*:716 (1974).

77. Schober, O., Basaller, C., Lehr, L., and Hundeshagen, H. Altered potassium homeostasis in Crohn's disease. *Eur. J. Nucl. Med., 8*:245 (1983).

78. Kessler, I. I. Cancer mortality among diabetics. *JNCI, 44*:673 (1970).

79. Colt, E. W. D., Dunner, D. L., Wang, J., Ross, D. C., Pierson, R. N., and Fieve, R. R. Body composition in affective disorder before, during, and after lithium carbonate therapy. *Arch. Gen. Psychiatry, 39*:577 (1982).

80. Edmonds, C. J., Smith, T., Griffiths, R. D., Mackenzie, J., and Edwards, R. H. T. Total body potassium and water, and exchangeable sodium, in muscular dystrophy. *Clin. Sci., 68*:379 (1985).

81. Nerup, J. Addison's disease—clinical studies. A report on 108 cases. *Acta Endocrinologica, 76*:127 (1974).

82. Viukari, M. Epilepsy, schizophrenia, and sodium-potassium A. T. P.-ase, *Lancet, 7753*:749 (1972).

83. Levi, R. N. and Waxman, S. Schizophrenia, epilepsy, cancer, methionine, and folate metabolism, *Lancet, 7293*:11 (1975).

84. Tsuang, M. T., Woolson, R. F., and Fleming, J. A. Schizophrenia and cancer death. *Lancet, 8166*:480 (1980).

85. Palo, J. Malignant diseases among patients with multiple sclerosis, *J. Neurol, 216*:217 (1977).

86. Doshay, L. J. Problem situations in the treatment of paralysis agitans. *JAMA, 156*:680 (1954).

87. Jansson, B. and Jankovic, J. Low cancer rates among patients with Parkinson's disease. *Ann. Neurol.*, *17*:505 (1985).

88. Scotto, J., Fears, T. R., and Fraumeni, Jr., J. F., *Incidence of Nonmelanoma Skin Cancer in the United Staes*, U.S. Department of Health and Human Services, NIH Publ. No. 83-2433, (1983).

89. National Institutes of Health, *End Results in Cancer*, Report No. 4. NIH Publ. No 73—272, (1972).

90. Granerus, A.-K., Jagerburg, R., and Svanborg, A. Kaliuretic effect of L-dopa treatment in parkinsonian patients. *Acta Med. Scand.*, *201*:291 (1977).

91. Sundström, S., Henrikson, R., and Lindström, P. Dopamine increases potassium efflux in the rat parotid gland by stimulating noradrenaline release from sympathetic nerve endings. *Brain Res.*, *337*:155 (1985).

92. Bishop, J. B. Viruses, genes, and cancer. II. Retroviruses and cancer genes. *Cancer*, *55*:2329 (1985).

2
Quantitative Theories of Carcinogenesis

DUNCAN J. MURDOCH and DANIEL R. KREWSKI *Health and Welfare Canada, Ottawa, Ontario, Canada*

KENNY S. CRUMP* *K. S. Crump/Clement, Inc., Ruston, Louisiana*

I. INTRODUCTION

The first substantial advance in defining the mechanism of carcinogenesis was reported by Berenblum [1], who demonstrated that chemical carcinogens may initially induce an apparently reversible change in the target cells followed by a partially reversible developmental phase ultimately leading to the expression of a tumor. This initiation/promotion model was subsequently established in the induction of mouse skin lesions [2-4] as well as in other tissues [5]. Since that time, much progress has been made in identifying the mechanisms of carcinogenesis [6] and in the development of biologically based mathematical models for the process of carcinogenesis [7,8].

This chapter reviews quantitative theories of carcinogenesis. In Section II, we consider the multistage model of carcinogenesis proposed by Armitage and Doll [9] and subsequently developed [10,11] to accommodate the effects of time-dependent exposure patterns. Extensions to the multistage model to cover the case of joint exposures to multiple agents are also considered [12,13]. In Section III, we consider stochastic models of carcinogenesis based on the birth, death, and mutation of cells within the target tissue. This class of models was originally proposed by Knudson [14] and was later refined by Moolgavkar and Venzon [15].

Current Affiliation:
Executive Vice President, Clement Associates, Inc., Ruston, Louisiana.

Because many carcinogens require some form of metabolic activation to exert their effects, pharmacokinetic models are discussed in Section IV [16]. These models specify certain kinetic processes for the uptake, activation, detoxification, and elimination of the agent of interest, and may be used to relate the delivered dose to the target tissue and the substance to which an individual is exposed via oral, dermal, or inhalation routes. These models are of particular interest when one or more of the component processes is saturable, since the relationship between internal and external exposure may then be nonlinear.

Because human exposure to most environmental carcinogens is low, the risks associated with long-term low-level exposure are of particular concern in human health risk assessment. Most theories of carcinogenesis do not admit the possibility of threshold doses below which tumor induction may not occur [17–19], so even low levels of exposure may not be free of some attendant degree of risk. Since a number of general theoretical considerations suggest that dose response curves for carcinogenesis may be linear at low doses, the plausibility of this assertion is examined in Section V.

II. THE MULTISTAGE MODEL

A. Derivation

Several models of cancer developed in the early 1950s were based on the assumptions that cancer originates in a single cell lineage and that a number of distinct events are required to occur for cancer to be initiated [9,20–23]. These models were proposed to explain the observation that, for many carcinomas, the age-specific cancer incidence rate increases as age raised to some power. The events in these models may be thought of as mutations, but this interpretation is not crucial. For most consequences, it makes no essential difference mathematically whether the events occur in a specific order [9] or in random order [22].

These models have been modified and extended. In an effort to explain the age-incidence patterns in human data with models having fewer stages than is required by simpler models, Armitage and Doll [24] permitted cells in intermediate stages to multiply more rapidly than nontransformed cells. Neyman and Scott [25] used a modified two-stage model to describe the tumor response in mice subject to a time-varying dosing regimen. Crump et al. [26] introduced the effect of a carcinogenic dose into the model of Armitage and Doll [9, 27]. Whittemore and Keller [28] used a multistage formulation to explain the joint effect of two chemicals—one a tumor initiator and the other a tumor promoter. Moolgavkar and Venzon [15] proposed and studied a two-stage model, noting that such a model is consistent with the development of homozygosity at a genetic locus, and that the existence of more than two rate-limiting steps has never been convincingly demonstrated. Moolgavkar [29] presents a discussion of this model in relation to human carcinogenesis. (See Section III for further details.)

In the multistage model of Armitage and Doll [27], it is assumed that cancer is initiated by a single cell, that a cell (and its daughters) must pass sequentially through $k \geqslant 1$ distinct stages to become an observable cancer, and that the cells in the target tissue compete independently to initiate the first cancerous lesion. Further, it is assumed that the waiting times between the events delimiting the stages are independently distributed for each cell and have exponential distributions:

$$P(T_i \leqslant t) = 1 - \exp(-\lambda_i d) \tag{1}$$

where T_i is the length of the ith stage and $1/\lambda_i$ is the mean length. The probability distribution for the waiting time until cancer is observed, $P(T \leqslant t)$, where $T = T_1 + \cdots + T_k$, is given by the convolution of the exponential distributions of the lengths of the k stages.

If the λ_i's are all equal to some constant λ, then

$$P(T \leqslant t) = \lambda^k \int_0^t \frac{x^{k-1} \exp(-\lambda x) \, dx}{(k-1)!} \tag{2}$$

This case ($\lambda_i = \lambda$ for all i) would arise if cancer is caused by the cell suffering k "hits" (from molecules of a carcinogenic compound or from radiation) and if the hits are realizations of a Poisson process. (A Poisson process is essentially one in which the events—hits in this case—are independent and the time between hits has an exponential distribution as described earlier [30].) Poisson processes occur under fairly general conditions and have been used to model diverse types of data, from radioactive decay to the number of chocolate chips in a cookie.

The key assumptions leading to a Poisson process are three: (1) events are independent; (2) it is extremely unlikely that two events will occur simultaneously; and (3) the probability of an event occurring in a fixed interval of time is proportional to the length of time (a linearity assumption). These assumptions are all reasonable when considering molecules or radioactive particles hitting a sensitive locus on a DNA molecule. The assumption that exactly k identical hits (identical in terms of their mean occurrence times) must be

received to cause cancer and that the cancer will then be observable
is less easily accepted. However, if we imagine k equally accessible
loci on the DNA, each of which must be altered by a hit for cancer
to occur, then the requirement of k identical hits is reasonable.

Van Ryzin and Rai [31] introduced the effects of exposure into
(2) by assuming that λ is proportional to the dose level d. For a
fixed time t (as in bioassay experiments in which all animals are
terminated at a common time) this leads to the gamma-multihit model

$$P(T \leqslant t) = \int_0^{\beta d} \frac{x^{k-1} \exp(-x) \, dx}{(k-1)!} \tag{3}$$

where $\beta = \lambda t$.

The probabilities considered thus far are those of a single cell
initiating cancer. The gamma-multihit model has been applied to
model the occurrence of cancer in tissues, but it is not clear that
the derivation described thus far should apply to whole tissues as
it does to individual cells. When n different cell lines compete in
producing the tumors, the probability of cancer in a tissue is given
by

$$1 - \exp[-nP_d(t)] \cong 1 - \exp(-\theta d^k) \tag{4}$$

where $\theta = n\beta^k/k!$, which is a Weibull distribution. Thus, the
Weibull distribution appears to have a stronger rationale than the
gamma multihit.

Since there are a large number of cells in a target tissue and
since the probability of cancer induction is generally much less than
1, our assumption that cells act independently in initiating cancer
forces us to conclude that the probability of any particular cell
initiating cancer is very small. Thus, one or more of the values λ_i
must be very small so that the overall waiting time is large. If
all of the λ_i are small enough so that $\exp(-\lambda_i t) = 1$, then

$$P(T \leqslant t) = \left(\prod_{i=1}^{k} \lambda_i \right) \frac{t^k}{k!} \tag{5}$$

This implies that the age-specific incidence rate of cancer is proportional to t^{k-1}. This relationship holds approximately for many
cancers—particularly carcinomas in other than sex organs—with the
exponent varying between 3 and 6 [32]. For this result to be consistent with (5), the number of stages k must be between 4 and 7.
Such a large number of rate-limiting stages does not have experimental verification and seems somewhat implausible. Armitage and Doll

[24] and Moolgavkar [29] have thus proposed modifications of the multistage process that would require fewer stages to predict an exponent between 3 and 6.

When the λ_i take larger values, approximation (5) begins to break down. Moolgavkar [33] has derived an infinite series representation of $P(T \leqslant t)$, in which (5) corresponds to the first term. A hypothetical example of a seven-stage model for a malignant tumor in humans is presented in which the largest λ_i is 0.009 transitions per cell per year, where retention of the second term in the expansion reduces the predicted incidence by 30% at age 75.

Once a cell line has reached the kth stage and become cancerous, there is an additional waiting time, often called the induction period, until the cancer is clinically observable. With the λ_i allowed to be nonequal, we can let the induction period correspond to the kth stage, or we can let it have an arbitrary distribution function $F(t)$. In the latter case, the probability $P_0(t)$ that a particular cell initiates a tumor observed by time t is given by the convolution of F with the distribution given in (2); that is,

$$
P_0(t) \cong \left(\prod_{i=1}^{k} \lambda_i \right) \int_0^t \frac{F(t-u)u^{k-1}}{(k-1)!} \, du \tag{6}
$$

If F has a small standard deviation relative to $1/\lambda_i$, then an increase in incidence proportional to a power of time can be approximated, but with the apparent exponent considerably larger than $k - 1$ as predicted by (6). Crump [34] showed, for example, that an incidence rate proportional to $t^{5.5}$ could be approximated by a four-stage model with a constant 20 year induction time.

The probability, $P(t)$, of observing a tumor in a target tissue containing n cell lines is

$$
\begin{aligned}
P(t) &= 1 - [1 - P_0(t)]^n \\
&= 1 - \exp\{n \log[1 - P_0(t)]\} \\
&= 1 - \exp\{-n[P_0(t) + P_0(t)^2/2 + \cdots]\} \\
&\cong 1 - \exp[-nP_0(t)] \tag{7}
\end{aligned}
$$

because $P_0(t)$ is a very small number (so that $P_0(t)^2$ and higher powers of $P_0(t)$ are negligible). With (6) this gives the multistage model

$$
P(t) = \exp\left\{ -n\left(\prod_{i=1}^{k} \lambda_i \right) \int_0^t \frac{F(t-u)u^{k-1}}{(k-1)!} \, du \right\} \tag{8}
$$

With a constant latency period t_0, we have the Weibull distribution

$$P(t) = 1 - \exp\left\{-n\left(\prod_{i=1}^{k} \lambda_i\right) \frac{(t - t_0)^k}{k!}\right\} \tag{9}$$

Crump et al. [26] introduced a constant dose d into the model by assuming that the intensity λ_i of each stage is linearly related to d as

$$\lambda_i = \alpha_i + \beta_i d \tag{10}$$

This leads to the multistage model,

$$P_d(t) = 1 - \exp\left\{-n\left[\prod_{i=1}^{k} (\alpha_i + \beta_i d)\right]\int_0^t \frac{F(t - u)u^{k-1} \, du}{(k - 1)!}\right\} \tag{11}$$

For a fixed time period t, this reduces to

$$P_d = 1 - \exp\left\{-n\left[\prod_{i=1}^{k} (\alpha_i + \beta_i d)\right]\right\} \tag{12}$$

Note that α_i and β_i determine the probabilities of cell transformation and must be nonnegative for all i. If there is a positive background rate of occurrence (i.e., a positive probability of observing tumors with d = 0), then $\alpha_i > 0$ for all i; if there is a dose effect, then $\beta_j > 0$ for some j. These conditions imply that for small values of d,

$$P_d \cong \prod_{i=1}^{k} \alpha_i \left[1 + \left(\sum_{i=1}^{k} \frac{\beta_i}{\alpha_i}\right) d\right] \tag{13}$$

This gives the important result that, whenever there is background carcinogenesis, the dose-related carcinogenic response is expected to vary linearly with dose d at low doses.

If we expand the polynomial

$$n \prod_{i=1}^{k} (\alpha_i + \beta_i d) = q_0 + q_1 d + \cdots + q_k d^k \tag{14}$$

then we get the form of the multistage model commonly used for extrapolation to low doses in cancer risk assessment [34]:

$$P_d = 1 - \exp\{-(q_0 + q_1 d + \cdots + q_k d^k)\} \tag{15}$$

The requirement that $\alpha_i \geqslant 0$ and $\beta_i \geqslant 0$ for all i places complicated constraints upon the coefficients q_i [35]. However, the set of all q_i which satisfy these constraints also satisfies the simple constraints $q_i \geqslant 0$ for all i, and so these simpler constraints are generally used when applying the model. This model has been widely applied to the estimation of carcinogenic risk at low doses from animal data [34].

B. Time-Dependent Exposure

Generalizations of the multistage model to allow for situations in which dosing cannot be assumed to be constant throughout life have been developed recently [10,11]. At the cellular level it is assumed that the transition rates between stages (10) depend on the instantaneous rate of exposure $d(t)$, that is,

$$\lambda_i(t) = \alpha_i + \beta_i d(t) \tag{16}$$

[11]. In cases where the applied dose changes rapidly, it may be more appropriate to interpret $d(t)$ as the delivered dose to the site of action, since (16) would unrealistically predict an immediate drop in $\lambda_i(t)$ following cessation of exposure. Under this model, equation (5) generalizes to

$$P(T \leqslant t) \cong 1 - \exp\left(-\int_0^t \cdots \int_0^{u_2} [\alpha_1 + \beta_1 d(u_1)] \cdots \right.$$

$$\left. [\alpha_k + \beta_k(d(u_k)] du_1 \cdots du_k \right) \tag{17}$$

If several stages are dose related, the carcinogenic response predicted by (17) is complicated. Under the assumption that at most two stages are dose related, however, an explicit form of (17) has been given by Crump and Howe [11].

If only one stage is dose related, then the age at dosing can, depending on the stage involved, have a market effect on the response rate. For example, if the first stage is dose related, then dosing early in life is much more effective than dosing later in life, whereas the reverse is true if the last stage is dose related. This may be expected, because if a large number of cells progress to the second stage early in life, many of them will have time to pass through the remaining stages required to complete the carcinogenic process. On the other hand, there will be many cells in stage k − 1 later on in life which are susceptible to dosing if the last stage is dose related.

Day and Brown [10] examined the carcinogenicity of several different chemicals administered to mice, including benzo[a]pyrene (BP), fraction G of T57 cigarette smoke (GT57), 2-acetylaminofluorene (2-AAF), and DDT. They found that on cessation of dosing, liver tumors due to 2-AAF and skin tumors due to BP continued to increase in incidence almost as rapidly as if dosing had been continued. On the other hand, the incidence of bladder tumors due to 2-AAF, liver tumors due to DDT, and skin tumors due to GT57 were sharply reduced upon cessation of dosing in comparison with continuous dosing. This appears to indicate that if the multistage model correctly describes these tumors, an early stage of the carcinogenic process is dose dependent for 2-AAF in the liver and BP on the skin, whereas a late stage is affected by the other chemical-site combinations.

Day and Brown [10] also considered epidemiological studies relating human lung cancer to smoking, all forms of cancer other than leukemia to radiation, lung cancer to asbestos, cancer of the nasal sinus to nickel, and bladder cancer to unknown occupational carcinogens. They classified the carcinogens into those affecting an early stage (radiation, asbestos, and the unknown cause of the bladder cancers) versus those affecting a late stage (smoking and nickel), based on the incidence of cancer after dosing ceased.

C. Mixed Exposures

When an individual is exposed to more than one chemical, the multistage model may be extended in several ways. For two carcinogens, Thorslund and Charnley [13] assumed that the transition intensities (10) are linear in d_1 and d_2, the doses of these two substances, with

$$\lambda_i = \alpha_i + \beta_{i1}d_1 + \beta_{i2}d_2 \tag{18}$$

Hamilton and Hoel [12] considered the inclusion of cross-product terms as

$$\lambda_i = \alpha_i + \beta_{i1}d_1 + \beta_{i2}d_2 + \sigma_i d_1 d_2 \tag{19}$$

and pointed out that in cases where the two chemicals act on different stages, these two models are indistinguishable.

III. BIRTH-DEATH-MUTATION MODELS

Moolgavkar and Venzon [15] and Moolgavkar and Knudson [36] have developed a series of stochastic models for carcinogenesis based on mutations occurring during cell division. In one form, two mutations occurring at the time of cell division are necessary for a normal cell to become malignant. Specifically, three possible changes to a normal cell are considered. First, it may divide normally, producing two normal daughter cells. Second, it may mutate on division, producing one normal cell and one damaged, or intermediate, cell. Third, it may die. The probability of any other change (such as the production of two intermediate cells at once) is assumed to be negligible. The same three processes compete for the fate of the intermediate cell, but here normal division produces two more intermediate cells and mutation produces an intermediate cell and a malignant cell. The malignant cell goes on to produce a tumor.

It is assumed that cell division, mutation, and cell death follow Poisson processes, with the intensities of normal division, mutation, and death being L, N, and D for normal cells and α, β, μ for intermediate cells, respectively. The time from the development of a malignant cell to growth of a clinically detectable tumor is assumed to be fixed (and in certain cases the growth may be assumed to be instantaneous). This assumption is not necessary in the derivation of the model, but in application some such assumption is necessary, since it is impossible to observe the birth of a malignant cell.

Let X(t), Z(t), and W(t) denote the number of normal, intermediate, and malignant cells at time t. Further, let

$$\Psi(x, z, w, t) = \sum_{i,j,k} P[X(t) = i, Z(t) = j, W(t) = k \mid$$

$$X(0) = 1, Z(0) = 0, W(0) = 0] x^i z^j w^k \qquad (20)$$

be the generating function for the number of cells of each of the three types at time t, starting with one normal cell at time 0. Next let

$$\Phi(z, w, t) = \sum_{j,k} P[Z(t) = j, W(t) = k \mid Z(0) = 1, W(0) = 0] z^j w^k$$

$$\qquad (21)$$

be the generating function for the number of intermediate and malignant cells at time t, starting with one intermediate cell at time 0. Equation (20) gives rise to an integral equation for $\Psi(x, z, w, t)$ consisting of four terms, corresponding to the three possible changes to a normal cell and to no change at all. This can be written as

$$\Psi(t) = \int_0^t \{L\Psi^2(t - u) + N\Psi(t - u)\Phi(t - u) + D\}e^{-Ku} du + xe^{-Kt}$$

$$(22)$$

where $K = L + N + D$, and the dependence of Ψ and Φ on x, z, and w has been suppressed. Similarly, assuming tumors arise instantaneously from malignant cells, we have

$$\Phi(t) = \int_0^t \{\alpha\Phi^2(t - u) + \beta w\Phi(t - u) + \mu\}e^{-\gamma u} du + ze^{-\gamma t}$$

$$(23)$$

where $\gamma = \alpha + \beta + \mu$. The solution to (23) and a series expansion of the solution to (22) are given in [15]. Alternatively, these functions can be approximated directly by numerical means such as Euler's method.

Given these generating functions, the hazard function for the appearance of the first malignant cell at time t is

$$H(t) = \frac{-\Psi'(1, 1, 0, t)}{\Psi(1, 1, 0, t)}$$

$$(24)$$

This follows from (20), since $\Psi(1, 1, 0, t) = P[W(t) = 0]$.

The number of normal cells in a tissue is often so large that the stochastic model is unnecessary, and X(t) can be treated as a deterministic function. In this case, an explicit form of (24) is available.

$$H(t) = -N \left[\int_0^t X(s)\{\alpha\Phi^2(t - s) - (\alpha + \beta + \mu)\Phi(t - s) + \mu\} ds \right]$$

$$(25)$$

Numerical approximations to (24) and (25) for particular parameter values are given in [15], and applications of the model to human lung cancer and breast cancer are given in [36]. These authors have found that this simple two-stage model is sufficiently flexible to fit the age-incidence curves of many forms of cancer.

IV. PHARMACOKINETIC MODELS

In many cases, the substance to which an individual is exposed may not be the active agent in the process of carcinogenesis, in that some form of metabolic activation may be necessary before damage occurs. For example, Gehring et al. [37] showed that the amount

of vinyl chloride metabolized is more linearly related to tumor incidence than is actual exposure. More recently, Andersen et al.
[38] have demonstrated that the carcinogenicity of methylene
chloride may be due to the metabolic product glutathione S-trans-
ferase.

A. Kinetic Laws

Pharmacokinetic models for metabolic activation are typically composed of many steps, with each step following a simple kinetic law.
The most common of these laws may be illustrated by considering
elimination of a substance X from one compartment in the body.

Let $x(t)$ be the total amount of X in the compartment at time
t. Under zero-order kinetics, elimination takes place at a constant
rate regardless of the amount in the body. Thus, in the absence
of uptake or any other route of elimination, $x(t)$ varies according
to

$$\frac{dx}{dt} = -k \tag{26}$$

where $k > 0$ is the rate constant of the reaction. Zero-order
kinetics may apply in situations where the substance abounds or is
being continuously replenished, so there is no need to consider the
effect of exhausting the supply. If the volume of the compartment
is v, then the concentration [X] in the compartment $x(t)/v$, and we
see that, provided the volume is fixed, it follows a similar law with
rate constant k/v.

First-order or linear kinetics occur when the rate of elimination
is proportional to concentration with

$$\frac{dx}{dt} = -kx(t) \tag{27}$$

First-order kinetics result from the application of the law of mass
action to an irreversible reaction with only one input; they are commonly used in pharmacokinetic models to describe flows between compartments in the body or simple chemical transformations of substances.

Second- or higher-order kinetics may be used when the reaction requires the interaction of two or more particles. For example, if X reacts with Y to be eliminated, the law of mass action predicts that

$$\frac{d[X]}{dt} = -k[X][Y] \tag{28}$$

In the case when $Y = X$ (i.e., X reacts with itself to be eliminated),
this gives rise to

$$\frac{dx}{dt} = -kx^2(t) \tag{29}$$

Saturable or Michaelis-Menten kinetics follow the Michaelis-Menten equation

$$\frac{dx}{dt} = - \frac{Vx(t)}{K + x(t)} \tag{30}$$

where V is the maximum velocity of the reaction and K is the level of x that produces half of this velocity. This equation describes the approximate behavior of systems with enzyme kinetics and was first presented in 1913 [39]. Briefly, it was derived as follows.

Consider the inversion of a sugar X into X* by means of the enzyme E according to the reaction

$$X + E \underset{1}{\overset{}{\rightleftarrows}} XE \underset{2}{\overset{}{\rightarrow}} X^* + E$$

Assume that reaction 1 proceeds much faster than reaction 2 so that the former is essentially at equilibrium. Then the law of mass action implies

$$[X][E] = k_1[XE] \tag{31}$$

Now assume the total concentration of free and bound enzyme is fixed; i.e.,

$$[E] + [EX] = C \tag{32}$$

Then

$$[X](C - [XE]) = k_1[XE] \tag{33}$$

which implies

$$[XE] = \frac{C[X]}{k_1 + [X]} \tag{34}$$

Now the law of mass action implies that the velocity of reaction 2 is $k_2[XE]$, so

$$\frac{d[X]}{dt} = - \frac{k_2C[X]}{k_1 + [X]} \tag{35}$$

and hence

$$\frac{dx}{dt} = \frac{k_2 vCx}{k_1 v + x} \tag{36}$$

This is the Michaelis-Menten equation with $V = k_2 vC$ and $K = k_1 v$. For small concentrations Eq. (30) is approximately the same as Eq. (27) for first-order kinetics, with rate constant $k = V/K$; for high concentrations it approximates Eq. (26) for zero-order kinetics with maximum flow V. An alternative parametrization is

$$\frac{d[X]}{dt} = \frac{k[X]}{1 + s[X]} \tag{37}$$

where $s = 1/K$ may be thought of as the saturability of the reactions, since $s = 0$ corresponds to linear kinetics, and $s > 0$ corresponds to Michaelis-Menten kinetics [8]. This chapter uses (37) to avoid having to treat linear kinetics separately from Michaelis-Menten kinetics.

B. Metabolic Activation

To model complete systems, we combine the laws described earlier into networks describing all the relevant processes in the metabolism of the substance of interest. Compartments are used to represent physical compartments, chemical or physical states of the substance, or amounts of any other entity that is formed in commensurate amounts as the substance is consumed. For example, Gehring and Blau [40] developed the compartmental model for carcinogenesis shown in Fig. 1.

Here, C stands for the chemical as absorbed, C_e for the chemical excreted from the body directly, RM for a reactive metabolite formed after activation of the chemical, CBN for reactive metabolite that is covalently bound to nongenetic material (and hence immobilized), IM for inactive metabolite that has undergone detoxification, CBG for reactive metabolite that is covalently bound to genetic material, causing damage, CBGR for covalently bound genetic material that has been repaired, and RCBG for replicated covalently bound genetic material—a tumor precursor. Paths labeled with names are assumed to follow Michaelis-Menten kinetics; those that are unlabeled follow linear kinetics. Dosing is unspecified but is assumed to be made to compartment C. This model leads to a system of eight differential equations, one for each compartment. For example, the equation describing the rate of change of the amount of RM is

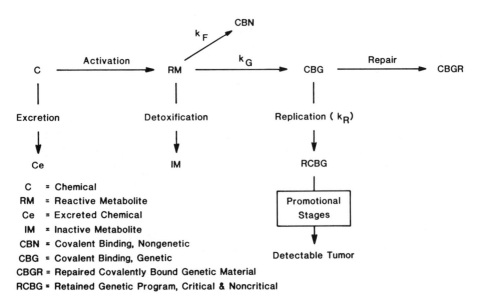

FIGURE 1   A compartmental model for carcinogenesis. From Ref. 40.

$$\frac{dx_{RM}}{dt} = \frac{k_a C}{1 + s_a C} - \frac{k_d x_{RM}}{1 + s_d x_{RM}} - k_F x_{RM} - k_G x_{RM} \qquad (38)$$

where the subscript a indicates the activation path, d indicates the detoxification path, F indicates the nongenetic binding path, and G indicates the genetic binding path.

Models such as this do not generally have explicit solutions because the differential equations describing them include nonlinear Michaelis-Menten terms. However, it is often sufficient to find the steady-state solution because many reactions approach equilibrium very quickly.

For example, consider the steady-state solution for the Gehring and Blau model. Because it contains no loops, the solution can proceed sequentially from compartment C onwards. Thus the only factors affecting the steady-state solution for compartment C are the dosing rate (which is assumed to be fixed independent of x_C) and the rates of activation and excretion, which depend on x_C but not on the contents of any other compartment. Once the steady-state solution for C is found, it may be used to calculate the input rate to compartment RM. The only other factors affecting x_{RM} are the rates of binding and detoxification, which depend only on x_{RM}. By this means, the complete solution may be calculated.

To illustrate, we assume that x_C is set to the steady-state level of that compartment, and we solve for the steady-state level of x_{RM}. By equation (38) if $dx_{RM}/dt = 0$,

$$0 = \frac{k_a x_C}{1 + s_a x_C} - \frac{k_d x_{RM}}{1 + s_d x_{RM}} - k_F x_{RM} - k_G x_{RM} \tag{39}$$

Since x_C is dependent of x_{RM}, we may simplify (39) by putting the input $I = k_a x_C/(1 + s_a x_C)$. We may also sum the two linear terms into a single linear term with coefficient $k = k_F + k_G$. Thus we can rewrite (39) in the generic form for a compartment with any independent input, any number of linear exits, and a single Michaelis-Menten exit:

$$0 = I - \frac{k_d x_{RM}}{1 + s_d x_{RM}} - k x_{RM} \tag{40}$$

Rearranging (40) gives the quadratic equation

$$0 = -s_d k x_{RM}^2 + (I s_d - k_d - k) x_{RM} + I \tag{41}$$

for x_{RM}. Since all of the constants k_d, s_d, k, and I are positive, the right side of (41) is a parabola opening downward that is positive when $x_{RM} = 0$. Thus, there is a unique positive solution

$$x_{RM} = \frac{(I s_d - k_d - k) + \{(I s_d - k_d - k)^2 + 4 s_d k I\}^{1/2}}{2 s_a k} \tag{42}$$

A linear equation arises if there is no Michaelis-Menten exit, whereas a quadratic equation results if there are two Michaelis-Menten exits and no linear ones such as for compartment C. The steady-state solution to the latter case is

$$x_C = \frac{[I(s_a + s_e) - k_a - k_e] + \{[I(s_a + s_e) - k_a - k_e]^2 + 4I(s_a k_e + s_e k_a - I s_a s_e)\}^{1/2}}{s_a k_e + s_e k_a - I s_a s_e} \tag{43}$$

Cubic or higher-order equations arise when there are two Michaelis-Menten exits together with linear ones, or more than two

Michaelis-Menten exits. In these cases numerical approximations will often be easier to obtain than explicit solutions.

Systems involving loops are much more difficult to solve except in certain special cases; hence they are not often used. The most important special case is the completely linear system, for which the solution involves inverting a matrix of rate coefficients.

The steady-state solutions of systems involving Michaelis-Menten kinetics can play many forms of dose dependence. Section VIII shows that all such solutions are linear in the low-dose limit, but the behavior at higher doses can be quite curvilinear. This is evident in the Gehring and Blau model [16], and may be illustrated by the simple model of Krewski et al. [8] shown in Fig. 2.

In this model, dosing is applied to compartment X. The raw chemical may be activated to form reactive metabolite Y, or it may be eliminated. Activation is governed by Michaelis-Menten kinetics, and elimination is linear. The reactive metabolite may be detoxified or eliminated, with Michaelis-Menten detoxification and linear elimination. Tissue damage is assumed to be proportional to the level of reactive metabolite present.

Using formula (42), we obtain the steady-state solution for x_X:

$$x_X = \frac{(ds_a - k_a - k_x) + \{(ds_a - k_a - k_x)^2 + 4ds_a k_x\}^{1/2}}{2s_a k_x} \qquad (44)$$

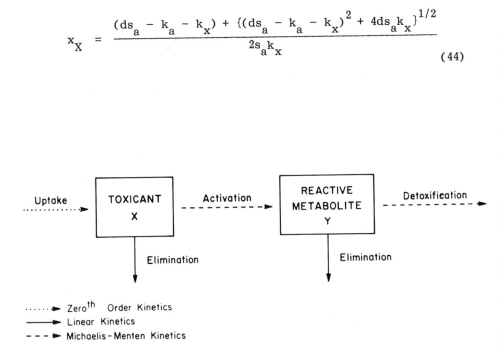

FIGURE 2   A simple two-compartment model for metabolic activation. From Ref. 8.

The steady-stage solution for x_Y is then

$$x_Y = \frac{\left\{ \begin{array}{c} k_a s_a x_X - (k_d + k_y)(1 + s_a x_X) + \{[k_a s_d x_X - (k_d + k_y)(1 + s_a x_X)]^2 \\ + 4k_a k_y s_d x_X (1 + s_a x_X)\}^{1/2} \end{array} \right\}}{2k_y s_d (1 + s_a x_X)}$$

(45)

Depending on the value of the pharmacokinetic constants in (44) and (45), the relationship between the delivered dose to the target tissue x_Y and the administered dose d may be linear, concave, convex, or sigmoid (Fig. 3). The linear relationship occurs when all of the processes follow first-order kinetics. Saturating the activation process results in a concave relationship, whereas the opposite situation occurs when elimination is saturable. When both of these processes are saturable, the relationship may be sigmoid.

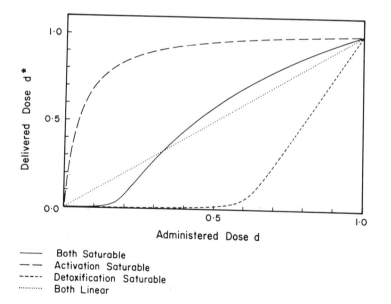

FIGURE 3 Relationship between the dose delivered to the target tissue and the administered dose with saturable activation and detoxification.

V. RISKS AT LOW DOSES

Because human exposure to most environmental carcinogens is low, the shape of the dose-response curve in the low-dose region is of particular concern (Fig. 4). Low-dose linearity corresponds to a finite slope $P'(0) > 0$ at the origin, whereas sublinearity and supralinearity result when this derivative is 0 and $+\infty$, respectively. The multistage model, for example, is low-dose linear provided $q_1 > 0$ in (15). In the remainder of this section, we discuss several general theoretical results on the shape of the dose-response curve in the low-dose region.

A. Additive Background Models

Suppose the background response rate $P(0)$ is nonzero. The class of additive background models [41] is characterized by the relationship

$$P(d) = H(d + \delta) \tag{46}$$

where δ denotes the effective background dose of the chemical and H is a strictly increasing function with continuous bounded derivatives up to second order. Under model (46) we may write

$$P(d) = H(\delta) + dH'(\delta) + o(d) \tag{47}$$

Thus the excess risk over background $P(d) - P(0)$ is linear in d to order $o(d)$, regardless of any other properties of the dose-response

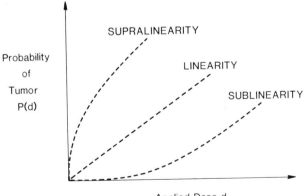

Applied Dose d

FIGURE 4   Linearity, sublinearity, and supralinearity at low doses.

curve. This result may be extended to the case of mixtures of n chemicals, provided that the dose-response curve can be written as

$$P(d_1, \cdots, d_n) = H(d_1 + \delta_1, \cdots, d_n + \delta_n) \tag{48}$$

where H is now strictly increasing in all of its arguments and is subject to the same smoothness condition on its derivatives. For two chemicals (47) becomes

$$P(d_1, d_2) = H(\delta_1, \delta_2) + d_1 \left.\frac{\partial H}{\partial d_1}\right|_{d=0} + d_2 \left.\frac{\partial H}{\partial d_2}\right|_{d=0} + o(d_1, d_2) \tag{49}$$

from which it can be seen that when d_1 and d_2 are low, the dose-response curve is linear in each of them and is additive in their mixture.

B. Michaelis-Menten Systems

In this section we derive the low-dose slope of the concentration in a single compartment in an arbitrary system of n compartments in which transitions from compartment to compartment follow either linear or Michaelis-Menten kinetics. Let $x(t; d) = [x_1(t; d), \ldots, x_n(t; d)]$ be a vector representing the amount of some substance in the n compartments at time t under a constant dose rate d. Let $p = (p_1, \ldots, p_n)$ be the fraction of the dose applied to each of the n compartments, so the actual dose to compartment i is dp_i.

The general Michaelis-Menten system can then be written as

$$\frac{\partial x_i(t; d)}{\partial t} = \sum_{\substack{j=1 \\ j \neq i}}^{n} \sum_{m=1}^{n_{ji}} \frac{k_{jim} x_j}{1 + s_{jim} x_j} - \sum_{j=1}^{n} \sum_{m=1}^{n_{ij}} \frac{k_{ijm} x_i}{1 + s_{ijm} x_i} + dp_i \tag{50}$$

where k_{ijm} and s_{ijm} are, for $j \neq i$, the Michaelis-Menten coefficients for the mth path from compartment i to compartment j, and k_{iim} and s_{iim} are the coefficients of the elimination paths from compartment i. [Note that under linear kinetics it is sufficient to have just one path between each pair of compartments (i.e., $n_{ij} = 1$), since several linear paths behave the same as one path with the appropriate coefficient. Michaelis-Menten paths cannot, in general, be combined in this way.]

We assume, for convenience, that initially the system contains none of the substance of interest; i.e., $x_i(0; d) = 0$ for all i. It then follows that $x_i(t; 0) = 0$ for all i and t. [The case of non-zero starting values is developed in essentially the same way, with $x_i(t; d)$ replaced by the excess due to dosing, $x_i(t; d) - x_i(t; 0)$.] By definition,

$$\frac{\partial x_i(t; 0)}{\partial d} = \lim_{d \to 0} \frac{x_i(t; d)}{d} \tag{51}$$

Letting $y_i(t; d) = x_i(t; d)/d$, we have

$$\frac{\partial y_i(t; d)}{\partial t} = \frac{1}{d} \frac{\partial x_i(t; d)}{\partial t}$$

$$= \frac{1}{d} \left\{ \Sigma\Sigma k_{jim} x_j - \Sigma\Sigma k_{ijm} x_i - \Sigma\Sigma \frac{k_{jim} x_j^2}{1 + s_{jim} x_j} \right.$$

$$\left. + \Sigma\Sigma \frac{k_{ijm} x_i^2}{1 + s_{ijm} x_i} + dp_i \right\}$$

$$= \Sigma\Sigma k_{jim} y_j - \Sigma\Sigma k_{ijm} y_i$$

$$-d \left\{ \Sigma\Sigma \frac{k_{jim} y_j^2}{1 + ds_{ijm} y_i} - \Sigma\Sigma \frac{k_{ijm} y_i^2}{1 + ds_{jim} y_j} \right\} + p_i \tag{52}$$

Since (52) is of the form of a Michaelis-Menten system, $\partial y_i(t; d)/\partial t$ is nonnegative when $y_i(t; d) = 0$, implying that $y_i(t; d) \geqslant 0$ for all t, and

$$\sum_i \frac{\partial y_i(t; d)}{\partial t} \leqslant \sum_i p_i = 1 \tag{53}$$

Thus $\Sigma y_i(t; d)$ and, hence, each $y_i(t; d)$ are bounded above by t. Rewriting the equation for $y_i(t; d)$ as

$$\frac{\partial y_i(t; d)}{\partial t} = L_i(y) - dQ(y) + p_i \tag{54}$$

where $L_i(y)$ represents the first two linear terms and $Q(y)$ the quadratic terms, we have

$$y_i(t; d) = y_i(0; d) + \int_0^t L_i[y(s; d)] \, ds$$

$$- d \int_0^t Q_i[y(s; d)] \, ds + tp_i \tag{55}$$

Now, the boundedness of y implies that Q_i is also uniformly bounded. Hence, as $d \to 0$, the integral involving Q_i vanishes, as we see that in the low-dose limit

$$y_i(t; 0) = y_i(0; 0) + \int_0^t L_i[y(s; 0)] \, ds + tp_i \tag{56}$$

We may also write this in the form

$$\frac{\partial y_i(t; 0)}{\partial t} = L_i(y) + p_i \tag{57}$$

demonstrating that $y(t; 0)$ satisfies a linearized form of the system equations governing $x(t; d)$.

For those systems where steady-state solutions exist, a similar argument shows that at steady state y satisfies

$$0 = L_i(y) - dQ_i(y) + p_i \tag{58}$$

whence $\lim_{d \to 0} y$ satisfies

$$0 = L_i(y) + p_i \tag{59}$$

the linearized steady-state solution.

In conclusion, we have shown that $y_i(t; 0)$, the low-dose slope of $x_i(t; d)$, obeys a linearized version of the kinetics of $x_i(t; d)$, with a normalized dose. Since the amount of the substance of interest in any compartment of a linear system can never return to zero once positive, we see that the low-dose slope of $x_i(t; d)$ is finite and nonzero for all $t > 0$ (including $t = \infty$ when a steady-state solution exists), and hence $x_i(t; d)$ is low-dose linear.

C. Heterogeneous Populations

In most populations the probability of response to a given dose may vary from individual to individual. There may be particularly susceptible subpopulations. In this case there are two kinds of dose-response curves that may be defined: that of each individual, and that of the population, which is the probability of a randomly chosen individual responding at a given dose. These curves may be qualitatively different.

For example, suppose that each individual in a population responds according to the one-stage model

$$P(d) = 1 - \exp(-q_1 d) \tag{60}$$

Assume that q_1^{-1} varies within the population according to a gamma-mixing distribution with shape $1/2$. It is then easily shown that the population has the supralinear dose-response curve

$$P(d) = 1 - \exp(-2\sqrt{d}) \tag{61}$$

More generally, it can be shown that supralinearity will occur if and only if the mixing distribution of q_1 has infinite expectation [8]. Another general result, showing that the power of dose that best approximates the population dose-response curve in the low-dose region is always less than that of any member of the population, is given in the Appendix.

VI. SUMMARY AND CONCLUSIONS

The process of human carcinogenesis is complex and may be modulated by a variety of dietary, hormonal, immunological, or other physiological factors. The multistage model of carcinogenesis which has evolved over the last three decades is based on the premise that neoplastic changes may occur after the completion of a sequence of k irreversible changes in the genetic composition of a cell, with the transition intensity functions for each stage linearly related to dose. The clinical observation of such lesions may, however, be delayed until the tumor has progressed to a detectable size, with the latter process possibly dependent on the promotion of the lesion by factors other than the proximate carcinogen. With k sufficiently large, the multistage model provides a satisfactory explanation for the power law for the age incidence of many forms of human cancer, and it may be extended to accommodate variable exposure patterns and joint exposure to multiple agents.

The class of birth-death-mutation models described by Moolgavkar and Venzon [15] also provides a good description of the age incidence of human cancer. In contrast to the multistage model, only two stages (the formation of initiated cells and, following promotion, subsequent conversion to malignant cells) are postulated. Unlike the multistage model, these models may involve a stochastic component describing tissue growth.

Because many carcinogens require some form of metabolic activation to their active form, pharmacokinetic models may be of considerable value in describing and understanding the carcinogenic process. If metabolic activation involves one or more rate-limiting kinetic processes, the relationship between the applied dose and the dose received by the target tissue may be nonlinear. In this case, elucidation of the underlying pharmacokinetic processes can be of use in more clearly defining the dose-response curve expressed in terms of the reactive metabolite.

Because human exposure to most environmental carcinogens is low, determination of the shape of the dose-response curve in the low-dose region is critical for purposes of carcinogenic risk assessment. Under the multistage model with transition intensity functions which are linear in dose, the dose-response curve will be linear at low doses. This same result also obtains under the two-stage birth-death-mutation models, whenever the transition intensity functions for the formation of intermediate and mutant cells are again linear functions of dose. Provided that saturable kinetic processes are adequately described by Michaelis-Menten kinetics, the incorporation of metabolic activation into the risk assessment process will not alter the shape of the dose-response curve at low doses, because in this case the dose delivered to the target tissue will be directly proportional to the applied dose in the low-dose region.

Low-dose linearity may also be established under a general class of additive background models in which spontaneous lesions are considered to be due to a background carcinogen, the dose of which combines additively with the applied dose. The same additive background model applied to joint exposures predicts not only low-dose linearity but additivity of the component excess risks at low doses.

Supralinearity at low doses may be shown to occur in heterogeneous populations for which the individual dose-response curves are all linear, but in which there is a large proportion of individuals with steep low-dose slopes. However, this mathematical possibility exists only when the distribution of the individual low-dose slopes has infinite expectation. More generally, it can also be demonstrated that the low-dose shape of the population dose-response curve in a heterogeneous population (as measured by the power of dose giving the best approximation to this curve in the low-dose region) will be at least as small as that for the different individuals within the population.

In conclusion, much progress has been made in understanding the mechanism of carcinogenesis since the early work in this area about 40 years ago. However, many of the plausible mathematical models of carcinogenesis which have been developed require further validation using appropriately designed toxicological or epidemiological studies. Although the prediction of carcinogenic risks associated with low levels of exposure is not amenable to direct investigation because of the low response rates involved, the assumption of low-dose linearity appears to be both prudent and reasonable in the absence of firm biological evidence to the contrary.

APPENDIX: POPULATION HETEROGENEITY

Let (Ω, F, G) be a probability space. Here F is a σ-algebra over the set Ω, and G is a probability measure defined on F. Assume that for each $\omega \in \Omega$, the dose-response curve $P(d|\omega)$ has low-dose shape $\beta(\omega) > 0$ defined by

$$\lim_{d \to 0^+} \frac{P(d|\omega)}{d^{\beta(\omega)}} = c(\omega) \tag{62}$$

where $0 < c(\omega) < \infty$ [35]. Here, Ω indexes subgroups of the population having the same dose-response curve $P(d|\omega)$, and G defines the relative proportion of each subgroup within the population. Thus, the dose-response curve for the population as a whole is

$$P(d) = E_G[P(d|\omega)] \tag{63}$$

Suppose that $P(d)$ has low-dose shape $\beta_0 > 0$; i.e.,

$$\lim_{d \to 0^+} \frac{P(d)}{d^{\beta_0}} = c_0 \tag{64}$$

$(0 < c_0 < \infty)$. We will show that the low-dose shape of the population curve is smaller than that of almost any member of the population. To this end, we may write

$$c_0 = \lim_{d \to 0^+} \frac{P(d)}{d^{\beta_0}} = \lim_{d \to 0^+} \int \frac{P(d|\omega)}{d^{\beta_0}} \, dG(\omega)$$

$$= \lim_{d \to 0^+} \int \frac{P(d|\omega)}{d^{\beta(\omega)}} \, d^{\beta(\omega) - \beta_0} \, dG(\omega) \tag{64}$$

Let $B_\varepsilon = \{\omega: \beta(\omega) < \beta_0 - \varepsilon\}$ for some fixed $\varepsilon > 0$. We will show that this set is negligible in size. Since the integrand in (64) is positive with $d^{\beta(\omega)-\beta_0} > d^{-\varepsilon}$ for $d < 1$ on B_ε, we have

$$c_0 > \lim_{d \to 0^+} d^{-\varepsilon} \int_{B_\varepsilon} \frac{P(d|\omega)}{d^{\beta(\omega)}} \, dG(\omega) \tag{65}$$

Now let $C_M = \{\omega: P(d|\omega)/d^{\beta(\omega)} < M \text{ for } d < 1\}$. Then given any ω, we can find M such that $\omega \in C_M$, since for d bounded away from zero the numerator of $P(d|\omega)/d^{\beta(\omega)}$ is bounded by 1 and the denominator is bounded below; for d near zero it follows from (62) that the whole fraction remains bounded. Thus C_M increases to Ω and $M \to \infty$.

Further restricting the integral in (65) to C_M and applying the dominated convergence theorem yields

$$c_0 > \lim_{d \to 0^+} d^{-\varepsilon} \int_{B_\varepsilon \cap C_M} \frac{P(d|\omega)}{d^{\beta(\omega)}} \, dG(\omega)$$

$$= \lim_{d \to 0^+} d^{-\varepsilon} \int_{B_\varepsilon \cap C_M} c(\omega) \, dG(\omega) \tag{67}$$

where the integral on the right side of (67) is independent of d. Since c_0 is finite and $d^{-\varepsilon}$ diverges as $d \to 0^+$, this integral must be exactly 0. Because $c(\omega) > 0$, however, we must have $\Pr(B_\varepsilon \cap C_M) = 0$ for all ε and M. This implies that

$$\Pr(B_\varepsilon) = \lim_{M \to \infty} \Pr(B_\varepsilon \cap C_M) = 0 \tag{68}$$

Thus, all sets B_ε are essentially empty, and

$$\beta_0 \leq \text{ess inf}\{\beta(\omega): \omega \in \Omega\}$$

$$= \sup\{\beta^*: \Pr[\beta(\omega) < \beta^*] = 0\} \tag{69}$$

The example in Section V.C in which $\beta = 1$ for all individuals in the population, but the population as a whole was supralinear, shows that the inequality is necessary.

REFERENCES

1. Berenblum, I. The cocarcinogen action of croton resin. *Cancer Research*, 1:44–48 (1941).

2. Berenblum, I. and Shubik, P. The role of croton oil applications, associated with a single painting of a carcinogen, in tumour induction of the mouse's skin. *British Journal of Cancer*, 1:379–382 (1947).

3. Berenblum, I. and Shubik, P. A new, quantitative, approach to the study of the stages of chemical carcinogenesis in the mouse's skin. *British Journal of Cancer*, 1:383–391 (1947).

4. Berenblum, I. and Shubik, P. The persistence of latent tumour cells induced in the mouse's skin by single application of 9:10-dimethyl-1:2-benzathracene. *British Journal of Cancer*, 3:384–386 (1949).

5. Pitot, H. C. and Sirica, A. E. The stages of initiation and promotion in hepatocarcinogenesis. *Biochimica et Biophysica Acta*, 605:191–215 (1980).

6. Clayson, D. B., Krewski, D., and Munro, I. C. The power and interpretation of the carcinogenicity bioassay. *Regulatory Toxicology and Pharmacology*, 3:329–348 (1983).

7. Armitage, P. Multistage models of carcinogenesis. *Environmental Health Perspectives*, 63:195–201 (1985).

8. Krewski, D., Murdoch, D. J., and Dewanji, A., Statistical modelling and extrapolation of carcinogenesis data, in *Modern Statistical Methods in Chronic Disease Epidemiology* (R. L. Prentice and S. Moolgavkar, eds.), Wiley, New York, pp. 259–282 (1986).

9. Armitage, P. and Doll, R., The age distribution of cancer and a multistage theory of carcinogenesis. *British Journal of Cancer*, 8:1–12 (1954).

10. Day, N. E. and Brown, C. C., Multistage models and primary prevention of cancer. *Journal of the National Cancer Institute*, 64:977–989 (1980).

11. Crump, K. S. and Howe, R. B., The multistage model with a time-dependent dose pattern: applications to carcinogenic risk assessment. *Risk Analysis*, 4:163–176 (1984).

12. Hamilton, M. A. and Hoel, D. G., Detection of synergistic effects in carcinogenesis. Unpublished manuscript (1979).

13. Thorslund, T. W. and Charnley, G., Use of the multistage model to predict the carcinogenic response associated with

time-dependent exposure to multiple carcinogenic agents. Unpublished manuscript (1986).

14. Knudson, A. G., Mutation of cancer: statistical study of retinoblastoma. *Proceedings National Academy of Science U.S.A.*, 68:820–823 (1971).

15. Moolgavkar, S. and Venzon, D., Two-event models for carcinogenesis: Incidence curves for childhood and adult tumors. *Mathematical Biosciences*, 47:55–77 (1979).

16. Hoel, D. G., Kaplan, N. L., and Anderson, M. W., Implication of nonlinear kinetics on risk estimation in carcinogenesis. *Science*, 219:1032–1037 (1983).

17. Brown, C. C., Mathematical aspects of dose-response studies in carcinogenesis—the concept of thresholds. *Oncology*, 33: 62–65 (1976).

18. Cornfield, J., Carcinogenic risk assessment. *Science*, 198: 693–699 (1977).

19. Brown, C. C., Fears, T. R., Gail, M. H., Schneiderman, M., Tarone, R. E., and Mantel, N., Letter to the editor and reply by J. Cornfield. *Science*, 202:1105–1108 (1978).

20. Iversen, S. and Arley, N., On the mechanism of experimental carcinogenesis. *Acta Pathologica et Microbiologica Scandinavica*, 27:773–803 (1950).

21. Arley, N. and Iversen, S., On the mechanism of experimental carcinogenesis. *Acta Pathologica et Microbiologica Scandinavica*, 30:21–53 (1952).

22. Nordling, C., A new theory on the cancer inducing mechanism. *British Journal of Cancer*, 7:68–72 (1953).

23. Fisher, J. and Holloman, J., A hypothesis for the origin of cancer foci. *Cancer*, 4:916–918 (1951).

24. Armitage, P. and Doll, R., A two-stage theory of carcinogenesis in relation to the age distribution of human cancer. *British Journal of Cancer*, 11:161–169 (1957).

25. Neyman, J. and Scott, E., Statistical aspects of the problem of carcinogenesis, *Fifth Berkeley Symposium on Mathematical Statistics and Probability*, University of California Press, Berkeley, California, pp. 745–776 (1967).

26. Crump, K., Hoel, D., Langley, C., and Peto, R., Fundamental carcinogenic processes and their implications for low dose risk assessment. *Cancer Research*, 36:2973–2979 (1976).

27. Armitage, P. and Doll, R., Stochastic models for carcinogenesis. *Fourth Berkeley Symposium on Mathematical Statistics and Probability*, University of California Press, Berkeley, California, pp. 19–38 (1961).

28. Whittemore, A. and Keller, J., Quantitative theories of carcinogenesis. *SIAM Review*, 20:1–30 (1978).

29. Moolgavkar, S., Carcinogenesis modeling: From molecular biology to epidemiology. *Annual Review of Public Health*, 7: 151–169 (1986).

30. Kalbfleisch, J. G., *Probability and Statistical Inference I*, Springer-Verlag, New York (1979).

31. Van Ryzin, J. and Rai, K., The use of quantal response data to make predictions, in *The Scientific Basis of Toxicity Assessment*, (H. Witschi, ed.), Elsevier North-Holland, New York, pp. 273–290 (1979).

32. Doll, R., The age distribution of cancer: Implications for models of carcinogenesis. *Journal of the Royal Statistical Society, Series A*, 134:133–166 (1971).

33. Moolgavkar, S., The multistage theory of carcinogenesis and the age distribution of cancer in man. *Journal of the National Cancer Institute*, 61:49–52 (1978).

34. Crump. K., An improved procedure for low-dose carcinogenic risk assessment from animal data. *Journal of Environmental Pathology and Toxicology*, 5(4/5):339–348 (1984).

35. Krewski, D. and Van Ryzin, J., Dose response models for quantal response toxicity data, in *Statistics and Related Topics* (M. Csorgo, D. A. Dawson, J. N. K. Rao, A. K. Md. E. Saleh, eds.), North-Holland, Amsterdam, pp. 201–231 (1981).

36. Moolgavkar, S. and Knudson, A. G., Jr., Mutation and cancer: A model for human carcinogenesis. *Journal of the National Cancer Institute*, 66:1037–1051 (1981).

37. Gehring, P. J., Watanabe, P. G., and Park, C. N., Resolution of dose-response toxicity data for chemicals requiring metabolic activation: example—vinyl chloride. *Toxicology and Applied Pharmacology*, 44:581–591 (1978).

38. Andersen, M. E., Clewell, H. J. III, Gargas, M. L., Smith, F. A., and Reitz, R. H., Physiologically based pharmacokinetics and the risk assessment process for methylene chloride. *Toxicology and Applied Pharmacology*, 87:185–205 (1987).

39. Michaelis, L. and Menten, M. L., Die Kinetik der Invertinwirkung. *Biochemische Zeitschrift*, 49:333–369 (1913).

40. Gehring, P. J. and Blau, G. E., Mechanisms of carcinogenesis: dose response. *Journal of Environmental Pathology and Toxicology*, *1*:163–179 (1977).

41. Hoel, D. G., Incorporation of background in dose-response models. *Federation Proceedings*, *39*:67–69 (1980).

3
Tumor Growth Models and Cancer Chemotherapy

GEORGE W. SWAN   *Consultant, Biomedicine and Bioengineering,*
Edmonds, Washington

I. INTRODUCTION

This chapter gives mathematical models of tumor growth and its treatment with a chemotherapeutic agent. Our method is to start off with simple mathematical models and go on to the more complicated ones. The simple models involve just the total number of cells making up the tumor. The latter involve descriptions of the cell cycle, and this automatically increases the complexity of the mathematical models. Deterministic formulations are used throughout, except for occasional features that seem to require a random component. No attempt is made at completeness. Rather, an attempt is made to bring to the reader's attention those models that presently seem worthy of future consideration.

We regard a tumor as being a homogeneous collection of cells. The spatial arrangement of these cells is not taken into consideration. These are obvious simplifications to the true state of affairs, where a tumor is heterogeneous and the cellular arrangement at a specific anatomical location may be important to its growth. If our interest lies in the overall gross behavior of the tumor, then the simpler models may be adequate. There is no point in working with a complex model if a simpler one will provide just as much insight. As the mathematical model becomes more complicated, insight into the interaction between its parts, and consequences of assumptions, may be lost.

Each mathematical model involves a differential equation of some particular type and describes the dynamic (time-varying) course of development of the cell populations. The descriptions therefore involve transient behavior and are not restricted to end-stage results and data. Differential equations are used because they are fundamental in providing a unifying description of various concepts of tumor growth. It would be possible to develop each of the models directly in terms of difference equations, but there does not appear to be any major compelling reason to proceed in that manner.

Our approach is as follows. We start off with the simplest mathematical model of tumor cell population growth and proceed to the more complicated models involving age and/or maturity structure. Wherever possible, we show how any available experimental or human data are used with the mathematical model. Since space is limited, we restrict attention to our preference as to what appear to be the main models. Many models are discussed from a variety of sources, and we try to unify the presentation by standardizing notation as far as possible. This means that the notation used to describe any particular model may differ greatly from that used in the original publication.

We start off in Section III with a discussion of the exponential growth model and relate it to clinical results. This is the simplest mathematical model of tumor growth. That is followed in Section V by the Verhulst-Pearl-Reed model (the logistic model), which is perhaps the simplest extension of the exponential growth model that retains biological significance.

The Gompertz model is considered in Section VI. A casual observer might be excused for believing that every investigation in cancer growth involves a Gompertz equation! Since there is a large amount of published work involving this equation, we devote a corresponding amount of space to discussing it, even though it is an empiricism.

Other mathematical models that could be useful in describing tumor growth are introduced in Section VII.

A cell spends a certain time in a given state. Examination of a population of cells in the biological system shows that a number of them will be in the same state. Cells subsequently divide, and subpopulations are formed. The measurement of time parameters, and the study of the growth characteristics of these biological populations are known as cellular growth kinetics. Section VIII deals with cytokinetics, the growth kinetics of cells.

An introduction to the mathematical modeling of cell populations with age structure is presented in Section IX. The main feature is the derivatization of the basic von Foerster equation. A different approach is in Section X, where Rubinow's equation is derived. His equation involves an interpretation of the growth of cellular populations that depends on each cell reaching a certain maturity.

Section XI deals briefly with an introduction to cancer chemotherapy.

The developments in cell kinetics offered promise of being able to improve cancer chemotherapy. A wealth of data and information has been obtained, and much of this is amenable to mathematical modeling. In Section XII.A we present a basic mathematical model involving age structure and ideas from cell kinetics studies for the description of a growing tumor and its treatment with an anticancer drug. The model incorporates some simple concepts from the pharmacokinetics of the anticancer drug. The section following presents the solution to this model.

There is a mixture of the equations with age structure and maturity variable in Section XIII, which describes the population growth of neutrophils. A novel approach to the chemotherapy for acute myeloblastic leukemia is presented.

The author believes that engineering optimal control theory is providing important results in the therapy of various diseases and that it can play a role in improving cancer chemotherapy. Section XIV provides an introduction to this area. A simple mathematical model for the control of multiple myeloma is examined in order to illustrate various features of the modeling process. Extensions of the model and some recent developments are described. Future prospects for optimal control theory in cancer chemotherapy problems are assessed.

Section XV goes through each of the previous sections and highlights problem areas that are suitable for future investigation.

II. MISCELLANEOUS DEFINITIONS AND NOTATION

The following descriptions are used in Section III. A cancer cell is assumed to be spherical. The radius of the cell is r, its diameter is D, and its volume $V = (4/3)\pi r^3$. A "typical" cancer cell is assumed to have a diameter of 10 μ and weigh 10^{-9} g (one micron (μ) is one-thousandth of a millimeter).

Throughout the chapter we use the following notation: Let

L(t) = level of tumor burden at time t

This may be interpreted as the number of cells composing the tumor, or L could denote the volume of the tumor. When we need to distinguish between cell number and tumor volume, we use the symbol V to represent the latter. At time t = 0 the initial size of L is given by L(0), or just L_0. The notation $\dot{L}(t)$ means dL(t)/dt.

Define t_c to be the length of time between the birth of a cell
and mitosis. This is also referred to as the intermitotic (or cell
cycle or cell regeneration) time. Define t_d to be the doubling time,
the time for a tumor population of cells to double in size.

Clinicians generally regard a tumor with 10^9 cells present as the
minimal lesion that can be detected by a sign or symptom.

III. SIMPLE MODEL: EXPONENTIAL GROWTH

The following list of assumptions is taken as being representative of
the simple model:

 1. Each cancer cell is no different from its neighbor.
 2. There is no cell death.
 3. There is no restriction on the supply of essential nutrients
    (such as oxygen) to each cancer cell.
 4. There is no spatial restriction on the cancer cells.

One consequence of the first assumption is that each cancer cell
has the same intermitotic time. The last assumption means that with
each division of a cell into its two offspring there is room available
for them in three-dimensional space. These assumptions indicate
that a cancer cell grows, then divides to become 2 cells, each of
which divides to produce 4 cells. In turn these 4 cells become 8,
16, etc.

Let L_1 denote the number of cells in the first generation, L_2
the number in the second generation, and so on, with L_i denoting
the number of cells in the ith generation. It follows that

L_0 = initial number of cells = 1

L_1 = number of cells after 1 doubling = 2

L_2 = number of cells after 2 doublings = $2L_1 = 2^2$

.

.

.

L_i = number of cells after i doublings

   = $2L_{i-1} = 2^i$, i = 0, 1, 2, . . .   (1)

The counter i, which is also the number of mitoses, is related to
the time t by the equation

$$t = i \, t_c \tag{2}$$

with t_c denoting the (constant) intermitotic time. Thus a different way of writing (1) is in the form

$$L(t) = 2^{t/t_c} \tag{3}$$

where, for convenience, we introduce $L(t) \equiv L_i$. In this mathematical model the intermitotic time is the same as the tumor doubling time $(t_c = t_d)$, so

$$L(t) = 2^{t/t_d} = \exp\left[(\ln 2)\, \frac{t}{t_d} \right] \tag{4}$$

The results leading to (1) are applicable at the end of discrete intervals of time. This is also reflected in the mathematical statement that $L_i = 2L_{i-1}$ is a linear difference equation. Strictly, then, the time t in (2) and (4) takes on discrete values. This simple model is an example of a discrete-time model.

Since $\ln L_i = i \ln 2$, a plot of this equation on semilogarithmic paper, with the number of doublings as abscissa, gives a straight line of slope $\ln 2$. The straight line is a direct consequence of our basic four assumptions.

The simple model appears to have been first examined in [1]. Collins and co-workers started with two assumptions for the growth of a hypothetical tumor: (i) one cell divides to become two, and each of these divides to become four, eight, etc.; and (ii) there is a constant growth rate. They do not define what they mean by "growth rate." However, the inference is that growth rate is the same as the slope of the straight line. Specifically, on p. 990, they state that the growth rate is expressed as doubling time.

Define the quantities V_0, V_1, ... as follows:

V_0 = volume of 1 cancer cell = $\left(\frac{\pi}{6}\right)(10\ \mu)^3 = \left(\frac{\pi}{6}\right)10^{-6}\ mm^3$

V_1 = volume after 1 doubling = volume of 2 cells = $2V_0$

V_2 = volume after 2 doublings = volume of 4 cells = $2^2 V_0$

V_i = volume of tumor after i doublings

= volume of 2^i cells = $2^i V_0$

A single cancer cell grows into a nodule of volume V_i containing 2^i cells after i doublings. The number of cells in this nodule, L_i, is directly proportional to the volume V_i with $L_i = k V_i$, where k is a constant of proportionality. Now $2 = L_1 = k V_1 = 2k V_0$, so $k = 1/V_0 = (6/\pi)10^6\ mm^{-3}$.

Write $V(t) \equiv V_i$; then $V(t) = 2^{t/t_d} V_0$ and

$$\ln V(t) = \left(\frac{\ln 2}{t_d}\right) t + \ln V_0 \tag{5}$$

which, on semilogarithmic paper, is represented as a straight line with slope $(\ln 2)/t_d$. Serial measurements of $V(t)$ for a particular tumor allow the doubling time t_d to be determined. The volume doubling time is the same as the number of cells doubling time t_d.

It is convenient to think of V_i as being spherical with a corresponding diameter. For example, when there are 10^6 cells in the nodule, the volume is given by $(\pi/6)$ mm^3 and corresponds to a sphere of diameter 1 mm. When $L_i = 10^6 = 2^i$, from (1), then $i = (6 \ln 10)/\ln 2 \approx 20$ doublings. A tumor with 1 billion (10^9) cells, at essentially 30 doublings from one cell, corresponds to a nodule with diameter of 1 cm and weighing 1 g. Approximately 40 doublings from one cell give 10^{12} cells or a 1-kg tumor nodule.

According to the present model, the tumor originates $20t_d$ before any macroscopic lesion appears and $30t_d$ before a significant radiographic density becomes visible. If we assume that there is just one primary extrapulmonary neoplasm, then it is already inoperable $30t_d$ before detectable pulmonary metastases appear. The model also predicts that $30t_d$ is a minimal time estimate (unless the preclinical growth rate exceeds the observed clinical growth rate), since a dormancy state may exist during which the initial tumor cell remains latent before successive mitotic divisions are triggered [2].

As noted earlier, it takes 30 doublings to reach a nodule of diameter 1 cm. A further 10 doublings produces approximately 1 kg of cancer tissue (10^{12} cells). Although a cancer patient may live beyond this point, death is near, since after five more doublings the weight of the tumor is (approximately) equal to half the weight of a 70-kg human. The model thus predicts that the total maximum duration of cancer is about the time required for 40 doublings in volume. If 1 mm is regarded as the limit for the earliest possible sign of a symptom (20 doublings), then half of the growth of the tumor occurs in a period of undetected growth. This period is also referred to as the silent interval or the period of occult growth. The innocuous equation (2) packs a powerful punch! For example, with "large" values of t_d, it shows that the occult period could be long. Examination in [2] of good data from a small group of patients indicates that tumors were in existence a decade before they were first picked up on chest radiographs. Schwartz noted that, on the average, less than one-fifth of the tumor's total growth was evident clinically; for 6 of the 13 neoplasms examined the observation fraction was less than one-tenth.

The simple exponential model [1] produces quantitative results. The conclusions deduced from the model had considerable impact on clinical thinking and were at the focus of a number of subsequent investigations, e.g., [3-6].

It is convenient now to regard t as a continuous variable. The way of expressing L(t) in the forms in (4) indicates that this simple model can be interpreted as geometric growth or in terms of a type of exponential growth. For exponential growth it is important to note that the

$$\text{specific growth rate} = \frac{1}{L} \frac{dL}{dt} = \text{constant} \tag{6}$$

Throughout this chapter when reference is made to the work of various (nonmathematically oriented) researchers who use the words "growth rate," it is *always* to be understood that it is the *specific* growth rate that they mean. For example, introduce

$$k = \frac{\ln 2}{t_d} \tag{7}$$

Then (4) can be written as L(t) = exp(kt). The quantity k is the specific growth rate constant for exponential growth. Some clinicians (loosely) refer to k as being the fraction of the population that is dividing per unit time.

One of the earliest papers that discusses exponential growth is by Mayneord [7], who expected the growth of a spherical mass to be represented by exponential growth. However, his paper actually deals with the study of the growth of a spherical surface layer of tumor cells. Logarithms of measurements of tumor area are reported in [8], and straight lines were produced. Mottram was dealing with exponential growth, although he does not use that term. These papers indicate that the concept of a tumor possibly growing at a constant growth rate did not originate with [1]. The investigators [1] preferred to use the words "constant growth rate" in describing and discussing their model. In a subsequent paper [9] the authors do refer to the simple model in terms of exponential growth. Schwartz [2] indicates that he is dealing with an exponential growth model.

It is apparent here that we are considering the tumor as growing from a single cell. This clonal nature of the growth of human tumors is supported by evidence from various studies; see [10]. Four major areas of support are presented in [11], p. 41.

A. Clinical Results

The authors [1] present a discussion of the simple theoretical model. But even more important they give observations on a wide selection of human tumors from 24 adults and 206 cases of Wilms' tumor in children. (Nephroblastomas, often called Wilms' tumors, are rapidly

developing tumors of the kidneys and affect children before their
fifth year.) It is generally acknowledged that their clinical data are
very good. The patients included in their investigation had primary
tumors at various anatomical locations which had metastasized. Interestingly, metastatic growth occurred in the lung, and this appeared
to be the site of choice for tumor growth. Why? No one knows. However, in [12], p. 45, Steel notes that the lung provides an excellent
blood supply and little physical resistance to tumor growth. This
anatomical site, more than any others, should therefore readily support exponential growth. Accordingly, then, it is important to ap-
preciate the limitations of the work by Collins and co-workers [1].
Their findings may not be applicable to nonpulmonary tumors. This
point is elaborated on more fully in the next section.

The progressive growth of pulmonary metastases can be documented from successive roentgenograms or radiographs (which are
x-ray or γ-ray photographs). At the end of known intervals of time,
measurements on the two-dimensional plate of the outline of the tumor
give estimates of its gross diameter. Then the magnitude of the tumor
volume is calculated and equation (5) allows the doubling time to be
determined. The evaluation of 24 patients with measurable pulmonary
metastatic cancer shows a tumor-doubling time range of between 11
days and 164 days with a median of 42 days. This means that the
periods of time taken by the metastatic tumors to reach the size of a
nodule 1 mm in diameter show variations from seven months to nine
years. The model allows for extrapolation backwards in order to provide a date of tumor origin for each metastasis. In this way Collins
and co-workers [1] indicate that pulmonary metastases were established
earlier than the first sign of symptom of the primary lesion in all but
1 of the 24 adult cases studied. One remarkable case is documented:
The line joining seven separate measurements made over a period of
three years was straight. The line was extrapolated backward and
showed that a 1-mm nodule existed in the lung 11 years before it was
detected clinically and 7 years before the "acorn-sized" primary tumor
was discovered.

The second set of clinical investigations in [1] deals with the time
at which tumor recurrence occurs in children with nephroblastomas
(Wilms' tumors). For their series of 206 children they predicted a
post-operative period of risk of recurrence that is equal in duration
to the age of the patient at the time the diagnosis was made plus nine
months. All recurrences fell within this period. The simple model, for
all these cases, predicts a period of risk beyond which no recurrence
will develop. This is not a statistical assessment but is, as Collins
and co-workers note, a tentative, simple criterion for "cure" and applies to each individual.

Again, it is important to emphasize and keep in mind that Collins
and his colleagues did no analysis on primary bronchogenic neoplasms.
A subsequent paper [13] presents the measured doubling times of 25

pulmonary metastases from carcinoma of the colon and rectum. The doubling times range from 34 to 210 days with a median of 96 days. Similar values are obtained [14] from a series of 18 patients with this type of tumor. Also in [9] there is a list of nine separate investigations that support the use of the exponential growth model. They examined all available cases of measurable lung nodules, multiple as well as solitary, having serial radiographs, and the rates of enlargement were recorded in terms of doubling time.

The paper [2] presents a study of 12 patients with autochthonous (primary) pulmonary neoplasms. Their radiographs were able to be measured serially, and tumor volumes were calculated as per the simple model. The doubling times were obtained by use of (5). This work appears to support the validity and wide applicability of the exponential growth model in describing the pulmonary tumors. It is noteworthy that Schwartz [2] regarded a 1-cm nodule as the smallest pulmonary lesion detectable on a radiograph even though he claimed that for lung metastases "1 mm reproducibility was generally obtainable." Yet there are difficulties in interpreting his calculated values. For example, on p. 1279 he gives data for patient A. R. From these data and (5) the doubling time of 56 days can be obtained, and this agrees with the value on p. 1280. But it does not appear to be possible to obtain his other values for the times $t_{1.1}$ and $t_{1.D}$. Also, in [4], p. 76, it is noted that "half the growth curves are slightly but unmistakably convex upwards on a semilogarithmic plot." What this means is that the established growth patterns were not always exponential, as claimed by Schwartz.

B. Assessment of the Simple Exponential Growth Model

In this section we attempt to construct a better understanding of the relevance of the exponential growth model to human tumor growth kinetics. First, the model is only as good as its assumptions. Data are obtained from the shadows of tumors on radiographs obtained sequentially. Such data are obtained over the clinical course of the disease, and this is where the mathematical model is applied. Perhaps one is not justified in making an extrapolation backwards in time, since generally there are no observations available to test the theory. In other words, just because exponential growth appears to be applicable for some tumors during the clinical phase, this does not mean that such growth is true during the phase of occult growth. This means that care is needed when developing any mathematical model of cancer growth; predictions from such models may never be able to be evaluated by clinical studies.

Discussions on the difficulties associated with obtaining good measurements of tumors are presented, for example, in [4] and [12], Chapter 1.

Much discussion on the possible exponential growth behavior of
human tumors is presented in [3–6]. Also, Chapter 1 of [12] deals
extensively with this type of growth. Many researchers devote considerable effort to the discovery of doubling times which they believe
are appropriate to the particular tumor under investigation. Even
though only a few measurements are made or the length of observation
of the tumor is short, nevertheless the data, in a number of cases,
are capable of being represented by an exponential growth function.
The preponderance of data come from observations of primary and
metastatic pulmonary lesions.

In [15] is presented a very detailed and precise study of the
growth of lung metastases. The authors of [15] indicate that some
tumors appear to exhibit exponential growth only over part of their
range of growth. When a change in growth rate occurs, it is sometimes possible to relate it to a particular feature in the patient's case
history, such as changes in hormonal status at menopause. That
such curves have been found is a clear warning on the dangers of
extrapolation of a supposedly exponential curve.

C. Mathematical Models and Exponential
Growth of Cancer

If the assumption is that there is strict growth of the population of
cells, then the simplest mathematical model is described by the equation $\dot{L}(t) = aL(t)$, i.e., exponential growth at rate a. The solution of
this equation grows like e^{at}. If cell mortality is now included in the
mathematical model as a first-order process, then $\dot{L}(t) = aL - bL$ and
the solution grows at a slower rate than before, assuming that $a > b$.
Instead of $a - b$, a single constant c could be used. Accordingly,
when someone says that growth is exponential, the gross characteristics of this growth are embodied in one equation of the type $\dot{L}(t) = aL$,
where a may or may not explicity contain a contribution from cell
mortality.

However, when dealing with mathematical models of tumor growth
kinetics, it is generally a good idea to explicitly show the form of the
loss term. In [15] it is shown that human tumors in clinically advanced stages of disease possess rates of cell loss that are almost the
same as the rates of cell production. This means that in those tumors
with high rates of cell production there are corresponding high rates
of cell loss, whereas in slowly proliferating tumors the rates of cell
loss are low. More information on cell loss in tumors is needed in order
to develop better models.

A number of interesting papers have appeared in which exponential
growth of the tumor is a key feature in the investigation. Here is a
partial listing of some of them.

In the discrete-stage model of [16] and [17] the expected subpopulations for large values of t are exponential. A more complicated

mathematical model considers that the times spent by a cell in the various stages are independent random variables with arbitrary distributions. This means that we need to consider a general multitype age-dependent branching process (e.g., [18]). It turns out that the expected total population size exhibits asymptotic exponential behavior. Later in this chapter we examine continuous-time age structure models; see (51). Again the population exhibits asymptotic exponential behavior.

An interesting analysis of cancer growth occurs in [19]. This work appears to have been overlooked. One particularly noteworthy feature of Berglas's book is the detailed appendix on mathematical formulations of cancer growth, which includes a discussion of a treated tumor. He derives the result

$$L(t) = L(0) \, 2^{t/t_d} \tag{8}$$

the slight extension of (3) to the case where the initial number of cells $L(0)$ is different from unity. Then, as any sensible applied mathematician would do, he shows graphs of (8) for various values of the doubling time t_d. A further extension of (8) takes into consideration the effect of cell mortality. Other parts of Berglas's work have now been superseded.

Mathematical developments for models of tumor growth are presented in [20]. Four cases are examined: (1) The total volume of the tumor is involved in the growth process. (2) A constant percentage of the tumor is involved in the growth process. (3) Growth is restricted to a spherical shell of constant thickness (compare [7]). (4) A constant number of cells of the tumor take part in the growth process. In the analysis of *human* tumor response to chemotherapy an exponential growth model is used in [21]. A model for the growth kinetics of exponentially growing populations where all the cells have a probability of division is developed in [22].

In [23,24] are developments of matrix models of heterogeneous, cultured cell populations on exponential growth. However, the structures of certain matrices containing transitional probabilities are wrong in some elements. A correction of these errors subsequently appeared [25]. But the work [26-29] dealing with cancer control makes extensive use of the incorrect matrices and therefore many of their results cannot be right. The Hahn model and extensions of it are based on exponential growth of cellular populations.

In Section VIII.B we examine the important cell kinetics procedure that leads to the percentage labeled mitoses curve. Such curves are investigated for exponentially growing populations in [30]. In the special model [31], which highlights the growth of cells in the G_0 phase of the cell cycle, the populations of cells are assumed to be growing exponentially. The growth of the experimental tumor.—mouse leukemia L1210—is modeled via exponential growth in [32].

The standard four-phase model of the cell cycle (see Section VIII.A) is combined with exponential growth to obtain values of cell kinetics parameters in [33] and [34]. Exponential growth of the tumor volume is used in the studies [35,36] of different treatment modalities. The assumption of exponential growth is used in [37]. The exponential growth model is compared with other models in [38]. Exponential growth is used in the model for tumor resistance to drugs in [39]. Leukemic growth in humans is described by exponential growth in [40].

Perhaps the large number of papers involving exponential growth is not too surprising. The models in these papers can be regarded as representing a first approximation to tumor growth. Even though the mathematics in these papers may appear to be formidable, the net result is that exponential growth frequently appears in the model descriptions.

IV. GROWTH FRACTION

It is convenient when discussing models of tumor growth to use the concept of growth fraction. This concept is due to Mendelsohn [41, 42]. The growth fraction (GF) of a population of growing cells is defined as

$$GF = \frac{\text{number of cells in cycle}}{\text{total number of cells}} \tag{9}$$

The number of cells in cycle is interpreted as the number of new proliferating cells. The general growth equation is

$$\dot{L}(t) = a(GF) L \tag{10}$$

For example, when the number of cells in cycle is assumed to be the same as the total number of new cells, then GF = 1; this gives the situation of exponential growth.

More information on the concept of growth fraction is provided in Section VIII.A.

V. THE VERHULST-PEARL-REED EQUATION

Assume that the rate of growth and multiplication of a cancer cell is determined by some quantity g. For our discussion knowledge of the exact nature of g is not required. Also, assume that each cell of the tumor exerts an inhibitory effect, due to a factor h, upon every other cell through the medium of a certain chemical substance. If the tumor comprises L cells, then the rate of multiplication of each cell is proportional to pg − q(L − 1)h, where p and q are constants of proportionality, and L − 1 denotes the inhibitory effect upon a cell by the other L − 1 cells. The equation for L is

$$\dot{L}(t) = L[pg - q(L - 1)h]$$

Let two new (positive) constants a and b be defined by a = pg + qh, b = qh. Then

$$\dot{L}(t) = (a - bL)L \qquad L(0) = L_0 \qquad (11)$$

The material leading to this derivation of (11) is in [43]; see also [44], Chapter 18. The initial condition is prescribed by the number of cells L_0 at time t = 0.

When b = 0, (11) reduces to the equation for exponential growth. Equation (11), therefore, can be regarded as representing an extension of exponential growth. Note that the gross effects of the growth of a tumor are assumed to be described by (11). For example, the effects of growth with or without cell mortality are already built into (11) through the nature of the first term.

Perhaps the earliest investigation of an equation like (11) is in [45]. The equation subsequently was rediscovered and reported in [46,47]. Equation (11) also represents growth in number of various biological organisms. Derivations of (11) together with its biological relevance are provided in the excellent book [48]. These investigators deal with ecological and biological studies; the symbol L denotes the number of individuals in the growing population. For some unknown reason (11) is also known as the logistic equation, and the graph of its solution (12) is called the logistic curve.

It is possible to obtain an exact solution to (11). The simplest and quickest way of doing this is to introduce the nonlinear transformation y(t) = 1/L(t), which allows (11) to be reduced to a linear differential equation for y(t). From its solution construct

$$L(t) = \frac{L_0 e^{at}}{1 - bL_0/a + (bL_0/a)e^{at}} \qquad (12)$$

For b sufficiently small (12) behaves like an exponential function. The initial slope is $\dot{L}(0) = (a - bL_0)L_0$. Hence, if $L_0 > a/b$, the graph of L versus t decreases monotonically until L reaches a/b.

In fact $L = a/b$ is the horizontal line asymptotic to the graph, and that behaves like a decaying exponential curve. More frequently, $\dot{L}(0) \ll a/b$. The graph is a sigmoid with positive slope throughout. The slope reaches its maximum size for $L = a/2b$ and then decreases to zero as the curve approaches the asymptote $L = a/b$. There is thus a point of inflection at $L = a/2b$ on the rising curve, which means that there is a change in the curvature of the graph. With this mathematical model a/b is regarded as being the greatest size of the tumor.

Although applications of the logistic equation to problems involving the population dynamics of various species in ecology are well known, less attention appears to have been devoted to the use of the equation in tumor growth dynamics. References 43 and 44 drew attention to the possibility of (11) being of use in cancer research.

A. Experimental Tumors

From a review of the data (and plots of these data) in many papers dealing with experimental tumors, it is easy to be convinced that they could be fitted by an appropriate logistic curve. This approach has been suggested recently by the author [49]. Steel [12], p. 20 and Tubiana [6] refer to [50], which indicated that the growth of certain experimental tumors could be well fitted to the logistic equation. However, they suggested no further developments.

Reference 51 is noteworthy for several reasons. First, it details contributions from Soviet scientists in the area of experimental tumor growth kinetics up to the date of the original Russian version published in 1977. Second, it uses mathematical models to understand cancer growth. These are nonbiostatistical models. A solution of the form (12) is referred to in [51] as the autocatalysis form.

Various papers that give data on experimental tumors are presented briefly in [51]. Then Emanuel gives (with no explanation of details of the derivation, fitting procedure used, data used, etc.) the form (12) that he claims represents the data. For example, Ref. 52 contains data on the average diameters of Walker carcinoma 256 one and two weeks after rats were inoculated with the tumor material. In this case the corresponding form of (12) that is suggested is

$$D(t) = \frac{a}{b} [1 + (ab^{-1}D_0^{-1} - 1)\exp(-at)]^{-1}$$

with $D(t)$ denoting the diameter of the tumor at time t (in days) and D_0 representing the diameter of the initial inoculum. From p. 33 of [51] the following values are deduced: $a = 0.18$, $a/b = 5.5$, and $ab^{-1}D_0^{-1} = 19.22$. But if we use these values to calculate $D(t)$, the data of [52] do not appear to be recovered. This suggests that the autocatalysis form given for this tumor is wrong. (Other discrepancies exist but are not discussed here.)

Similarly, on p. 33 of [51] is an expression of type (12) with given numerical values for each of the constants. This expression is supposed to represent data in [53], but it does not seem to. So, although there are solutions of type (12) used in [51], it would appear that they need to be carefully checked out.

B. Human Tumors

From the point of view of applications of an equation like (11) and its solution (12) in the studies of human cancer growth, very little has so far appeared. This would appear to be an oversight. Reference 49 asks for more effort in the use of (11) with studies of human tumors.

A detailed study of instantaneous tumor cell kill, due to radiation insult, followed by logistic growth of normal tissues is presented in [54], pp. 72–84.

The volume of a growing tumor is assumed [38] to be represented by a logistic equation of the type

$$\dot{V}(t) = (m - nV)V \qquad V(0) = V_0 \tag{13}$$

where m and n are positive constants, and

$$V(t) = V_0 \exp(mt) \left[1 - nV_0 m^{-1} + nV_0 m^{-1} \exp(mt) \right]^{-1} \tag{14}$$

The fit of (13) and (14) to the human data given in [2] on primary bronchogenic tumors is demonstrated in [38]. This is done in two stages in order to obtain good starting values for the fitting of the nonlinear expression (14). First the Gompertz equation (see discussion in the next section) is fitted to a given set of data. Then the derivative form of the Gompertz equation is used to generate numerical values for the derivative. These values are used with (13) in a linear least squares fit of (13) to the data in order to obtain starting values for m and n for the nonlinear regression approach.

In this detailed numerical study and comparison of mathematical models, Vaidya and Alexandro show that the use of the logistic equation gives the *closest* fit to the human tumor data for all the patients considered. This is an interesting conclusion, since the data were also fitted to an exponential curve. It would be useful to have an analysis performed of the fitting of the logistic equation to data from human tumors at various anatomical sites.

Recently, the author [49] used the logistic equation in studies of the use of optimal control theory to improve cancer chemotherapy. Parameter values are based on data for multiple myeloma. See Section XIV.B for more information.

C. Extensions of the Logistic Equation

The equation

$$\dot{L}(t) = aL - bL^{\gamma} \qquad L(0) = L_0 \qquad \gamma > 0 \qquad (15)$$

is an extension of (11). As noted in [55], p. 5, when $1 < \gamma < 2$, the curve generated by (15) is rapidly growing and this feature may be applicable in the modeling of these human tumors that are rapidly growing, such as acute leukemia and lymphoma. Values of $\gamma > 2$ give curves that are slowly growing and lie far to the right of the logistic curve ($\gamma = 2$). Slowly growing human tumors, such as adenocarcinoma of the colon and lung, may be able to be modeled by such curves. Redefine the dependent variable and change the time variable by the transformations

$$y(\xi) = \frac{b}{a} L^{\gamma-1}(t) \qquad \xi = (\gamma - 1)at \qquad (16)$$

Substitution of these transformations into (15) gives

$$\frac{dy}{d\xi} = y - y^2 \qquad y(0) = y_0$$

In other words, the canonical form of the logistic equation is recovered. This means that when the appropriate solution to the logistic equation is found the transformations in (16) produce the solution to (15). Hence it is appropriate to just restrict attention to (11).

It is straightforward to deduce that an extension of the case of logistic growth is provided by the equation

$$\dot{L}(t) = [\lambda(t) - \mu(t)L(t)]L(t) \qquad L(0) = L_0 \qquad (17)$$

where λ and μ are functions of t. Are there cellular populations whose growth may be described by an equation like (17)? The coefficients could be periodic functions of t. Write $y(t) = 1/L(t)$ to simplify (17). Then deduce that

$$L(t) = \frac{\rho(t)}{C + \int^{t} \mu(\xi)\rho(\xi) \, d\xi} \qquad \rho(t) = \exp\left[\int^{t} \lambda(\xi) \, d\xi\right]$$

(18)

where C is an integration constant. Other extensions are possible; e.g., [54], p. 13.

Presently there does not appear to be any application of an equation like (17) to describe tumor growth.

In a fascinating paper [56] dealing with population dispersal, a nonlinear diffusion equation of the type

$$\frac{\partial L}{\partial t} = (1 - L)L + \kappa \frac{\partial^2 L}{\partial x^2}$$

is introduced. Here κ is a constant, x is a spatial coordinate, and $L(x, t)$ denotes the number in the population at time t and position x. More recently, the researchers in [57] consider tissue growth in a constant environment, and attempt to model the growth of cancerous tissue that is being attacked by immune cytotoxic cells. They derive the equation

$$\frac{\partial p}{\partial t} = \lambda p(1 - p - q) + \frac{\lambda a^2}{2} \frac{\partial}{\partial x}\left[(1 - q)\frac{\partial p}{\partial x} + \frac{\partial q}{\partial x}\right]$$

where λ, a are constants and x is a spatial coordinate. By definition

$$p(x, t) = \frac{P(x, t)}{L} \qquad q(x, t) = \frac{Q(x, t)}{L}$$

where $P(x, t)$ denotes the population of cells of the tissue that can replicate and $Q(x, t)$ denotes those that cannot; $P(x, t) + Q(x, t) \leqslant L$, the greatest number of cells which a spatial element of size Δx may contain. When $q = 0$, then Skellam's equation is recovered.

The noteworthy feature in both of these mathematical models is the occurrence of quadratic nonlinearities, i.e., logistic terms.

VI. THE GOMPERTZ EQUATION

Gompertz [58] presents a study on human mortality. His analysis leads to curves that can be produced from the equation

$\dot{x}(t) = rx \ln(\theta/x)$, with $r < 0$. This equation and the properties of
its solution have been used by actuaries in numerous studies. It is
still used in the actuarial field. This is all the more surprising
since the Gompertz equation is an empiricism. One of the reasons
for its continued popularity is the property that the solution of the
equation provides a mathematical expression which often gives a good
fit to real data, that is, data that are not artificially constructed.

The *growth* form of the Gompertz equation takes the basic form

$$\dot{L}(t) = \alpha L \ln \left(\frac{\theta}{L}\right) \qquad L(0) = L_0 \qquad (19)$$

where α and θ are positive constants. Equation (19) enjoys wide
application in biology and medicine. For example, it is used to
describe the growth of normal embryos, visceral organs, animal
populations and the growth of cell populations in experimental and
human tumors! For a partial bibliography of papers that relate to
those items, see [59]. A number of details on the history and
usage of the Gompertz equation in a variety of biological growth
situations is presented in [60].

Let $L(t)$ denote the number of cells in a growing tumor, and
let θ denote the greatest size of this tumor. Then, it is *assumed*
that (19) represents the growth of the cellular population. Instead
of L the volume $V(t)$ is often used, and then

$$\dot{V}(t) = \alpha_1 V \ln \frac{V_m}{V} \qquad V(0) = V_0 \qquad (20)$$

where V_m is the greatest volume of the tumor. Since equations (19)
and (20) are empiricisms, there are no biological interpretations of
the parameters α and α_1.

To obtain the exact general solution of (19), introduce the nonlinear transformation $y = \ln(\theta/L)$ to give $\dot{y}(t) = -\alpha y$. Hence, deduce that

$$L(t) = \theta \exp \left\{ -\left[\ln \left(\frac{\theta}{L_0}\right) \right] \exp(-\alpha t) \right\} \qquad (21)$$

The structure of this expression (often called the Gompertz function)
shows that L is described by an exponential growth that is constrained by an exponentially decreasing growth rate. Note that the
form (21) shows clearly how α, L_0, and θ enter into the expression.
The curve of L versus t as given by (21) has a positive slope
throughout and has a change of curvature for $L = \theta/e$. Since θ is
about 10^{12}, the change of curvature is occurring near the end of

the range of L. The greatest value for L is θ, sometimes called the saturation level, and the growth curve is asymptotic to θ. The growth curve is sigmoid. In fact it is just one example from a family of mathematical equations that possess growth and saturation behavior of the sigmoid type.

Many investigators decide that they do not prefer the single non-linear differential equation (19). Instead, they say that Gompertz growth is defined by the pair of linear differential equations

$$\dot{L}(t) = \sigma(t)L \qquad \dot{\sigma}(t) = -\alpha\sigma \qquad (22)$$

with $L(0) = L_0$ and $L(\infty) = \theta$. Of course, the solution of this two-point boundary value problem gives the same expression for L as shown in (21). There is no apparent reason for making the selection indicated in (22). Observations of a number of tumors indicate that the growth rate decreases with time. In the first equation in (22) the growth rate is $\sigma(t)$. The second equation in (22) is just *one* of the many possible selections that can be made to conform with the observations; it is *not* unique.

On comparing (19) with (10), we see that GF is a function of $\ln(\theta/L)$. Thus GF is zero when $L = \theta$, and so it is not possible to realize growth above θ in any situation. There is no plausible biological control mechanism with this characteristic. Another difficulty with (19) is that it shows the overall rate expression $\alpha \ln(\theta/L)$ to be a nonseparable combination of the growth fraction and the inherent growth rate (i.e., the growth rate when all cells are in cycle).

From (21) differentiation with respect to t and rearrangement of the results gives

$$\ln\left[\frac{\dot{L}(t)}{L}\right] = \ln\left[\alpha \ln\left(\frac{\theta}{L_0}\right)\right] - \alpha t \qquad (23)$$

which shows that the natural logarithm of the specific growth rate is a linear function of t. This is a useful result when used to fit the model to data. Assume that a tumor grows from one cell that divides to form two cells. Also assume that $L_0 = 1$, and hence the theoretical doubling time is obtained from (21) as

$$t_d = \alpha^{-1} \ln\left[\frac{\ln \theta}{\ln(\theta/2)}\right] \qquad (24)$$

This result is often used by various researchers. But there are difficulties with the derivation just given. There is no reason to believe that the derivative in (19) is meaningful when the cell population numbers are low. Consequently an error (of unknown size) is committed when L_0 is selected to be unity. At best, (24) is some approximation to the doubling time.

The similarity in the behavior of the solutions of the Gompertz and logistic equations is examined by Winsor [61], who noted that "when approximately 30-40 per cent of the total growth has been realized we may use the Gompertz curve with the expectation that the approximation to the data will be good." Perhaps this quote from Winsor is one other reason why many investigators prefer to use the Gompertz equation.

A nonsymmetric asymptotic regression equation to fit a large selection of data is introduced in [62]. The main reason for this equation is to take care of problems (such as inadequate fit to the last part of the growth curve by the tumor data) that occur when trying to fit the regular Gompertz function. A comparison of the fit to the Gompertz and other models to experimental and human tumor data is given in [38].

The researchers in [63], on using the data for 11 patients as described in [64], indicate that there is a quantitative relationship between the initial size and the final size of the human tumor multiple myeloma given by

$$\ln \left(\frac{\theta}{L_0} \right) \ = \ 28.5 \pm 0.6 \tag{25}$$

Surely this conclusion is not surprising? Does not the data just mean that there is a representative (average) value of $\ln(\theta/L_0)$? Certainly that is the point of view taken in [65], where, on p. 321, an average value of $\ln \theta = 29$. The Swan-Vincent paper was published independently of any knowledge of the Brunton-Wheldon paper. No matter what tumor system is fitted with the Gompertz model, there will always be a particular average value for $\ln(\theta/L_0)$ peculiar to that system. Yet the contributions [66-68] claim that there is more to the relation (25). An assessment of the Brunton-Wheldon work is in [69]. In particular, various limitations on the use of the Gompertz equation and the dangers of using extrapolations of that model to deduce results of biological interest are in [69]. Steel concludes that within a given species there is a wide range of growth restraint on the tumor that is somehow linked to the species or body weight of the host.

Once more it is important to stress that there is no biological basis for support of the use of the Gompertz equation in any of the investigations with which this author is familiar. That fact is to be kept in mind when examining the growing number of papers that deal with experimental and human tumors and make use of the Gompertz growth equation. (Added in press: See [261].)

A. Experimental Tumors

By far the greatest number of applications of the Gompertz growth equation in cancer research occurs in the investigation of experimental tumors. The following brief synopsis is a partial representation of papers in this active area.

The first paper that uses the Gompertz equation in connection with the growth of an experimental tumor appears to be Ref. 70. Tumor material was inoculated into the testicles of rabbits, and the volume of the primary tumor was obtained at autopsy. Plots of volume (in cm^3) versus days are given in [70].

The follows a gap of 30 years. In a paper which generated much interest, Laird [71] does not present any motivation for her introduction of the Gompertz equation. She analyzes 10 mouse tumors, 8 rat tumors, and 1 rabbit tumor, and gives numerical values for the constants in the equation. One interesting feature is that she also gives a table of the times required for the first doubling of tumor size and the approximate number of doublings to the upper limit; see also [72]. A study of four tumor types in rats is in [73]. Reference 74 indicates that certain rat tumors are well fitted by Gompertz equations. The fit of the Gompertz function to data on transplantable and spontaneous rodent tumors is described in [75].

The landmark paper [76] deals with comprehensive growth curves and kinetic parameters for a series of experimental tumor systems. In it are described the best-fitting Gompertz curve for (1) a C3H mouse mammary tumor, and (2) the L1210 ascites tumor (often used as an experimental model for human leukemia). Reference 59 considers treatment (chemotherapy, surgery, radiation) of tumors that causes cell death in a relatively short interval. The tumor is assumed to grow according to a Gompertz equation before and after treatment. The displacement in time between the two growth curves is related to the tumor cell kill, and a comparison is made between the theoretical results and bioassay values. For 8 cases of B-16 melanoma in BDF$_1$ mice and 10 cases of transplantable mammary carcinoma 13672 in Fisher 344 rats, Ref. 77 describes the use of a least squares procedure to fit volume data to the Gompertz curves; see also [78] and [79]. In connection with these latter papers, see [80] and [81].

During this decade the number of papers on Gompertz models continues unabated. In a study of the growth of multicellular spheroids from tumor and transformed cells, [82] describes the fit of volume data to a Gompertz equation. Gompertz growth for a rat glial tumor line in culture is examined in [83].

B. Human Tumors

The first paper that deals with the fit of a Gompertz equation to
data from the growth of a human tumor is [64]. Tables of data on
patients with IgG multiple myeloma are presented. The equilibrium,
or saturation, value of θ is about 4×10^{12} cells for each patient.
The parameter α in (19) ranges from 0.004 to 0.026 per day with an
average value of $\alpha = 0.015$ days^{-1}. Sullivan and Salmon also discuss
the use of the Gompertz equation during treatment of this disseminated tumor.

Data from two female patients are analyzed in [84]. Case 1 involves the examination of the clinical growth curves of skin metastases from a breast carcinoma. In the second case history the
patient has multiple lung metastases from a leiomyosarcoma of the
uterus. Computed volumes of these solid tumors are obtained, and
fits to Gompertz equations are assessed. Reference 68 examines
sequential chest roentgenograms for 10 selected cases of testicular
tumor (a solid neoplasm) and gives fits of the Gompertz equation to
the patient data. Other work on testicular tumors is in [85].

The author makes use of the Gompertz equation in studies of the
chemotherapy of human multiple myeloma [49,65,86–88]. The growth
of 12 human malignant melanomas in athymic nude mice is described
in [89], where Gompertz curves are fitted to the volumetric growth
data.

VII. EXAMPLES OF OTHER GROWTH EQUATIONS

A survey of growth equations used in biology is presented in [90].
The equation $\dot{L}(t) = kL^{2/3}$ is based on the diffusion of products
through the surface of a solid tumor (see [91]); for applications of
this equation see [92] and [93]. A mathematical model based on the
growth of a spherical shell surrounding the tumor is in [7]. Models
of this type are generally discounted in favor of more appropriate
ones. We now examine some areas of investigation that give rise to
certain growth equations that may be appropriate in some areas of
cancer research.

A. Nonlinear Rate Equations

An equation of the logistic type (11) occurs in chemical physics,
where it is known as a rate equation. The coefficients in (11) are
then referred to as rate constants. The growth curves given by
the logistic and Gompertz equations are similar, the basic difference
being that equation (12) is symmetric about the point of inflexion,
whereas (21) is not. Reference 94 reviews mathematical models involving nonlinear rate equations that are used to describe either

the growth of a single species or the interaction between a number of populations. An extension of this work appears in [95], but it is not yet clear whether this material has relevance for cancer growth models. However the techniques described in [94] and [95] may be useful in future developments.

B. Thermodynamic Considerations

The main paper that deals with thermodynamics and cancer is [96]. As a first approach to setting up a thermodynamic theory, Salzer bases his analysis on an extension of the ideas of Gibbs. Consequently he postulates the existence of a differential relation of the form

$$dE = TdS - p\, dv + \sum_{i=1}^{n} \mu_i\, dm_i + b \tag{26}$$

which can be applied to many cells, including cancer cells. Here E, T, S, p, v, respectively, denote the internal energy, the temperature, the entropy, the pressure, and the volume. The m_i denote chemical substances, and b is "something characteristic of biology." Salzer presents a wide-ranging discussion of the possible application of (26) in cancer growth and therapy.

Other thermodynamic theories of growth in biology are in [60]. Zotin's approach is through the framework of linear and nonlinear irreversible processes. Reference 97 discusses the validity of the notion that entropy is a measure of biological order and its relation to the spontaneous creation of order. But how is biological order quantitated? How is this order coupled with the entropy production (or dissipation) of a living system? Some work in these areas is in [98]. A fascinating series of books edited by Lamprecht and Zotin [99–101] concentrate on the thermodynamics of biological processes. It is evident that the whole subject is still in its infancy. Unfortunately these papers and books do not provide any useful growth equation that could be used to describe tumor growth kinetics.

C. Bertalanffy's Equation

Of the differential equations introduced in [102], the most general one is

$$\dot{V}(t) = aV^m - bV^n \tag{27}$$

where V is the tumor volume. The first term on the right is expected to govern the characteristics of the anabolic process (leading
to constructive metabolism), and the second term governs the cata-
bolic or degradative process; see also [103]. The use of (27) has
fallen in favor of other growth equations. Yet in [38] the Bertalanffy
equation (27) gives the best fit to the data on animal tumors used
in their paper.

D. Allometric Growth Equations

Growth according to the first term in (27) is called allometric. Such
allometric growth is widespread in biology and other areas. However, there is a consensus of opinion that allometric growth is
basically an empiricism. The search for a basis for allometric growth
continues unabated. Various investigators show that the standard
growth equations (exponential, logistic, etc.) are particular cases
of certain general equations. For example, Savageau, on p. 5416 of
[104], makes the bold claim that his basic growth equation

> is *not* simply another empirically derived formula but is
> based upon the nature of the elemental mechanisms in
> synergistic systems. In principle, this theory allows
> overall properties of growing systems to be related to
> the parameters of the underlying processes.

However, in essence, he really does not do anything different from
other workers even though his starting point is more complicated
mathematically. See also [105] and [106].

E. Heterogeneous Tumor Growth Model

The growth of a heterogeneous neoplasm is considered in [107],
where Kendal introduces the equation [compare (10)]

$$\dot{L}(t) = aG \tag{28}$$

where G is proportional to the number of cells capable of growth.
Consider a population of L cells where the jth cell has the potential
to take on one of q_j possible states, $j = 1, 2, \ldots, L$. For example, different phases of the cell cycle and different phenotypes
specify distinct states. The number of states within the population
is described by a measure of the intraneoplastic diversity, P, defined by

$$P = q_1 q_2 \cdots q_L$$

It was shown in [108] that there is a qualitative relationship between the degree of tumor heterogeneity and the growth rate. This implies that P is related to the growth rate of the tumor population.

Kendal introduces an "index" G and assumes that it is a function of P. But what form does this function take? In this development of the mathematical model, this is a crucial point, for on it depends the growth characteristics of the tumor. To make progress, one needs an assumption. Kendal assumes, with no biological or mathematical justification, that G is "additive." That is, for two populations P_1 and P_2,

$$G(P_1 P_2) \;=\; G(P_1) + G(P_2) \tag{29}$$

Mathematically, (29) is an example of a functional equation. In this case the general solution of (29) is obtained by inspection and is the function given by $G = k \ln P$, where k is a constant. Equation (28) shows that

$$\dot{L}(t) \;=\; ak \ln P \tag{30}$$

and this is the equation for general growth of the heterogeneous tumor mass.

Let the population consist of L identical and noninteracting cells. Assume that each cell has the ability to take on one of m states. The number of combinations of states is $P = m^L$. In this case (30) becomes $\dot{L}(t) = ak(\ln m)L$, an equation for exponential growth.

It is reasonable to ask what requirement P satisfies to produce other standard growth equations. Say it is desired to deduce the Gompertz equation (19). Equate the right side of (30) to the right side of (19) to give $P = (\theta/L)^{\alpha L / ak}$. Select $ak = \alpha$ (for convenience); then

$$P \;=\; \left(\frac{\theta}{L}\right)^{L} \tag{31}$$

This is a peculiar result. Equation (31) indicates that P is inversely proportional to the total number of possible intercellular interactions. Kendal's approach is to first assume the result (31) and then derive (19).

If the right side of (30) is equated to $\alpha L - \beta L^2$ (for logistic growth), the following result is obtained

$$P \;=\; \exp\left(\frac{\alpha L - \beta L^2}{ak}\right) = m^{L - (\beta/\alpha)L^2} \tag{32}$$

where $\alpha = ak \ln m$.

F. Fischer's Equation

Solid tumors are known to contain well-oxygenated and hypoxic cells. The poorly oxygenated cells do not reproduce. To account for the growth of the well-oxygenated cells, Fischer introduced the following growth equation [109]:

$$\dot{L}(t) = \lambda L \exp(-\mu L) \tag{33}$$

where λ and μ are considered to be constants. There is no explicit solution to this equation. Detailed applications of this equation in radiotherapy treatment models are provided in [54].

G. General Observations on Growth Equations

One characteristic of a general growth equation of the form

$$\dot{L}(t) = Lf(L) \tag{34}$$

for nonconstant $f(L)$ is that df/dL be negative. The models in (11), (19), (33), and (39) satisfy that restriction.

None of the models so far considered in this review provides any understanding of the basic underlying *mechanisms* which give rise to and control the growth of the cell population. (An exception is Salzer [96], discussed earlier; however, his work is still at the embryonic stage.) This comment also applies to most mathematical models dealing with tumor growth, and is especially true for the cell cycle models in Section VIII.

The correct approach to the formulation of basic equations that describe the general behavior of the dynamics of a continuous medium is presented in [110]. What is needed is the generation of similar equations for biological media. A start in this direction is provided by [111,112]. These approaches and related ones ought to provide the background information necessary to describe mechanisms of biological growth, including tumor growth kinetics. Certainly these papers provide a good reference point for the development of future work.

VIII. CYTOKINETICS

The past 35 years have seen three major developments in cytokinetics, the analysis of the cell cycle behavior of cell populations. The first of these began with the demonstration that DNA is synthesized in interphase and the cell cycle could be divided into G_1, S, G_2, and M phases [113]. The second began with the introduction of tritiated thymidine [114,115] and its extension to detailed kinetic analysis

[116]. The third major development began with the procedure of flow cytometry [117,118].

These three areas have influenced the growth of mathematical modeling in cytokinetics. In the following sections we give a brief synopsis of these areas and the relevance to tumor growth kinetics, if any. The three developments, in general, try to quantitate key parameters, such as the fraction of cells in the G_1, S, G_2, and M phases of the cell cycle, and help further our understanding of what is going on through the cycle.

A. The Cell Cycle

A new trend in the mathematical modeling of the cellular populations started in the fifties with the introduction of a conceptual model for the cell cycle. The classical idealized model of the life cycle of a *normal* proliferating cell from one mitosis to the next is divided into the four distinct portions (called phases) G_1, S, G_2, and M. This conceptual model is due to Howard and Pelc [113] and describes the active part of the cell cycle. The following identification of each phase is due to Baserga [119]:

G_1 (gap 1): Here proteins and ribonucleic acid (RNA) are synthesized. It is also called the predeoxyribonucleic acid (pre-DNA) phase.

S: DNA synthesis takes place; DNA is duplicated, and RNA protein synthesis continues.

G_2 (gap 2): Post-DNA synthesis phase (no net synthesis of DNA; RNA and protein synthesis continues).

M: Mitosis (prophase, metaphase, anaphase, telophase); no DNA synthesis, protein synthesis is minimal, and RNA synthesis is negligible during all except early prophase and late telophase.

It is generally assumed that this conceptual model is appropriate to describe the gross characteristics of a proliferating cancer cell. However, for cancer cells, it is suggested in [120] and [121] that there is an actual resting period G_0 from which cells can be triggered into the mitotic cycle. Yet it is difficult to distinguish between an extended G_1 phase and G_0 from experimental measurements. Naturally this leads to differences in opinion. Thus some mathematical models of the cell cycle include a completely separate G_0 state, whereas others do not. Even at the present time this dilemma is unresolved.

As might be expected, many papers and books deal with the cell cycle and the growth of tumors. References 12 and 122–132 are relevant to our study here. A particularly useful critical

evaluation of the concept of the cell cycle is presented in [133].
(Note added in press: See also [257-261, 263].)

B. Experimental Techniques for Cell Kinetics

Important techniques are available for the study of cell population
kinetics. The main ones in use through the mid-1970s are described
in [12]. Generally, these techniques are used to solve experimental
tumor growth problems, although, where appropriate, they can also
be used in studies involving human tumors.

The thymidine labeling technique plays a key role. In this
technique the isotope tritiated thymidine ^{3}H-TdR is injected into
animals or humans, where it becomes incorporated into the cell nuclei
that are synthesizing DNA. It is possible to recognize labeled cells
in autoradiographs of sections or smears of tissue. A whole new
technology based on this technique has developed over the past 30
years. We select a few concepts necessary for the present chapter.
At the end of this section we draw attention to the dramatic new
area involving bromodeoxyuridine.

The labeling index (LI) is defined to be the ratio of labeled
cells (L_S) to the total cells (L) in autoradiographs of tissue removed about 1 hr after injection of the isotope. The labeling index
can give some information on the rates of cell proliferation. A comparison of values of LI in the same tissue before and after chemotherapy may suggest changes in the proliferative population.

The percent labeled mitoses (PLM) technique is important for
estimating the mean duration and variability of the cell cycle and
its constituent phases. A single injection of ^{3}H-TdR is made, and
subsequent tissue samples are excised. Then autoradiographs are
prepared, and mitotic figures are scored as labeled or unlabeled.
From this information a curve can be produced that gives the plot
of the PLM data against time after thymidine administration. The
PLM curve is now known as the FLM curve. The fraction

$$FLM(t) = \frac{\text{no. of labeled mitotic cells at time t after } {}^3H\text{-TdR pulse}}{\text{total number of mitotic cells at the same time}} \qquad (35)$$

is defined to be the fraction labeled mitoses FLM(t) curve. Assume
that a pulse of ^{3}H-TdR is given to the cells. Since there are no
labeled cells initially then the FLM curve must start at zero. The
curve continues with positive slope, the value of FLM increasing because the number of labeled cells is also increasing. Eventually the
value of the fraction reaches unity and thereafter decreases. Then,
as time increases, the curve decreases until it reaches a minimum
before increasing once more to a new local maximum, which has a
value less than the previous one. Theoretically, the curve continues

in this manner with successive peaks and valleys. In practice, repeated cell division weakens the label, and this means that only the response from a few cycles appears meaningful.

Historically, the FLM method has provided the most extensive information about cell cycle traverse in asynchronously growing cell populations. Many papers deal with methods that give expressions for the FLM function. No attempt is made here at completeness. The interested reader is referred to Refs. 12, 30, 34, 127, 131, and 134–140.

The experimental FLM data give information about the DNA histogram. Theoretical attempts at generating DNA histograms that resemble those obtained experimentally involve analysis of the G_1, S, G_2, and M phases (denoted by 1, 2, 3, and 4, respectively) of asynchronously growing cell populations. The time t_i spent by a cell in phase i, i = 1–4, is assumed to be a random variable with an arbitrary distribution function f_i. A further assumption is that the time spent by a cell in one particular phase is independent of the time spent in any other phase. Approaches that have been used to describe the probability density functions of the phase durations include normal, log-normal, and gamma distributions. A mathematical expression for the FLM function can be determined. Techniques such as maximum likelihood, least squares, or Monte Carlo are then used to fit the theoretical FLM functions to the experimental curves. See, for example, [30,34,134–140]. Later, see the material leading to (59) or (71), we introduce the probability distribution function $f_i(a_i)$ where a_i is an age variable corresponding to phase i.

However, it is evident that there are a number of major difficulties associated with the theoretical and experimental methods for the determination of the FLM curves; see, e.g., [141,142]. For example, the distinction between labeled and unlabeled mitotic cells often is not apparent and this can give an incorrect estimation of cell cycle parameters [143]. There is variation in the rate of DNA synthesis by cells in S phase, with the result that some S-phase cells (usually those in early and late S phase) are more lightly labeled than others [144]. Reference 145 also highlights difficulties in using the tritiated thymidine technique.

The fraction (35) gives the continuous labeled curve and is a function of the time elapsed since the start of injections with triated thymidine given with intervals considerably shorter than the assumed mean value of the transit time in S phase. A useful method for evaluating continuous labeling data is in [146].

A new procedure called RCS_i (radioactivity per cell in a narrow window of S phase) is introduced in [147]. It eliminates some of the technical problems associated with the FLM procedure and is faster and more accurate. An extension of the RCS_i procedure is described in [148].

The whole issue of [149] is devoted to the technology required for the quantification of bromodeoxyuridine (BrdUrd) incorporated into cellular DNA. The BrdUrd is used as a label, and its presence in cellular DNA is detected immunochemically. For example, techniques [149] are now available (1) to provide an estimate of the cell cycle traverse rates from a single cell sample and (2) to measure the resistance of a tumor population to chemotherapy. These two areas are of considerable importance in clinical studies. It is apparent that there will be an explosion in the number of papers dealing with this new extremely powerful technique.

C. Flow Microfluorometry

The early flow microfluorometers used a monodisperse cell suspension stained with a fluorescent dye. The cell suspension is constrained so that cells flow in single file through a tiny orifice. The output of the nozzle orifice crosses a quiescent region and intersects the light from a laser. Each cell, when excited by the laser beam, yields a short fluorescent light pulse whose duration is determined by cell speed and dimensions. Subsequently the light pulses are analyzed by a multichannel pulse height analyzer. The distribution of the fluorescent stain content over the cell population gives a histogram. A brief historical account and the then current description of cell analysis and cell sorting by this new type of high-speed flow of cells is in [150]. The abbreviation FMF designates flow microfluorometry or variants of it. The FMF approach gives detailed information on the frequency distribution of cellular DNA. The FMF technique is also known by the words "flow cytometry."

Over the past decade numerous papers have appeared dealing with cell cycle analysis (and sorting) by FMF; see [151–154]. Early detailed reviews of this dramatic new area are in [155] and [156].

In [156] the authors discuss a basic equation of FMF studies, namely

$$DNA_M(y) = \int_0^\infty DNA_T(x)P(x - y, kx) \, dx$$

where $DNA_T(x)$ is the theoretical fraction of the cell population with DNA content x, $DNA_M(y)$ is the measured fraction of the fraction of the population with fluorescence y (assumed to be linearly related to DNA content), and $P(x, y)$ is the probability that a cell of DNA content x will be detected with fluorescence y. This is an integral equation of the first kind. Equations of this general type occur in diverse applications in the physical sciences. The important feature is that the problem of trying to determine the kernel function (the so-called inverse problem) is usually ill conditioned. For this problem this means that there are probably greatly differing theoretical content distributions which give rise to the *same* experimental distributions. This is such an important point that it seems curious that there does not appear to be anything published on it since 1978.

A summary of the use of FMF analysis is presented in [157] through the computer program DRUGFIT. A variety of mathematical models have been proposed by investigators to approximate the DNA histograms obtained by FMF: They are reviewed in [155, 156]. Reference 158 compares 12 methods using the same set of data. Reference 159 also deals with some of the mathematics involved in dealing with FMF analysis.

An interesting review of the display and analysis of flow cytometric data is in [160]. Applications of flow cytometry in cancer research and clinical oncology are included as part of the very detailed review in [161], which covers the principles, advantages, limitations, and major applications of flow cytometry in research and clinical diagnosis.

D. The Cox-Woodbury-Myers Model

Models of tumor growth based on biological reasoning are preferred over those not capable of biological justification. Cox, Woodbury, and Myers [162] derive an interesting mathematical model of tumor growth that is based on biological premise. Their model is now examined.

Assume that each tumor cell secretes a growth-inhibiting molecule I at a constant rate into the extracellular space, in which it can diffuse freely. Assume that degradation and/or secretion of I takes place by a nonsaturable first-order process:

$$\frac{d}{dt} [I] = P \frac{L}{v} - F[I] \qquad (36)$$

where [ ] indicates concentration. Here, P denotes the cellular rate of secretion of I (mg cell^{-1} sec^{-1}), L is the number of cells in the population, v is the volume of distribution (ml), and F is the rate of degradation or secretion of I (sec^{-1}). The reaction is assumed to take place at a much faster rate than the growth rate of the general population. This means that d[I]/dt rapidly approaches zero and stays there. Hence (36) gives the equilibrium relation

$$[I] = \frac{PL}{vF}$$

Consider each tumor cell to have one receptor site R capable of combining with I. When the receptor R is unbound, the tumor cell traverses the cell cycle each generation time t_c and goes on to proliferate. However, when the receptor is bound by I, the tumor cell leaves the cell cycle to enter the (assumed) resting phase G_0, from which it may reenter the cell cycle if I becomes unbound. The following simple reaction accounts for this behavior:

$$[I] + [R] \underset{k_2}{\overset{k_1}{\rightleftharpoons}} [RI]$$

with k_1, k_2 denoting rate constants. For this reversible reaction

$$\frac{d}{dt} [RI] = k_1[I][R] - k_2[RI]$$

Assume, as before, that this reaction takes place quickly enough that equilibrium is reached. Then

$$\frac{[I][R]}{[RI]} = \frac{k_2}{k_1} = K \tag{37}$$

The total receptor concentration $[R_{tot}] = L/v$ is

$$[R_{tot}] = [R] + [RI]$$

and with (37), can be rearranged to produce

$$\frac{[R]}{[R_{tot}]} = \frac{1}{1 + [I]K^{-1}}$$

Recall that $[R]/[R_{tot}]$ is the percentage of cells that are in the proliferative cycle with growth fraction (GF). It follows that

$$\frac{dL}{dt} = \frac{[R]}{[R_{tot}]} \alpha L = \frac{\alpha L}{1 + [I]K^{-1}} = \frac{\alpha L}{1 + \beta L} \tag{38}$$

on using (10), and setting $\beta = P/KvF$. Equation (38) represents the first model derived by Cox and co-workers. Note that $(1 + \beta L)^{-1}$ is the growth fraction.

Now assume that cell loss from the tumor is a first-order process to a first approximation. The equation for the number of cells in the tumor is now

$$\frac{dL}{dt} = L\left[\frac{\alpha}{1 + \beta L} - \gamma\right] \tag{39}$$

where γ is the rate of loss per cell. Equation (39) represents the second model of Cox et al.

The models described by (38) and (39) are fitted to the experimental plasmacytoma data given by [76]. The cell loss model (39) gives a significantly better fit to the data. Also, Cox et al. demonstrate that the fit of the model (39) is at least as good, if not better, than the fit of the Gompertz model to the same data.

The cell loss model needs to be investigated further. In particular, for any tumor we need to know how to get information on the three parameters α, β, and γ, instead of just fitting the model to tumor data.

E. The Burns-Tannock Model

A novel model of the cell cycle is proposed in [31]. Burns and Tannock refer to the active part of the cycle $G_1 \to M$ as the C phase, which is assumed to have a constant duration T. There is a separate G_0 phase, which is entered by *all* dividing cells. Release of cells from this phase is assumed to be random with a constant probability per unit time γ; i.e., it is a Poisson process with parameter γ. For application to renewal tissue they assume that cells leave the population with constant equal probability per unit time irrespective of their position in the cycle. We take this as a Poisson process with parameter k.

Let x(t), y(t) represent the numbers of cells in C phase and G_0 phase, respectively. Then

$$\dot{x}(t) = \gamma y(t) - \gamma y(t - T)e^{-kT} - k\,x(t) \tag{40}$$

$$\dot{y}(t) = 2\gamma y(t - T)e^{-kT} - \gamma y(t) - k\,y(t) \tag{41}$$

The first term on the right side of (40) represents the rate of flow of cells from the G_0 phase into the C phase. The second term denotes the rate at which cells leave the C phase at mitosis. It is given by the product of the rate into the C phase at time T earlier and the probability of not being lost from the C phase for time T. The rate of flow of cells out of C phase is represented by the last term. For (41) the first term on the right is the same as the second term in (40) except that binary fission gives the factor 2. The last two terms denote the loss terms.

Equations (40) and (41) are examples of a time-lagged system; see [163-165]. Interestingly, in the present formulation (40) is uncoupled to (41). Burns and Tannock derive the labeled mitoses curve and the labeling index for continuous labeling and show that the predicted curves are in tolerable agreement with certain experimentally derived results.

A model that is formally the same as the Burns and Tannock model is proposed in [166]. Other related models involving a separate G_0 phase are considered in [167–170].

F. A Simple Cell Cycle Model

In this section we take the following model of the cell cycle. We assume a subpopulation of resting or quiescent cells with number of cells at time t denoted by $Y(t)$. These cells can be regarded as being in the G_0 phase of the cycle. The rest of the cycle G_1 to M is identified as giving rise to a subpopulation of reproducing cells. Let the number of cells in this second subpopulation at time t be denoted by $X(t)$. Assume that cell death is a first-order process. This model of the cell cycle allows for a development of a simple mathematical model.

Now, the equation for $X(t)$ is described by

$$\dot{X}(t) = \phi(t)Y - \sigma X - \gamma X \qquad X(0) = X_0 \qquad (42)$$

The first term on the right gives the rate of entry of cells from the quiescent population. The second term gives the rate at which cells leave the reproducing population to enter the quiescent state, and the third term represents the rate at which cells in the reproducing population are dying. Here $\phi(t)$ is a function of t, and σ and γ are constants. Also,

$$\dot{Y}(t) = 2\sigma X - \phi(t)Y - \gamma Y \qquad Y(0) = Y_0 \qquad (43)$$

The first term on the right indicates the rate of production of new cells assuming binary division. The second term gives the rate of loss of cells from the quiescent population into the reproducing population, and the third term represents the rate at which quiescent cells are dying.

The total population is $L(t) = X(t) + Y(t)$. Hence, adding equations (42) and (43) gives the general growth equation

$$\dot{L}(t) = \sigma X - \gamma L \qquad L(0) = L_0 \qquad (44)$$

To make progress at this point, we need an assumption that enables us to write a connection between X and L. There does not appear to be any clear-cut guidance on how to proceed.

Yet there is one approach that can be followed through mathematically, and its biological consequences can be examined. Inspection of (39) and (44) shows that both equations are identical when ever

$$X = \frac{\alpha}{\sigma} \frac{L}{1 + \beta L} \tag{45}$$

The expression for X is thus of Michaelis-Menten form, and X approaches the saturation level $\alpha/\sigma\beta$ as L increases. Also

$$\frac{dX}{dL} = \frac{X}{L} \frac{1}{1 + \beta L} = \frac{X}{L} \frac{\alpha/\sigma\beta - X}{\alpha/\sigma\beta} \tag{46}$$

with initial condition $X_0 = \alpha L_0 / \sigma(1 + \beta L_0)$. The quiescent population size is

$$Y = \frac{L(\sigma - \alpha + \sigma\beta L)}{\sigma(1 + \beta L)} \tag{47}$$

If L is known as an explicit function of t (in this example it is only known implicitly), then (45) and (47) give X and Y as explicit functions of t. That information could be used in (42) to give $\phi(t)$. Generally, though, equations (42–44) need to be integrated numerically and fit to data to ascertain values for $\phi(t)$ and the parameters. Within the context of the present discussion, no one has apparently used (45) in their studies of cell cycle behavior.

Other selections for X as a function of L can be made. For example, equate the right sides of (44) and (11), and note that $L < a/b$ for the logistic model. Here L(t) is known explicitly as a function of t, and so, in principle, an explicit expression for $\phi(t)$ can be found.

Reference 171 describes the fit of a growth equation for L(t) to the plasmacytoma data of [76]. Piantadosi notes that "In fairness, it should be mentioned that simpler (i.e., fewer parameter and/or closed form) models would fit these data as well." I believe that if a simple model is adequate, why complicate it?

G. More Complicated Models of the Proliferative and Quiescent Pools of Cells

Assume that cells progress through the cell cycle G_1 to M, there being no G_0 phase. Let $x_1(t)$ denote the number of cells in the G_1 phase, $x_2(t)$ the number in S, $x_3(t)$ the number in G_2, and $x_4(t)$ the number in M. The quantities $\beta_1, \ldots, \beta_4$ are associated with the rate of cell loss from each of the four phases, respectively.

The quantities $\alpha_1, \ldots, \alpha_4$ are associated with the cell growth rates for each phase. The α's and the β's have dimensions of $(\text{time})^{-1}$. Hence

$$\dot{x}_1(t) = 2\alpha_4 x_4 - (\alpha_1 + \beta_1)x_1 \qquad x_1(0) = x_{10} \qquad (48)$$

where the 2 indicates an assumption of binary fission (exponential growth assumption). Also, the first term gives the rate of production of new cells that come into the G_1 phase after mitosis. The second term is the rate at which cells are lost from the G_1 phase to go into S phase. The last term is the rate of cell loss due to death. We can proceed in this manner to write the remaining three equations:

$$\dot{x}_2(t) = \alpha_1 x_1 - (\alpha_2 + \beta_2)x_2 \qquad x_2(0) = x_{20}$$

$$\dot{x}_3(t) = \alpha_2 x_2 - (\alpha_3 + \beta_3)x_3 \qquad x_3(0) = x_{30}$$

$$\dot{x}_4(t) = \alpha_3 x_3 - (\alpha_4 + \beta_4)x_4 \qquad x_4(0) = x_{40} \qquad (49)$$

Equations (48–49) represent a system of ordinary differential equations. In the simplest case the α's and β's are assumed to be constants. This means that there are eight parameters in this mathematical model. Numerical solution is necessary.

When a quiescent pool is required to be included in the model, then there is no difficulty in doing this.

Some investigators are not content to have just four phases in the active part of the cycle, so they divide each of them into many component subphases. Thus the G_1 phase can be divided into n subphases where each subphase is considered to have its own subpopulation. Repeat this approach for S, G_2, and M, selecting, if desired, different numbers for the respective subdivisions. When this is completed, it is possible to write expressions for the differential equations that can be produced to describe the progress through each subphase of the active part of the cell cycle. Again, a quiescent pool, suitably divided into subdivisions can be incorporated into the model.

Cell cycle models of the above types may be found in [129, 172–174].

One reason cited for the selection of many subdivisions is the need to identify a control point in the cell cycle where something important happens to the cell. These control points, however, are not well defined. Additional subdivisions can be handled with a digital computer. Models with many subdivisions can be regarded as compartmental models. Briefly, a compartment is an amount of material that acts kinetically in a homogeneously distinct manner. The compartments may or may not be readily identified as having any physiological relevance. Analyses of compartmental models indicate that great care is needed in formulating and interpreting the mathematical models that arise. For general discussions on compartmental analyses see [175-177]. Interesting critiques and review of compartmental modeling are presented in [178,179].

H. Assessment of the Models of Tumor Cell Kinetics

One of the earliest reviews of the kinetics of cellular proliferation in spontaneous and induced tumors is in [180]. Other important reviews are contained in [6,12,124,132,181,182].

Since 1959 [116] there have been a tremendous number of papers dealing with the production of FLM curves from mathematical models of the cell cycle and from experimental data. There is even a major scientific journal, *Cell and Tissue Kinetics*. However, careful examination of all of this work reveals that the emphasis of cell kinetics has been in extending our knowledge of cell proliferation on both malignant and normal tissue of *animals*. There is a remarkable paucity of information available for *humans*.

Tannock [182] points out that there is a lack of data on cell cycle phase duration of recognizable granulocyte precursors in normal human bone marrow, a tissue that is frequently limiting for anticancer chemotherapy. He notes that labeled mitoses data are available for only two patients, and the cell cycle phase duration is not well defined [183,184].

If cell kinetics is to be useful in cancer research, then it should be able to be used in those situations of considerable interest, namely treatments by radiation or drug insult. Such treatment results in perturbation of tissue and alters the kinetics. Tannock expresses grave concern over the measurements of thymidine LI, FMF histograms, and other proliferative indexes obtained after treatment with radiation or toxic drugs, because many of the cells that appear morphologically intact will have been sterilized by the treatment. Furthermore, he believes that cell kinetics has no major part to play in directly predicting optimal drug scheduling in humans. He lists the following major reasons for his pessimism.

1. The dominant problem of intrinsic drug sensitivity and resistance
2. Extreme complexity of drug delivery, pharmacology and heterogeneity of the target population in man
3. Lack of knowledge about target clonogenic cells in man.
4. Lack of knowledge of perturbations in therapeutic index (ratio of tumor damage to normal tissue damage) as opposed to perturbations in tumor kinetics alone

5. Limited evidence for prediction of optimal treatment in
animals (where knowledge is great and complexity low)

We list these reasons because we firmly believe that they must be at
the forefront of future mathematical modeling attempts when dealing
with tumor growth and therapy for humans.

Tannock also makes a plea for models that describe *mechanisms*
that control cell kinetics.

I. Computer Models of Cell Kinetics

Early attempts at modeling the kinetics of cell populations by means
of digital computer programs occur in [185–188]. (Note added in
proof: Recent progress appears in [262].)

A different type of computer model is investigated in [189].
Düchting examines a cell-renewal control loop model based on a section of the erythropoietic system. This model is set up on a special
analog computer and includes a number of control loops. Extensions
of this work continue [190–194].

J. Cell Kinetics and Cancer Chemotherapy

We believe that cell kinetics provide a conceptual framework for drug
therapy. The basic information needed in cell kinetics is the length
of the transit time through each phase of the cell cycle. Such information can be obtained from the FLM curve. This information for
the specific phases is used with agents designed to destroy cells in
these phases. These agents are called phase specific. Information
for the complete cell cycle and its distribution provides estimates on
the duration of therapy.

The fraction of clonogenic cells in a tumor is also an important
piece of information in cell kinetics studies. (Clonogenic cells are
capable of indefinite proliferation; they are often called malignant
cells.)

Useful reviews of cell kinetics and cancer chemotherapy are given
in [195–199] and in [257–259].

Mathematical models of tumor growth that are based on cell kinetics
concepts therefore offer promise in understanding cancer chemotherapy.
Before examining several typical models, we need to provide some
background information on mathematical developments for cell populations involving age and maturity structure.

IX. CELL SYSTEMS WITH AGE DISTRIBUTION

The exponential, logistic, etc., models regard the number of cells as
being a function of time only. Many people believe that these models

are inadequate to represent cell populations because the variations due to cell age are not incorporated. The mathematical study of the age distribution in a cell population is generally recognized as starting with [200] and [201]. We follow part of the development of [202], where von Foerster derives the complete partial differential equation (incorporating a loss term) for the age density n(t, a), where a denotes the "age" variable. In practice, a is always interpreted as the chronological age of the cell or organism; but, nevertheless, a precise definition of a is lacking. The total number of cells in the population at time t is taken through all age classes and is defined as

$$
L(t) = \int_{a=0}^{\infty} n(t, a) \, da \tag{50}
$$

The number of cells which are in the age category a to a + Δa at time t is n(t, a)Δa. If it is assumed that age and time are measured in the same units, then, in a small time element Δt, the age of each cell is increased by Δt. The number of cells of age a + Δt at time t + Δt is equal to the number of cells that at time t are in the age category a to a + Δa, minus the number of cells lost in the same category. In symbols,

n(t + Δt, a + Δt)Δa = n(t, a)Δa − λ(t, a, . . .)n(t, a)ΔaΔt

The expression on the left is expanded into a Taylor series. In the limit as Δt → 0 we obtain

$$
\frac{\partial n(t, a)}{\partial t} + \frac{\partial n(t, a)}{\partial a} = -\lambda(t, a, \ldots)n(t, a) \tag{51}
$$

This partial differential equation is of the von Foerster type. The dots in λ indicate that n, L, etc., could be included. The present derivation of (51) is based on [203]. See also the follow-up paper [204]. To complete the mathematical description of (51), we include the birth rate

$$
n(t, 0) = \alpha(t) \tag{52}
$$

and the initial age distribution

$$
n(0, a) = \beta(a) \tag{53}
$$

Next we develop a general solution of (51−53) when λ is restricted. Thereafter, for a further restriction on λ, we show the form that the solution takes.

Assume that

$$\lambda(t, a, \ldots) = \lambda(t, a) \tag{54}$$

that is, λ is a function of t and a only. Equation (51) is called a hyperbolic equation. Such an equation possesses curves known as characteristics. Analyzing such characteristics for (51), we find that a key role is played by the transformations $\xi = t - a$ and $\zeta = a$. The functions

$$n(t, a) = n(\xi + a, \zeta) \equiv u(\xi, \zeta)$$

$$\lambda(t, a) = \lambda(\xi + a, \zeta) \equiv m(\xi, \zeta)$$

where the two new functions $u(\xi, \zeta)$ and $m(\xi, \zeta)$ are introduced for convenience. The transformations let us rewrite the given partial differential equation in a basic form. To show this, first construct the derivatives

$$\frac{\partial n}{\partial t} = \frac{\partial n}{\partial \xi} \frac{\partial \xi}{\partial t} + \frac{\partial n}{\partial \zeta} \frac{\partial \zeta}{\partial t} = \frac{\partial n}{\partial \xi} = \frac{\partial u}{\partial \xi}$$

$$\frac{\partial n}{\partial a} = \frac{\partial n}{\partial \xi} \frac{\partial \xi}{\partial a} + \frac{\partial n}{\partial \zeta} \frac{\partial \zeta}{\partial a} = -\frac{\partial n}{\partial \xi} + \frac{\partial n}{\partial \zeta} = -\frac{\partial u}{\partial \xi} + \frac{\partial u}{\partial \zeta}$$

Substituting these results into (51) and (54) gives

$$\frac{\partial}{\partial \zeta} \ln u(\xi, \zeta) = -m(\xi, \zeta)$$

Integrating this equation gives

$$\ln u(\xi, \zeta) = \ln f(\xi) - \int_{p(\xi)}^{\zeta} m(\xi, x) \, dx$$

where $f(\xi)$ is an arbitrary function of ξ. The function $m(\xi, \zeta)$ is defined only for $\xi + x \geqslant 0$ and $x \geqslant 0$. In terms of the original variables t and a this means that

$$n(t, a) = \alpha(t - a) \exp \left[-\int_{x=0}^{a} \lambda(t - a + x, x) \, dx \right]$$

$$\text{for } t > a \tag{55}$$

$$n(t, a) = \beta(a - t) \exp \left[- \int_{z=0}^{t} \lambda(z, z + a - t) \, dx \right]$$

$$\text{for } t \leqslant a \qquad (56)$$

These expressions are given in [203].

Now consider a further simplification in the form of λ:

$$\lambda(t, a) = \lambda(a) + c(t) \qquad (57)$$

The effect of the split is to show the contribution from the age-specific death rate $\lambda(a)$ and the rate of cell loss $c(t)$. This type of structure for λ is used in mathematical models of cancer chemotherapy involving concepts from cell kinetics and pharmacokinetics; see Sections XII.A and XII.B.

It is convenient to define

$$j(t) = \exp \left[- \int_{0}^{t} c(x) \, dx \right] \qquad (58)$$

Assume that the time spent by a cell going through its cycle is described by an independent probability density function $f(a)$. Material is presented in [205] on the growth of a population of cells subject to random fluctuations. Harris considers the situation of binary fission. If the cell has survived until age a, then the probability that the cell splits during the time interval $(a, a + da)$ is $f(a) \, \Delta a/[1 - \phi(a)]$, and $f(a)/[1 - \phi(a)]$ is the age-specific death rate. The quantity $\phi(a)$ is the cumulative distribution, defined by

$$\phi(a) = 1 - \int_{0}^{a} f(x) \, dx$$

In the current development the age-specific death rate is $\lambda(a)$. Hence

$$\lambda(a) = \frac{f(a)}{\phi(a)} \qquad (59)$$

Integrating both sides shows that $\ln \phi = - \int_{0}^{a} \lambda(x) \, dx$. We can now deduce that

$$\phi(a) = 1 - \int_{0}^{a} f(x) \, dx = \exp \left[- \int_{0}^{a} \lambda(x) \, dx \right] \qquad (60)$$

Also, by (57),

$$\int_0^a \lambda(t - a + x, x) \, dx = \int_0^a \lambda(x) \, dx + \int_0^a c(t - a + x) \, dx$$

$$= \int_0^a \lambda(x) \, dx + \int_0^t c(y) \, dy - \int_0^{t-a} c(y) \, dy$$

The rearrangement of the second integral on the first line comes about by setting $y = t - a + x$ and splitting up the range of integration. Hence, from (55), (58), and (60) we deduce that

$$n(t, a) = \frac{\alpha(t - a)\phi(a)j(t)}{j(t - a)} \qquad t > a \qquad (61)$$

Proceeding in a similar manner allows (56) to be written as

$$n(t, a) = \frac{\beta(a - t)\phi(a)j(t)}{\phi(a - t)} \qquad t \leqslant a \qquad (62)$$

Instead of using an age variable, S. Rubinow introduced the novel concept of using cell maturity. In the next section we examine the derivation of his basic equation. In Section XIII we apply a mixture of age and maturity variable equations to the analysis of a cancer chemotherapy problem.

X. CELL SYSTEMS WITH MATURITY VARIABLE

The concept of a maturity variable is introduced in [206] in the development of a theory of cell growth according to a maturity-time representation, where mitosis always occurs at the same maturity level. Two possible interpretations for the maturity variable are (i) cell volume and (ii) the amount of DNA in a cell. We adhere to Rubinow's notation. Let $n(\mu, t)$ denote the cell density function, with $n(\mu, t)\Delta\mu$ denoting the number of cells in the maturity level μ to $\mu + \Delta\mu$ at time t. A maturation "velocity" $\nu \equiv \nu(\mu, t, \ldots)$ is introduced, which is a prescribed quantity; also $\nu = d\mu/dt$ is the time rate of change of maturity μ at time t. Rubinow assumes that

$$n(\mu + \Delta\mu, t + \Delta t)\left[\Delta\mu + \frac{\partial \nu}{\partial \mu}\Delta\mu\Delta t\right] = n(\mu, t)\Delta\mu - \lambda(\mu, t, \ldots)\Delta\mu\Delta t$$

which expresses the assumption that the number of cells of maturity $\mu + \Delta\mu$ at time $t + \Delta t$ is equal to the number of cells matured from an earlier level μ minus the number of cells lost. Here, $\lambda(\mu, t, \ldots)$ denotes a loss function that can depend on μ, t, n, L, etc. A Taylor expansion of the first factor on the left of this equation gives, in the limit as $\Delta t \to 0$,

$$\frac{\partial n(\mu, t)}{\partial t} + \frac{\partial}{\partial \mu} [\nu n(\mu, t)] = -\lambda(\mu, t, \ldots) n(\mu, t) \quad (63)$$

This is Rubinow's equation [206].

At t = 0 there is the initial condition $n(\mu, 0) = g(\mu)$, say. The maximum maturation level is chosen to occur for $\mu = 1$, when all cells complete mitosis and give birth to p_1 new daughter cells. Hence, there is the following boundary condition to be applied:

$$n(0, t)\nu(0, t, \ldots) = p_1 n(1, t)\nu(1, t, \ldots)$$

The dots signify that ν can depend on n, L, etc. The total number of cells is defined to be

$$L(t) = \int_0^1 n(\mu, t) \, d\mu \quad (64)$$

A general solution to (63) in the special case where λ and g are functions of μ only is given in [206]. Another particular case occurs when $\nu \equiv 1$, $\lambda \equiv 0$, for then (63) gives

$$\frac{\partial n(\mu, t)}{\partial t} + \frac{\partial n(\mu, t)}{\partial \mu} = 0 \quad (65)$$

By inspection, an arbitrary function of $t - \mu$ satisfies this equation. Alternatively, we could introduce the transformations $p = t - \mu$, $q = \mu$ and deduce $\partial u/\partial q = 0$ from (65), where $n(\mu, t) = n(q, p + \mu) = u(q, p)$; then u is a function of p alone. [Compare the analysis leading to (55) and (56).] It is convenient to write the solution to (65) in the general case in the following forms:

$$n(\mu, t) = n(\mu - t, 0) \qquad t \leqslant \mu \quad (66)$$

$$n(\mu, t) = n(0, t - \mu) \qquad t > \mu \quad (67)$$

XI. CANCER CHEMOTHERAPY

Where do anticancer drugs come from? What is the history of their usage? The answers to questions like this lead one to a fascinating history of human endeavor. As noted in [207], the treatment of

cancer by anticancer drugs may be as ancient as medicine and surgery, going back at least 1500 years. In [208] there is documented
evidence of the use of diverse substances as chemotherapeutic agents
against various diseases. Examples include quinine, used as treatment for malaria, and emetine for amebic dysentery. Woven among
the various developments are the pieces of information that led to the
use of certain substances—metals, arsenic, etc.—against different
types of cancers. Renaissance writings, for example, note the use
of concoctions involving arsenic, zinc, silver, antimony, mercury,
and bismuth on local skin tumors.

    Yet it is not until 1942 that the first recorded clinical trial of an
anticancer drug took place. The drug nitrogen mustard was administered to a patient with advanced lymphosarcoma [209]. A few
years later Sidney Farber noted what he termed an "acceleration
phenomena" in a retrospective analysis of children with acute leukemia
treated with folate conjugates. This led to his report on the dramatic
responses in 10 of 16 children treated with the folate antagonist
aminopterin [210]. Much progress has been made since these early
studies. Many people believe that chemotherapy offers the hope of
an ultimate cure because of the ability of drugs to seek out tumor
cells that are not visible, or that are in pharmacologically protected
sanctuaries, and destroy them. Present drugs are cytotoxic, and
their use often creates toxicity such as nausea, alopecia, and leuko-
penia. Such toxicities need to be balanced with the long-term
amelioration of symptoms occurring due to the tumor. An important
survey of cancer chemotherapy is the recent position paper [211] for
the American Association for Cancer Research, Inc.

    The modern history of the chemotherapy of cancer is divided into
five epochs: (1) the realization that the chemotherapy of cancer is
a possibility (1935–1945); (2) discovery and evaluation of new antitumor agents (1945–present); (3) development of sanctuary therapy
with intrathecal methotrexate or craniospinal irradiation or both
(1957–1965); (4) development of intensive intermittent combination
therapy (1960–present); (5) development of combined modality (ad-
juvant) therapy (early era, 1955–1971; present era, 1971–present).
This division is suggested in [208].

    Many anticancer drugs appear to exert a lethal effect in several
phases of the cell cycle. Unfortunately, attempts to correlate the cell
cycle phase in which the drug is most lethal with the biochemical action of the drug in that phase have not been too successful. The
progression of cells through the cycle can be blocked or arrested at
particular points in the cycle by cytotoxic drugs. Such a progression
delay often can be reversed. Even within a particular phase, different agents may arrest cells at a different number of points [212].

    The level of concentration of drug used is an important factor.
A single drug may block progression at one point in the cycle and
so reduce its own effectiveness as a cytotoxic agent by protecting

a proportion of the cells and preventing their reaching the phase where it can exert its lethal effect. One consequence of this feature is that it suggests combination chemotherapy, that is, the use of distinct agents.

A natural consquence of these considerations is to try to synchronize cancer cells so as to place as many of them as possible into a sensitive phase of the cycle, and then a drug designed to act in that particular phase could possibly kill significant numbers of them. This approach is appealing because many less normal cells are in the sensitive phase. The name "blocker" is given to a drug that slows down rates of transit through the particular phases of the cell cycle. Evidence is accumulating, though, that synchronization does not appear to be clinically useful [6, 197, pp. 400, 401] and [199]. These remarks are included because they are directly relevant to a recent mathematical model [213] where a treatment plan is optimized to increase the degree of synchronization.

From the analysis of certain experimental results, Skipper et al. [214] proposed that the ability of a drug to eradicate malignant cells depends on the dose of the drug *and* on the number of tumor cells present. In addition, cell destruction by a cytotoxic agent is assumed to obey first-order kinetics. Their work leads to the statement: A given treatment destroys a constant fraction, not a fixed number, of the tumor cells present. For example, a treatment that reduces a tumor cell population from 1 million to 10 should reduce a population of 100,000 to 1. Later, in Section XIII we examine a mathematical model of cancer chemotherapy for AML in which the constant fraction cell kill hypothesis is used.

XII. CELL KINETICS AND CANCER CHEMOTHERAPY

This section is an overview of the mathematical model [215] that relates the cell kinetics of a tumor with its treatment using a drug. The analysis serves as a prototype for dealing with other models of this type. The tumor model used in [215] consists of three populations: proliferating (with G_1, S, G_2, and M phases), temporarily nonproliferating (with G_0 resting phase), and dead. The presence of dead cells affects the physical determination of tumor size for solid tumors and cell count for disseminated neoplasms. Figure 1 shows the tumor model.

The objectives of the mathematical model are to examine (1) the nature of the theoretical FLM function (see Section VIII.B) in terms of both proliferative and nonproliferative compartments and (2) the requirements for describing tumor behavior during periods of growth and drug treatment.

We assume the cells in each of the five phases are subject to two separate events. First, through natural causes cells may die

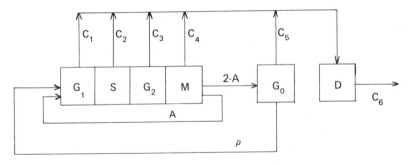

FIGURE 1   Model for tumor growth and drug treatment.   From Ref.
215.

and so are no longer considered. Second, the action of the drug
exerts an influence on the cells within each phase. These two
events are assumed to be combined into a single loss function appropriate to each separate phase. Thus there are five loss functions
for this tumor model. Cells that will die or are dead accumulate in
the death compartment, D. A certain proportion ρ of cells in G_0
may reenter the proliferative cycle at G_1 (by assumption). After
each binary fission, 2-A cells enter the nonproliferative compartment
G_0, and A cells continue in the proliferative cycle, $1 \leqslant A \leqslant 2$.

A. Development of a Basic Mathematical Model

At this point a decision is required on what type of mathematical
model is needed. If gross characteristics of the cell populations in
each phase are all that one needs, then an ordinary differential equation model like that in (48) and (49) with a G_0 phase included is
appropriate. However, such a model is unable to deal with more in-
depth details of the cellular kinetics features. Typical of some of
these details are the assumptions that go into the model to allow a
description of the nature of the loss of cells from each phase. These
more detailed assumptions can be incorporated into a mathematical
model with cellular age structure. Here we assume that a von Foerster
equation of the type (51) applies in each phase of the active part of
the cycle. Specifically, let $n_1(t, a_1)$ denote the cell density function
for cells in the G_1 phase, the age variable being a_1. In the same
way let $n_i(t, a_i)$, $i = 2, 3, 4$, denote the cell density functions for
the cells in the S, G_2, and M phases, respectively. Each phase has
its own cell density function and its own age variable. The von
Foerster equation has a general loss term on the right. For the
present investigation Chuang and Lloyd assume that the loss term is
of the separable form (57) so that

$$\lambda_i(t, a_i) = \lambda_i(a_i) + c_i(t) \qquad i = 1, \ldots, 4 \qquad (68)$$

This split shows the contribution from the age-specific death rate and the corresponding rate of cell loss from each phase.

The basic equations for the active phase are now

$$\frac{\partial n_i(t, a_i)}{\partial t} + \frac{\partial n_i(t, a_i)}{\partial a_i} = -[\lambda_i(a_i) + c_i(t)]n_i(t, a_i)$$

$$i = 1, \ldots, 4 \qquad (69)$$

From (50) we see that the expected cell populations within each phase are

$$L_i(t) = \int_0^\infty n_i(t, a_i) \, da_i \qquad i = 1, \ldots, 4 \qquad (70)$$

Assume that the transit times of cells in the proliferative phases are random variables with independently distributed probability density functions $f_i(a_i)$. Then, as in the analysis leading to (59) and (60),

$$\lambda_i(a_i) = \frac{f_i(a_i)}{\phi(a_i)} \qquad (71)$$

$$\phi_i(a_i) = 1 - \int_0^{a_i} f_i(x) \, dx = \exp\left[-\int_0^{a_i} \lambda_i(x) \, dx\right] \qquad (72)$$

The boundary condition is

$$\alpha_1(t) = n_1(t, 0) = A \int_0^\infty \lambda_4(a_4)n_4(t, a_4) \, da_4 + \rho L_5(t) \qquad (73)$$

The first term on the right denotes the contribution to the birthrate of cells in G_1, and comes from those cells that have just completed mitosis. The last term gives the contribution to the birthrate from those cells that leave the G_0 compartment and enter the proliferating state. Here $L_5(t)$ denotes the total number of cells in G_0 at time t, and ρ is a rate coefficient with dimensions of $(\text{time})^{-1}$. The remaining boundary conditions are the birthrates given by the equations

$$\alpha_{i+1}(t) = n_{i+1}(t, 0) = \int_0^\infty \lambda_i(a_i)n_i(t, a_i) \, da_i \qquad i = 1, 2, 3 \qquad (74)$$

The initial age distributions are

$$n_i(0, a_i) = \beta_i(a_i) \qquad\qquad i = 1, \ldots, 4 \qquad\qquad (75)$$

Equations (69), (73–75) specify the basic mathematical problem.

The expected number of cells $L_5(t)$ in the resting state at time t is described by the equation

$$\frac{dL_5(t)}{dt} = (2 - A) \int_0^\infty \lambda_4(a_4)n_4(t, a_4) \, da_4 - [\rho + c_5(t)]L_5(t) \qquad (76)$$

The first term on the right is the rate at which cells are being added to the population; the second term is the cumulated rate at which cells are being lost. To complete the mathematical description of (76), we need to prescribe the initial condition $L_5(0)$. This value depends on the particular tumor.

The death compartment consists of those permanently nonproliferating cells. Although these cells do not respond to chemotherapy, their presence is reflected in any physical determination of tumor size (for solid tumors) or cell count (leukemias). Let $L_6(t)$ denote the population size in the death compartment. We have

$$\frac{dL_6(t)}{dt} = -m_6 L_6(t) + \sum_{i=1}^{5} c_i(t)L_i(t) \qquad (77)$$

where m_6 is the rate constant for those death compartment cells that leave the tumor site.

Equations (69), (76), and (77) contain the cell loss functions $c_i(t)$. An interpretation of the cell kill hypothesis of [214] shows that cell loss functions depend on the drug concentration $v(t)$ at the tumor site. However, the hypothesis does not indicate the mathematical nature of the relationship between the $c_i(t)$ and $v(t)$. Generally it is assumed that the drug concentration needs to be above a certain minimum level in order to achieve a therapeutic effect. When the drug concentration is below a threshold level in the drug-sensitive phase of the cycle, it is assumed [215] that the cell loss is due to natural attrition. The implication of this assumption is that each of the cell loss functions is a constant c_i (the constants differ, depending on the phase) regardless of the level of the drug at the tumor site, this situation holding true up to the threshold concentration v_{min}. Again v_{min} will be different for each of the phases.

For drug concentrations above the threshold, Chuang and Lloyd assume that the cell loss function at time t is an increasing linear function of the drug concentration at the same time. Eventually a drug concentration level, v_{max}, is reached, beyond which it is assumed that cell loss is occurring at a constant rate. The collection of all these assumptions is contained in the following representation:

$$c_i(t) = \begin{cases} c_i & v(t) \leqslant v_{min,i} \\ \dfrac{d_i[v(t) - v_{min,i}] + c_i[v_{max,i} - v(t)]}{v_{max,i} - v_{min,i}} & v_{min,i} < v(t) < v_{max,i} \\ d_i & v_{max,i} \leqslant v(t) \end{cases} \qquad (78)$$

where the subscript $i = 1, \ldots, 5$. For drug concentrations above v_{max} the loss function is assumed to be a constant d_i with $d_i > c_i$. The middle portion of (78) looks complicated, but it is just the mathematical representation of the linear portion.

How do we get information on $v(t)$? One way to deal with this problem is to predict it from an analysis of the drug distribution in various compartments. These compartments may represent actual physiological structures (such as the liver, blood, etc.) or, as often happens, nonphysiological quantities. It is assumed [215] that the drug obeys first-order kinetics and is distributed through N compartments. A linear pharmacokinetics model then gives

$$v(t) = \sum_{j=1}^{N} B_j \exp(-\delta_j t) \qquad (79)$$

where the B_j and δ_j are obtained by using a least squares routine that fits (79) to data. The restriction to first-order kinetics is not necessary. Nonlinear pharmacokinetics can be incorporated into the model, if desired.

This completes the discussion on the formulation of the basic mathematical model.

B. Solution of the Basic Mathematical Model

In this part we outline the solution of the basic mathematical model and briefly describe how to apply the model to treat an experimental tumor.

Introduce [compare (58)]

$$j_i(t) = \exp\left[-\int_0^t c_i(x)\, dx\right] \qquad i = 1, \ldots, 5 \qquad (80)$$

Equation (76) is of first-order type with integrating factor

$$
\exp \int^t (\rho + c_5(x))\, dx \;=\; \frac{\exp(\rho t)}{j_5(t)}
$$

Hence the solution of (76) can be expressed as

$$
L_5(t) = e^{-\rho t} j_5(t)\left[L_5(0) + (2 - A)\int_{\tau=0}^t \frac{e^{\rho \tau}}{j_5(\tau)}\int_{a_4=0}^\infty \lambda_4(a_4)n_4(\tau, a_4)\, da_4\, d\tau \right]
$$

We can proceed in the same manner as in the steps leading to (61) and (62) to produce

$$
n_i(t,\, a_i) = \begin{cases} \dfrac{\alpha_i(t - a_i)\phi_i(a_i)j_i(t)}{j_i(t - a_i)} & t > a_i \\[4mm] \dfrac{\beta_i(a_i - t)\phi_i(a_i)j_i(t)}{\phi_i(a_i - t)} & t < a_i \end{cases} \qquad i = 1,\ldots, 4 \qquad (81)
$$

These relations indicate that a cell, which is in phase i with age $a_i < t$ at time t, must have entered phase i at time $t - a_i$ and have survived to age a_i, and a cell with age $a_i > t$ must have been in phase i with age $a_i - t$ at time zero and survived to age a_i.

Assume that the untreated tumor is growing exponentially. As initial age distributions, Chuang and Lloyd assume that

$$
\beta_i(a_i) = K_i\phi_i(a_i)\exp[-(c + c_i)a_i] \qquad i = 1,\ldots, 4 \qquad (82)
$$

where c is the specific growth rate of the tumor. Application of the boundary and initial conditions (73)–(75) to (81) gives a system of four integral equations for the birthrates $\alpha_i(t)$:

$$
\alpha_1(t) = Aj_4(t)\left\{ \int_{a_4=0}^t \frac{\alpha_4(t - a_4)}{j_4(t - a_4)} f_4(a_4)\, da_4 + \int_{a_4=t}^\infty \frac{\beta_4(a_4 - t)}{\phi_4(a_4 - t)} f_4(a_4)\, da_4 \right\}
$$

$$
+ \rho e^{-\rho t} j_5(t)\left[L_5(0) + (2 - A)\int_{\tau=0}^t e^{\rho \tau}\frac{j_4(\tau)}{j_5(\tau)} \right. \qquad (83)
$$

$$
\left. \cdot \left\{ \int_{a_4=0}^\tau \frac{\alpha_4(\tau - a_4)}{j_4(\tau - a_4)} f_4(a_4)\, da_4 + \int_{a_4=\tau}^\infty \frac{\beta_4(a_4 - \tau)}{\phi_4(a_4 - \tau)} f_4(a_4)\, da_4 \right\}\, d\tau \right]
$$

$$\alpha_{i+1}(t) = j_i(t) \left\{ \int_{a_i=0}^{t} \frac{\alpha_i(t - a_i)}{j_i(t - a_i)} f_i(a_i) \, da_i \right.$$

$$\left. + \int_{a_i=t}^{\infty} \frac{\beta_i(a_i - t)}{\phi_i(a_i - t)} f_i(a_i) \, da_i \right\} \qquad i = 1, 2, 3 \tag{84}$$

A starting function for any one of the $\alpha_i(t)$ is chosen. Then the system (83), (84) is solved in an iterative manner. The fast Fourier transform technique developed in [216] is used to deal with the convolution-type integrals.

When the birthrates are known, (70) and (81) give the sizes of the expected cell populations:

$$L_i(t) = j_i(t) \left\{ \int_{a_i=0}^{t} \frac{\alpha_i(t - a_i)}{j_i(t - a_i)} \phi_i(a_i) \, da_i \right.$$

$$\left. + \int_{a_i=t}^{\infty} \frac{\beta_i(a_i - t)}{\phi_i(a_i - t)} \phi_i(a_i) \, da_i \right\} \qquad i = 1, \ldots, 4 \tag{85}$$

$$L_5(t) = e^{-\rho t} j_5(t) \left[L_5(0) + (2 - A) \int_{\tau=0}^{t} e^{\rho \tau} \frac{j_4(\tau)}{j_5(\tau)} \right.$$

$$\cdot \left\{ \int_{a_4=0}^{\tau} \frac{\alpha_4(\tau - a_4)}{j_4(\tau - a_4)} f_4(a_4) \, da_4 \right.$$

$$\left. \left. + \int_{a_4=\tau}^{t} \frac{\beta_4(a_4 - \tau)}{\phi_4(a_4 - \tau)} f_4(a_4) \, da_4 \right\} d\tau \right] \tag{86}$$

$$L_6(t) = \exp(-c_6 t) \left[L_6(0) + \int_{\tau=0}^{t} \exp(c_6 \tau) \left\{ \sum_{i=1}^{5} c_i(\tau) L_i(\tau) \right\} d\tau \right] \tag{87}$$

The total population is then

$$L(t) = \sum_{i=1}^{6} L_i(t) \tag{88}$$

Consider the situation with the initial age distributions

$$n_2^*(0, a_2) = \beta_2(a_2) \qquad n_i^*(0, a_i) = 0 \qquad i = 1, 3, 4 \qquad (89)$$

and $L_5^*(0) = 0$. The asterisk denotes quantities associated with labeled cells. We can obtain a theoretical expression for the FLM function, on using (35), in the form

$$FLM(t) = \frac{L_4^*(t)}{L_4(t)} \tag{90}$$

The observed FLM curve is derived from the untreated tumor. For this situation $\beta_2(a_2)$ is assumed to have the form shown in (82), and the loss functions are given by $c_i(t) = \exp(-c_i t)$.

A summary is now presented of the steps involved in using the present mathematical model to describe the growth of an untreated tumor.

Select a distribution for the phase duration $f_i(a_i)$, $i = 1, \ldots, 4$. The mean and standard deviation must be specified or found from an analysis of the FLM curve.

The loss functions $c_i(t)$, $i = 1, \ldots, 5$, are taken as zero or as small positive constants c_i during growth. A value for c_6 (assumed to be a constant) needs to be obtained. An estimate could come from data on tumor regression in experimental animals.

The initial value $L_6(0)$ is estimated from experimental data at a time that corresponds to the state of the tumor at the beginning of the numerical simulation.

Specify the size of the rate constant ρ, the number of cells that enter the nonproliferative compartment (and so deduce the size of A), and $L_5(0)$.

In (82) one of the K_i values is to be determined from available data. We could base this determination on the experimental thymidine labeling index. From Section VIII.B we see that

$$LI = \frac{L_2(0)}{L(0)} \tag{91}$$

where $L(0)$ is given by (88). The Laplace transformation of a function $f(t)$ may be defined by the equation

$$F(s) = \int_0^\infty f(t)e^{-st} \, dt \tag{92}$$

Hence, from (70), (82), the first equation in (89), and (92), we get

$$L_2(0) = K_2 \Phi(c + c_2)$$

where $\Phi(s)$ is the Laplace transform of ϕ. This equation can be used to find K_2 when the measured LI and tumor size are known. If we set $t = 0$ in (83), (84) and use the Laplace transform (92), it is possible to deduce that

$$K_1 = AK_4 F_4(c + c_4) + \rho L_5(0)$$

$$K_{i+1} = K_i F_i(c + c_i) \qquad i = 1, 2, 3$$

Use these equations to form $K_4/K_1 = (K_4/K_3)(K_3/K_2)(K_2/K_1)$ and deduce that

$$AF_1(c + c_1)F_2(c + c_2)F_3(c + c_3)F_4(c + c_4) = 1 - \frac{\rho L_5(0)}{K_1}$$

This equation is used to determine the specific growth rate of the tumor c. The $f_i(a_i)$ are obtained by a curve fit of the theoretical FLM function to observed data.

It is possible to obtain expressions for the Laplace transforms $L_4^*(s)$ and $L_4(s)$ from (85). Numerical inversion of these transforms (see, e.g., [217]) allows for the calculation of $L_4^*(t)$ and $L_4(t)$. Equation (90) now gives the theoretical FLM function, which can be fitted to a given curve. As a result of this fitting procedure, we can obtain estimates of the cell cycle parameters.

A discussion of the basic mathematical model is present in [218]. Chuang gives information on a numerical simulation of the model to the treatment of L1210 mouse leukemia with the drug ara-C (arabinosylcytosine). For this tumor system (see Fig. 1), experimental data suggest that $\rho = 0.10$, $A = 1.99$, $c_i = 0$, $i = 1, \ldots, 4$, c_5 was not observed, and $c_6 \geqslant 0.01$; he selects $c_5 = 0.01$ hr^{-1} and $c_6 = 0.02$ hr^{-1}. In (78), $v_{max,2} = 1.5$ μg/ml, $v_{min,2} = 0.3$ μg/ml, and $d_2 = 0.8-1.2$ hr^{-1}. He considers the following case. An inoculum of 10^5 cancer cells is delivered to a BDF$_1$ mouse. On day 2 a 15-mg / kg dose of ara-C is given every 3 hr for a total of eight doses. Then the same process is repeated for days 6, 10, and 14. The model-estimated populations for G_1, S, G_2, and M are shown graphically. Tumor regression and regrowth are clearly shown. The cell kill during S phase makes the populations in the other

proliferating phases oscillate during the regrowth periods and with
a different time lag in growth. At the end of treatment on day 14,
the cells in each proliferating phase are reduced to less than one.
No details are provided of the fit of the FLM function to data and
the determination of other cell kinetic parameters. Interestingly, in
a different computer model [219] it is indicated that animals with
tumor populations of up to 10^6 cells could be cured within 14 days
of therapy on at least one schedule.

It is possible to examine other tumor models. For example, in
Fig. 1, the G_0 and G_1 compartments could be combined. Instead of
cells entering G_1 from G_0, cells could enter directly into S phase.
Chuang discusses these variations in [218].

The tumor model of Fig. 1 is used by the investigators in [220]
as the basis for their mathematical development of an expression for
a theoretical continuous labeling function. An experimental continuous labeling curve gives the fraction—number of labeled cells
per total number of cells—as a function of the time elapsed since
the start of injection with ^{3}H-TdR. They discuss the application of
their model to the partial or complete blocking effect in cancer
chemotherapy.

The availability of the basic mathematical model of this section
provides a useful starting point for the investigation of the growth
of tumor systems under conditions of no treatment and when there
is treatment with an anticancer drug. Unfortunately there does not
appear to be any more recent work in this area using these models
of Chuang and Lloyd. However, see [260].

XIII. A CHEMOTHERAPY MODEL FOR ACUTE MYELOBLASTIC LEUKEMIA

Neutrophil leukocytes (also referred to as granulocytes) are the
principal white cells in normal human blood [221]. Leukemia is
characterized by the uncontrolled proliferation and accumulation of
neutrophil leukocytes. It is natural then to consider the natural
history of the neutrophil and its precursors. This is examined in
detail in [222].

Acute myeloblastic leukemia (AML) occurs in children and mature
adults. It is characterized by (i) an overproduction of myeloblasts,
(ii) appearance of myeloblasts in the blood. The myeloblast is the
earliest cytologically identifiable neutrophil precursor normally found
in the bone marrow [223]. In addition, it is assumed [224] that there
exist side by side in AML two cell populations, the normal neutrophil
cell system, with total number of cells $L(t)$, and a population of
leukemic blood cells (LBC), their total number being denoted by
$L'(t)$.

In normal neutrophils [223] there is assumed to be a resting compartment G_0 to account for dynamic variations in the depletion of blood cells caused by unfavorable events. Cells are released at random at a rate α per unit time from G_0 and enter the proliferative part of the cycle to go through the G_1, S, G_2, and M phases. A cell that proceeds in this manner undergoes cell division later at a fixed time T_A. The subscript A denotes the active $G_1 \rightarrow M$ part of the cycle. After mitosis the two cells produced by the division enter the G_0 phase. The model [223] also assumes that there is a certain portion of cells that leave the G_0 compartment at random at a rate β per unit time and enter a maturation compartment m (see Fig. 2), which is a "pipeline" in which all cells mature for a fixed time T_m, and then enter the marrow reserve compartment R. This compartment is not a pipeline but a "random" compartment because all the cells are treated equivalently and can leave at random. Cells leave R and enter the blood compartment B at the fractional rate γ. The blood compartment is also a random compartment from which cells disappear or die at random at the fraction rate per unit time δ.

Let a, μ, and t, respectively, denote age, maturity, and chronological time. Let $n(\mu, t)$ denote the cell density function for the active compartment, $G_1 \rightarrow M$ phases combined. Then with $\nu \equiv 1$ and $\lambda \equiv 0$, equation (63) gives

$$\frac{\partial n(\mu, t)}{\partial t} + \frac{\partial n(\mu, t)}{\partial \mu} = 0 \qquad 0 < \mu < T_A \qquad (93)$$

The emphasis here is that maturity is the key feature for cells in the active compartment. Let $g(t, a)$ denote the cell density function for the G_0 compartment. Then from Fig. 2 and (51),

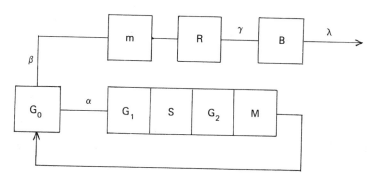

FIGURE 2　Normal neutrophil system.

$$\frac{\partial g(t, a)}{\partial t} + \frac{\partial g(t, a)}{\partial a} = -[\alpha(t) + \beta(t)] \, g(t, a) \qquad 0 < a \tag{94}$$

where emphasis is on the age of a cell in the resting compartment. Now let $h(\mu, t)$, $r(t, a)$, and $b(t, a)$, respectively, denote the cell density functions for the maturation, reserve, and blood compartments. We see that

$$\frac{\partial h(\mu, t)}{\partial t} + \frac{\partial h(\mu, t)}{\partial \mu} = 0 \qquad\qquad 0 < t < T_m$$

$$\frac{\partial r(t, a)}{\partial t} + \frac{\partial r(t, a)}{\partial a} = -\gamma(t) r(t, a) \qquad 0 < a \tag{95}$$

$$\frac{\partial b(t, a)}{\partial t} + \frac{\partial b(t, a)}{\partial a} = -\delta(t) b(t, a) \qquad 0 < a$$

where T_m is the time spent in the maturation compartment. The cell density functions satisfy the initial conditions

$$n(\mu, 0) \ = \ f_A(\mu) \qquad g(0, a) = f_G(a) \qquad h(\mu, 0) = h_m(\mu)$$

$$r(0, a) \ = \ f_R(a) \qquad b(0, a) = f_B(a) \tag{96}$$

It is assumed that the fractional loss rates α and β depend on the total population in all the compartments $L(t) + L'(t)$ [223, 224]:

$$\alpha(t) \ = \ \alpha_0 + \alpha_1 \left(\frac{L_e^{\nu}}{[L(t) + L'(t)]^{\nu} - 1} \right) \tag{97}$$

$$\beta(t) \ = \ \alpha_0 + \beta_1 \left(\frac{L_e^{\nu}}{[L(t) + L'(t)]^{\nu} - 1} \right) \tag{98}$$

where α_0, α_1, β_1, ν are constants, and L_e is the total population homeostatic level. Stability analysis indicates that $\alpha_1 > \beta_1$ [223]. The fractional loss rate in the blood (δ) is assumed to be a constant. To describe the control of release of cells from the marrow reserve compartment to the blood, we assume that

$$\gamma(t) \ = \ \begin{cases} \gamma_0 + \gamma_1 \left(\dfrac{L_b^{\rho}}{[L_B(t - t_R)]^{\rho} - 1} \right) & L_B(t - t_R) < L_b \\[4mm] \gamma_0 & L_B(t - t_R) \geqslant L_b \end{cases} \tag{99}$$

where γ_0, γ_1, L_b, ρ, and t_R are positive constants. The interesting feature here is the presence of the time delay t_R, which is suggested by various experiments—for example, the response to leukopheresis. The symbol L_b denotes the steady-state value of the population in the blood compartment.

As noted in [224], leukemic myeloblasts do not differentiate into more mature forms of neutrophil precursors. This suggests that the LBC behaves like a proliferative pool only (Fig. 3). All symbols associated with the leukemic blood cells are denoted with a prime ('). The LBC are assumed to leave the resting compartment G_0' at a fractional rate α' to enter the active part of the cycle or at a fractional rate β' to enter the blood compartment B'. Cells are assumed to leave the blood at random at a fractional rate δ'. Thus we have [compare (93)]:

$$\frac{\partial n'(\mu, t)}{\partial t} + \frac{\partial n'(\mu, t)}{\partial \mu} = 0 \qquad 0 < \mu < T_A' \qquad (100)$$

with initial condition $n'(\mu, 0) = f_A'(\mu)$ and boundary condition $n'(0, t) = \alpha'(t)L_0'(t)$, where $\alpha'(t)$ is prescribed and $L_0'(t)$ is found from the solution of (104). Integrating (100) with respect to μ gives

$$\dot{L}_A'(t) + n'(T_A', t) - n'(0, t) = 0 \qquad (101)$$

where

$$L_A'(t) = \int_0^{T_A'} n'(\mu, t) \, d\mu$$

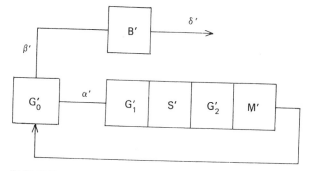

FIGURE 3   Leukemic state.

For $t < \mu$, $n'(\mu, 0) = f'_A(\mu)$; hence, from (66) we have

$$n'(\mu, t) = f'_A(\mu - t) \qquad t \leq \mu$$

It follows that $n'(T'_A, t)$ is

$$n'(T'_A, t) = \begin{cases} f'_A(T'_A - t) & t \leq T'_A \\ n'(0, t - T'_A) & t > T'_A \end{cases}$$

Hence, from the boundary condition on $n'(0, t)$ and the last display, (101) becomes

$$\frac{dL'_A(t)}{dt} = \alpha'(t)L'_0(t) - \begin{cases} f'_A(T'_A - t) & 0 < t \leq T'_A \\ \alpha'(t - T'_A)L'_0(t - T'_A) & t > T'_A \end{cases} \tag{102}$$

Also, compare (94),

$$\frac{\partial g'(t, a)}{\partial t} + \frac{\partial g'(t, a)}{\partial a} = -[\alpha'(t) + \beta'(t)]g'(t, a) \qquad 0 < a \tag{103}$$

with $g'(t, 0) = 2n'(T'_A, t)$. The factor 2 means that two cells are produced by division of the cells in the proliferative compartment when they reach age T'_A. Integrating (103) with respect to a gives

$$\frac{dL'_0(t)}{dt} = -[\alpha'(t) + \beta'(t)]L'_0(t) + 2 \begin{cases} f'(T'_A - t) & 0 < t < T'_A \\ \alpha'(t - T_A)L'_0(t - T'_A) & t \geq T'_A \end{cases} \tag{104}$$

where we set $g'(t, \infty) \equiv 0$ and define

$$L'_0(t) = \int_0^\infty g'(t, a) \, da$$

Finally,

$$\frac{\partial b'(t, a)}{\partial t} + \frac{\partial b'(t, a)}{\partial a} = -\delta'(t)b'(t, a) \qquad 0 < a \tag{105}$$

with $b'(t, 0) = \beta'(t)L_0'(t)$. Integrating (105) with respect to a and using $b'(t, \infty) \equiv 0$, we obtain

$$\dot{L}_B'(t) = \beta'(t)L_0'(t) - \delta'(t)L_B'(t) \tag{106}$$

where

$$L_B'(t) = \int_0^\infty b'(t, a) \, da \tag{107}$$

Equations (102), (104), and (106) describe the numbers of leukemic cells in the proliferative, G_0' and B' compartments, respectively, at time t, and f'(a) represents the initial distribution of leukemic cells in the active compartment as a function of age a.

The control functions α' and β' are defined [224] as

$$\alpha'(t) = \alpha_0' + \alpha_1' \ln \left[\frac{L_e'}{L(t) + L'(t)} \right]$$

$$\beta'(t) = \alpha_0' + \beta_1' \ln \left[\frac{L_e'}{L(t) + L'(t)} \right] \tag{108}$$

where $L'(t) = L_A'(t) + L_0'(t) + L_B'(t)$ is the total number of LBC.

At this stage we have derived a mathematical model that describes the growth kinetics of both the normal neutrophils and the LBC. It is possible now to explore the consequences of varying the parameters in the control functions. However, here, we wish to superimpose a chemotherapeutic drug treatment regimen on the mathematical model.

Assume that a dose of drug kills a fixed fraction of all cells in the DNA synthesis phase [214]. Also assume that 90% of all cells in the DNA synthesis phase are killed at the time the drug is administered. Results of calculations are presented in [225] for the administration of an agent n times with periodicity P followed by a rest period τ_R. Yet, it is not at all evident how these results were obtained. My own separate investigations indicate that, for Fig. 5 in [225], p. 1264, b should be labeled d and d should be labeled b. (A personal communication from Dr. Rubinow to me confirmed this.)

The L-6 protocol is the name given to drug doses of the cycle-specific drug ara-C in combination with 6-thioguanine that are administered sufficiently close together in time so that leukemic cells are prevented from completing DNA synthesis. One of the conclusions of [225] is that the L-6 protocol can be improved by varying the periodicities P and $P + \tau_R$, the duration of the rest period, and the number of courses of treatment.

It is interesting to compare this mathematical model with the one described in Section XII.A. There are no cell loss contributions from the proliferative compartment and no inclusion of the pharma-cokinetic behavior of the agents. These features are deemed to be important and were included in the Chuang and Lloyd model, dis-cussed earlier.

Further discussion on the two-population model is in [226].

Other works on modeling acute leukemic processes are in [40] and [227].

XIV. APPLICATION OF ENGINEERING OPTIMAL CONTROL THEORY IN CANCER CHEMOTHERAPY

It is apparent from the material presented in this chapter that there is no underlying guiding principle from which the basic equations of tumor growth dynamics can be deduced. Contrast this situation with a typical engineering problem, where equations are capable of being deduced from basic principles, such as conservation of mass, energy, etc. The early 1950s began an era of rapid technological change and aerospace exploration. Aerospace engineers needed solutions to optimal control problems. Up to this time a control system was re-quired to achieve some objective; now it was imperative that it do it optimally. One early, dramatic engineering application of an optimal control problem was to influence the motion of a satellite so that it would rendezvous with another object in space. This problem em-bodies the basic ideas of optimal control—the dynamical state equa-tions govern the motions of the objects in space, and the optimal trajectory (the path through space which allows the rendezvous to be successful conditional on the allowable time and/or fuel) must be discovered. Since 1950, engineering optimal control has enjoyed explosive growth, which continues even now. An extensive treat-ment of optimal control theory is in [228], and a useful introduction to some of the basic concepts is in [87], Chapter 1. We outline, in algorithmic style, some of the features of optimal control theory, then give an application to a cancer chemotherapy problem. The prospects for future therapy are assessed in Section XIV.C.

Assume that we are given a state equation

$$\dot{x}(t) = \phi(x, u) \qquad x(0) = x_0 \qquad (109)$$

for the state of the system $x \equiv x(t)$. The quantity $u \equiv u(t)$ is the control variable. Introduce a performance index

$$J(u) = \int_0^{t_f} \psi(x, u) \, dt \qquad (110)$$

which is some measure of performance of the system under investigation in $[0, t_f]$, where t_f is the final time. We want to determine the optimal control that minimizes the functional $J(u)$, subject to the constraint equation (109). Equations (97) and (98) provide examples of specified control variables. In contrast here, the control is to be found as the solution of an optimal control problem. The control u might represent a drug concentration, a voltage level, or some other variable of interest.

One way to proceed is to form the H-function, a function of t, as follows:

$$H(x, u, t) = \psi(x, u) + \lambda(t)\phi(x, u) \tag{111}$$

where $\lambda \equiv \lambda(t)$ is a multiplier called the costate variable. The minimization of $J(u)$ is equivalent to the minimization of H. Under the restriction that H is a continuous function of u in $[0, t_f]$ a necessary condition for H to possess a minimum is

$$\frac{\partial H}{\partial u} = 0 \tag{112}$$

Also, it can be shown [87,228] that

$$\dot{\lambda}(t) = -\frac{\partial H}{\partial x} \tag{113}$$

We refer to (113) as the costate equation. In addition,

$$H = 0 \tag{114}$$

along an optimal trajectory ([87], p. 11 or [228], p. 265).

In principle, then, we can use (109)–(114) to find the nature of the optimal control. Often this control will turn out to be a continuous function of t. This feature is of considerable significance to us in Sections XIV.A and XIV.B. When we know the optimal control, it can (theoretically) be placed in (109) and the corresponding optimal trajectory can be obtained.

It occurred to the author some years ago that many of the concepts of optimal control theory could possibly find application in cancer therapy and in other areas of biomedicine. This is borne out in the publications [49,54,55,65,86–88] and [229–235]. Chapter 6 of [87] gives a review of contributions from other investigators of the use of optimal control in cancer chemotherapy. They are not considered here.

A. Optimal Control in the Chemotherapy of Multiple Myeloma

The first known appplication of engineering optimal control theory to a cancer chemotherapy problem involving a human tumor is in [65]. Immunoglobulin G multiple myeloma (a disseminated bone marrow cancer) provides a unique characteristic: myeloma protein excreted in the urine can be assayed and related to the number of myeloma tumor cells. This allows [64] for estimates of the size of this tumor to be made at various times, if desired. A representation of this tumor by the mathematical model (19) is made in [65], where at time $t = 0$ the initial size is known from clinical observations. Under the action of a chemotherapeutic agent the perturbed equation of tumor growth is assumed to be of the form

$$\dot{L}(t) = \alpha L \ln \left(\frac{\theta}{L}\right) - \frac{k_1 vL}{k_2 + v} \qquad L(0) = L_0 \qquad (115)$$

The second term is a cell loss term of the E_{max} type; see [236], p. 307 for a recent discussion of this type of expression. The quantity v is a time-dependent control variable and represents the actual size of the drug level at the tumor site. However, the assumption is made that v is approximated to be the same as the amount of cycle nonspecific drug infused. Also, k_1 and k_2 are positive constants.

Instead of the notation used in [65] we introduce the transformations

$$\tau = \alpha t \qquad u = \frac{v}{k_2} \qquad x = \ln \left(\frac{\theta}{L}\right) \qquad p = \frac{k_1}{\alpha} \qquad (116)$$

Then (115) becomes

$$\frac{dx}{d\tau} = pu(1 + u)^{-1} - x \qquad x(0) = C \qquad (117)$$

where $C = \ln(\theta/L_0) > 0$. Equation (117) was fitted to data from a number of patients undergoing a standard intermittent melphalan, cyclophosphamide, and prednisone (MCP) treatment program. In this case the control u was specified as a decaying exponential. Values of the patient-dependent parameter p were obtained; see [65] for details. The mathematical model gave a tolerable fit to the patient data.

A performance index of the form

$$J(u) = \int_0^T u \, d\tau \qquad (118)$$

where T is a nondimensional length of treatment interval, is introduced as a measure of the contribution to toxicity. This expression is an approximation to the integral of the drug concentration in the plasma, often regarded by clinicians as a measure of the toxicity.

An optimal control problem can be formulated as follows: determine the optimal control u that minimizes the toxicity of treatment, subject to the growth kinetics of the tumor. That is, minimize (118) subject to the state equation (117).

On using (111) we form an H-function as

$$H(x, u, \tau) = u + \lambda[-x + pu(1 + u)^{-1}] \qquad (119)$$

From this equation and (112) we see that $1 + u = \pm(-\lambda p)^{1/2}$. Since u must be positive, this means that

$$u(\tau) = [-\lambda(\tau)p]^{1/2} - 1$$

The costate equation (113) becomes $d\lambda / d\tau = \lambda$ with $\lambda(\tau) = \lambda(0)e^{\tau}$. To find $\lambda(0)$ use (114) and (119) to produce the quadratic equation

$$(p - x_0) \lambda(0) + 2 p^{1/2}[-\lambda(0)]^{1/2} - 1 = 0$$

Of the two solutions

$$[-\lambda(0)]^{1/2} = [p^{1/2} - x_0^{1/2}]^{-1}$$

is appropriate, for it gives $u(0) > 0$ as long as $p > x_0$. The other solution of the quadratic gives $u(0) < 0$, which is not allowed. Hence

$$u(\tau) = \left[1 - \left(\frac{x_0}{p}\right)^{1/2}\right]^{-1} e^{\tau/2} - 1 \qquad (120)$$

which is a continuous function of τ. Furthermore, this control can be shown to be the optimal one. When (120) is substituted into (117), the resulting equation can be integrated to give

$$x(\tau) = p \left\{ 1 - \left[1 - \left(\frac{x_0}{p} \right)^{1/2} \right] \exp\left(\frac{-\tau}{2} \right) \right\}^2 \tag{121}$$

Eliminating $\exp(\tau/2)$ between (120) and (121) gives the feedback relation

$$u = \frac{(x/p)^{1/2}}{1 - (x/p)^{1/2}} \tag{122}$$

For a given value of the state, the optimal level of drug to be delivered is given by (122).

Although no upper constraint is placed on the control variable $u(\tau)$, computations [65] show that the levels of the (fictitious) drug used by the optimal control method are always much less than preassigned levels. This optimal control study demonstrates that

1. The drug is to be delivered at low dose in a continuous manner.
2. The accumulated amount of drug is about 1/40 of the accumulated amount with the standard discrete-dosage MCP program.
3. The number of cancer cells reach a plateau level in ·a time that is less than with the MCP program.
4. There is an interesting feedback relation.

No claim is being made that the mathematical model (115) is the one to describe the perturbed growth kinetics of this tumor. What is important here is to understand the importance of the four conclusions that the model generates.

Unfortunately, I was not aware of Refs. 237 and 238 until November 1985. Reference 237 reports on 45 patients with multiple myeloma, who were given long-term low-dose melphalan therapy over a seven-year period. The melphalan was administered orally on a daily schedule. The low dosage produced less toxicity but the same therapeutic effectiveness was achieved. Significant prolongation of survival was reported. In the discussion section of [238] some studies indicate that melphalan given continuously is inferior to intermittent high-dose therapy, whereas other studies found the reverse situation to be the case. It is interesting to compare the conclusions of these papers with conclusions (1) and (2) of the mathematical model which indicate that the continuous delivery of an anticancer drug would be a worthwhile therapeutic alternative to a regimen based on discrete doses of a drug.

Buckles [239] reports on the progress made in the development of reservoirs and pumps that could be used for the delivery of anticancer drugs. One major advance was developed by him and used on himself to deliver anticancer drugs in an unsuccessful attempt to deal with his own cancer. Reference 240 presents clinical results using these extracorporeal pumps. Significant benefits that accrue to patients using these pumps for continuous therapy involved the significant lessening of the degree of systemic toxicity and the side effects of conventional therapy. A review of the progress on *implantable* pumps for regional cancer chemotherapy appeared in [241]. Instead of having an anticancer drug be transported in the general circulation, recent emphasis is on delivering the drug to a specific region or site of the body—hence the term regional chemotherapy. For example, [242] and [243] deal with results of clinical trials on patients treated for the control of liver metastases via the continuous delivery of anticancer drug from a totally implantable device. More recently, Ref. 244 reported on the use of continuous chemotherapy of metastatic colorectal cancer. Also, there is an increasing usage of regimens based on continuous low-dose infusions (over 21 days) of ara-C for the treatment of pre-leukemic RAEB and for AML [245]. Low-dose treatment of leukemia with ara-C is reported in [246].

This increasing clinical evidence in support of the benefits of low-dose continuous anticancer drug delivery for regional chemotherapy is noteworthy. But, nevertheless, it is interesting that the optimal control model [65] gave conclusions that agree with some current approaches to chemotherapy treatment for certain human cancers, as evidenced by an increasing number of clinicians.

How the optimal control approach fits in with those therapies involving high drug doses with subsequent patient rescue is not clear.

B. Other Optimal Control Models

At the time of diagnosis a cancer patient may have about 10^{12} cancer cells present. One of the goals of cancer chemotherapy is to reduce this number to the 10^9 level; see Section II. Define

$$z = \ln\left(\frac{\theta}{L_d}\right) \qquad L_d = 10^9$$

Introduce the performance index

$$J(u) = \int_0^T [(x - z)^2 + \rho u^2]\, d\tau \tag{123}$$

where ρ is a positive constant. The first term is a measure of how close the model-derived value x is to the desired level z. The

second term, quadratic in the control variable, penalizes excess
amount of drug used. Also, x is a nondimensional variable related
to the level L by a prescribed equation. The previous section, in
(116), has an example of a given equation that connects x with L.
Determine the optimal control that minimizes the performance criterion
(123) subject to the state equation (117). This is a nontrivial problem. It is designated as the third optimal control problem in [88],
where its solution is developed both analytically and numerically. In
particular, the feedback relation is shown to be

$$2\rho \left(1 - \frac{x}{p}\right) u^3 + \rho \left(1 - 4 \frac{x}{p}\right) u^2 - 2\rho \frac{x}{p} u - (x - z)^2 = 0$$

$$(124)$$

For a given value of the state x this cubic gives a unique positive
solution for u.
  Instead of ρu^2 in (123) we could have made the selection βu.
This leads to a different optimal problem, which is solved in [88].
  There is no need to use the Gompertz form in (115). The
logistic form is used in [49]. A logistic growth equation with a
simple loss term is

$$\dot{L}(t) = a_1 L - b_1 L^2 - k_3 vL$$

$$(125)$$

whereas the logistic equation with the E_{max} loss term is

$$\dot{L}(t) = a_1 L - b_1 L^2 - \frac{k_1 vL}{k_2 + v}$$

$$(126)$$

I favor the use of the E_{max} term as being more representative of
the behavior one might expect of an anticancer drug. The determination of the optimal control that minimizes (123) subject to either
(125) or (126) is considered in detail in [49].
  That there appears to be the possibility of a feedback expression
in these particular optimal control problems led me to investigate the
general problem: determine the optimal control that minimizes

$$J(u) = \int_0^T [w(x) + \rho u^2] \, d\tau \qquad w(x) \geqslant 0$$

$$(127)$$

subject to the constraint equation

$$\frac{dx}{d\tau} = x[f(x) - ph(u)]$$

$$(128)$$

In [49] it is shown that this problem has the general feedback relation

$$F(x, u) = \frac{u^2}{2} + \frac{uf(x)}{ph'(u)} - \frac{uh(u)}{h'(u)} + \frac{w(x)}{2\rho} = 0 \qquad (129)$$

There are only certain optimal control models that produce feedback relations. We have provided two particular cases, (122) and (124), of the general result (129). The importance of these relations is that they give the level of control (possibly the optimal control) in terms of a function of the state x. If we know this state, then we know the control. That is a powerful conclusion. Frequently we need to solve (129) numerically to obtain values for the control. Examples of this procedure are in [49].

C. Future Prospects for Optimal Control Theory in Cancer Chemotherapy

The flow diagram of Fig. 4 was given in [247]. Consider the situation of a cancer patient. Assume that some type of biochemical marker [e.g., a monoclonal antibody (MoAb)] is used in diagnosing a particular cancer [248], and assume that it is possible to relate the MoAb to the level L of tumor cells present. We are given a mathematical model of the growth dynamics of the tumor [e.g., (128)] for a certain selection of the function f(x). This mathematical model also includes a prescribed form for the loss term h(u) in terms of the nondimensional level u of drug to be infused. Equation (128) contains at least one parameter p, which is probably patient-dependent.

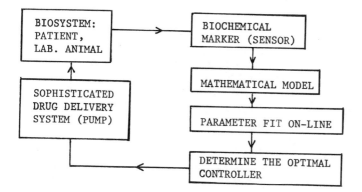

FIGURE 4   Closed-loop control system.

In the discussion section in [49] a method is suggested for obtaining p for a particular patient from on-line noise-corrupted measurements of x during treatment with a drug that is being delivered continuously. A performance criterion such as (127) is selected with w(x) chosen to give the output as close as possible to a desired level. This output is generated by the discrete-time version of (128). An example of a representative performance criterion is

$$J_k(u) = E[(x[(k + 1)\delta] - z[(k + 1)\delta])^2 + \rho u^2(k\delta)] \qquad (130)$$

where k is a counter, δ is a unit of τ, and E[$\cdot$] denotes the expectation operation [249]. The minimization of (130) with respect to u(kδ) provides the optimal input.

The on-line fit of the model to data and the determination of the optimal input is done by a microprocessor. The information on the optimal input is passed to a sophisticated drug delivery device which automatically infuses the desired amount of drug to the patient.

We use the word "drug" in this section in a broad sense to apply to an anticancer agent as well as to an immunotherapeutic agent. For example, it is reasonable that one should, with present knowledge, be able to do the following. Test a tumor sample in tissue culture or nude mice with an anticancer agent to find the most suitable one for the patient. Then develop a custom-made monoclonal antibody which can be injected into the patient to control the growth of the tumor. These ideas were presented in [247] in connection with Fig. 4.

Although the material in this section applies to cancer chemotherapy, a moment's reflection indicates that Fig. 4 applies equally well to other disease states for which a chemotherapy treatment is recommended; see also [234].

XV. FUTURE INVESTIGATIONS

As noted in Section III, the exponential growth model is used quite extensively in investigations of cancer growth problems. Because of the errors in [23], see Section III.C, it would be of interest to redo [23–29] and update this material. An improvement to exponential growth is the logistic model of Section V. There is a need to fit human and experimental tumor data to the logistic model. Mathematical models that show the use of the logistic equation in cancer chemotherapy problems need to be developed. Reference 49 shows a recent application in an optimal control problem.

No doubt many more papers using the Gompertz equation and function will appear. Since the Gompertz equation lacks a biological foundation, this would appear to be a waste of effort. (Note in press: See [261].)

Thermodynamic investigations are needed. As indicated in Section VII.B, they have been ignored in cancer research. Yet if more knowledge was available, it might be possible to exploit it in the development of new approaches to dealing with the cancer cell.

Perhaps investigators have been too hasty in throwing out Bertalanffy's equation (27). It is recommended that a current assessment be made of the applicability of his equation to human and experimental tumors.

It is known that a number (perhaps all?) of solid tumors are not homogeneous. As the tumor grows, changes take place in the tumor cells and layers of cells, different from their parents, occur. The heterogeneity of such tumors has received hardly any attention from modelers. A brief discussion is in Section VII.E. Much more remains to be done. The importance of the heterogeneous nature of tumors is stressed in [250], where each paper is devoted to this area. So [250] is a good place for mathematical modelers to start their investigations. This is an important area for future developments.

As indicated in Sections VII.G and VIII.H, we need to develop models that are concerned with mechanisms of cancer growth.

At the end of Section VIII.B we briefly introduce the new BrdUrd technique. It seems clear that mathematical models will be developed to provide much needed information on the use of BrdUrd in a number of cancer studies; see [149].

The tumor growth model of Cox et al. in Section VIII.D has not been applied to any human tumor data. No one has studied the use of the model in cancer chemotherapy problems. It would be interesting to use this model in optimal control problems (see Section XIV).

Section VIII.H assesses the models of tumor cell kinetics. Future work needs to progress along the directions outlined there. An additional problem with cell kinetics studies is that they provide very little information on tumor stem cells, which many believe are crucial to the growth of the tumor. Tumor stem cells are not able to be identified morphologically. Certainly, future efforts ought to be directed at including stem cell populations in the mathematical models.

The mathematical model developed in Section XII.A can be programmed for a digital computer, and the program is able to be run for different selections of parameter values. This approach is recommended. The pharmacokinetic model in Section XII.A needs to be updated. For example, the lumped compartmental description of [251] could be used. However, it is important to be aware of the many advances that have been made since 1970 in the mathematical modeling of clinical pharmacokinetics; see [236] and [252].

Also, the basic work of Section XIII needs to be updated to include more relevant pharmacokinetics.

The development of optimal control models in cancer chemotherapy offers much promise for improvements in therapy. Much remains to be

done here. Models that extend the work of [253], dealing with the
effect of the drug on the white blood cells, need to be introduced.
The damage to the normal cell population needs to be minimized.
Time lags could be incorporated into the models to better approximate
physiological reality. (A cancer chemotherapy model involving time
lags is in [254].) The recent progress in using on-line techniques
to study parameter determination and to derive the optimal control
from noise-corrupted observations needs to be put to work for the
cancer chemotherapy models. In connection with these studies we
need to develop models that can relate knowledge from tumor markers
to the number of tumor cells present. Since optimal control models
may be of most use in regional cancer chemotherapy, we need to explore this area in detail. One area of investigation involves the
treatment of brain tumors. A useful starting point is provided by
[255]. We need more studies on the choice of performance criterion
in the optimal control models.

No doubt these optimal control studies will be intimately connected
with the use of digital computers. Already there is much clinical
progress in using applied control to improve patient care in the noncancer setting [256]. Many of the techniques that improve therapy
for the patients described in [256] need to be carried over to the
treatment of the cancer patient.

The modeling of diffusion in tumors is discussed at length in
[55]. Since that time, many papers have appeared. This area is
one that needs to be updated.

Mathematical models of the immune system and how it interacts
with a growing tumor are of interest. Some were examined in detail
in [55]. Again, this area needs to be updated to take into consideration more recent developments.

The special issue of Ref. 262 deals with computer simulation and
modeling in cancer research. We need to continue developing appropriate models.

REFERENCES

1. Collins, V. P., Loeffler, R. K., and Tivey, H., Observations
    on growth rates of human tumors. *Am. J. Roentgenol. Radium
    Ther. Nucl. Med.*, 76:988 (1956).

2. Schwartz, M., A biomathematical approach to clinical tumor
    growth. *Cancer*, 14:1272 (1961).

3. Archambeau, J. O., Heller, M. B., Akanuma, A., and Lubell,
    D., Biologic and clinical implications obtained from the analysis
    of cancer growth curves. *Clinical Obstet. Gynecol.*, 13:831
    (1970).

4. Steel, G. G. and Lamerton, L. F., The growth rate of human tumours. *Br. J. Cancer, 20*:74 (1966).

5. Sommers, S. C., Growth rates, cell kinetics, and mathematical models of human cancers, in *Pathobiology Annual 1973* (H. L. Ioachim, ed.), Appleton-Century-Crofts, Meredith Corporation, New York, p. 309 (1973).

6. Tubiana, M., L. H. Gray Medal Lecture: Cell kinetics and radiation oncology. *Int. J. Radiation Oncology Biol. Phys., 8*: 1471 (1982).

7. Mayneord, W. V., On a law of growth of Jensen's rat sarcoma. *Am. J. Cancer, 16*:841 (1932).

8. Mottram, J. C., On origin of tar tumours in mice, whether from single cells or many cells. *J. Path. and Bact., 40*:407 (1935).

9. Nathan, M. H., Collins, V. P., and Adams, R. A., Differentiation of benign and malignant pulmonary nodules by growth rate. *Radiology, 79*:221 (1962).

10. Fialkow, P. J., Clonal origin of human tumors. *Biochim. Biophys. Acta., 458*:283 (1976).

11. Shackney, S. E., Cell kinetics and cancer chemotherapy, in *Medical Oncology* (P. Calabresi, P. S. Schein, and S. A. Rosenberg, eds.), Macmillan, New York, p. 41 (1985).

12. Steel, G. G., *Growth Kinetics of Tumours*, Clarendon Press, Oxford (1977).

13. Collins, V. P., Time of occurrence of pulmonary metastasis from carcinoma of colon and rectum. *Cancer, 15*:387 (1962).

14. Welin, S., Yonker, J., and Spratt, J. S., Jr., The rates and patterns of growth of 375 tumors of the large intestine and rectum observed serially by double contrast enema study. *Am. J. Roentgenol. Radium Ther. Nucl. Med., 90*:673 (1963).

15. Malaise, E. P., Chavaudra, N., and Tubiana, M., The relationship between growth rate, labelling index and histological type of human solid tumours. *Eur. J. Cancer, 9*:305 (1973).

16. Kendall, D. G., On the role of variable generation time in the development of a stochastic birth process, *Biometrika, 35*:316 (1948).

17. Kendall, D. G., Les processus stocastiques de croissance en biologie. *Ann. Inst. H. Poincaré, 13*:43 (1952).

18. Harris, T. E., *The Theory of Branching Processes*, Springer, Berlin (1963).

19. Berglas, A., *Cancer, Nature, Cause and Cure*, Institute
     Pasteur, Paris (1957).

20. Schwartz, H. and Wolff, G., Mathematische Betrachtungen zum
     Wachstum von Geschwülsten. *Acta Biol. Med. Germ.*, *13*:378
     (1964).

21. Priore, R. L., Using a mathematical model in the evaluation of
     human tumor response to chemotherapy. *JNCI*, *37*:635 (1966).

22. Elkind, M. M. and Whitmore, G. F., *The Radiobiology of
     Cultured Mammalian Cells*, Gordon and Breach, New York (1967).

23. Hahn, G. M., State vector description of the proliferation of
     mammalian cells in tissue culture. I. Exponential growth.
     Biophys. J., *6*:275 (1966).

24. Hahn, G. M. and Kallman, R. F., State vector description of
     the proliferation of mammalian cells in tissue culture. II. Ef-
     fects of single and multiple doses of ionizing radiations.
     Radiation Res., *30*:702 (1967).

25. Hahn, G. M., A formalism describing the kinetics of some mam-
     malian cell populations. *Math. Biosci.*, *6*:295 (1970).

26. Kim. M., Bahrami, K., and Woo, K. B., A discrete-time model
     for cell-age, size, and DNA distributions of proliferating cells,
     and its application to the movement of the labeled cohort.
     IEEE Trans. Biomed. Eng., *BME-21*:387 (1974).

27. Kim, M. and Woo, K. B., Kinetic analysis of cell size and DNA
     content distributions during tumor cell proliferation: Ehrlich
     ascites tumor study. *Cell Tissue Kinet.*, *8*:197 (1975). (See
     also pp. 387–390, same issue, for details on kinetic parameters.)

28. Kim, M., Bahrami, K., and Woo, K. B., Mathematical descrip-
     tion and analysis of cell cycle kinetics and the application to
     Ehrlich ascites tumor. *J. Theor. Biol.*, *50*:437 (1975).

29. Kim. M., Woo, K. B., and Perry, S., Quantitative approach to
     the design of antitumor drug dosage schedule via cell cycle
     kinetics and systems theory. *Annals Biomed. Eng.*, *5*:12
     (1977).

30. Trucco, E. and Brockwell, P. J., Percentage labeled mitoses
     curves in exponentially growing cell populations. *J. Theor.
     Biol.*, *20*:321 (1968).

31. Burns, F. J. and Tannock, I. F., On the existence of a G_0
     phase in the cell cycle. *Cell Tissue Kinet.*, *3*:321 (1970).

32. N. S. Ullman and Jacquez, J. A., Analysis of tests of chemo-
     therapeutic agents involving repeated drug treatment. *Bio-
     metrics*, *29*:677 (1973).

33. Bjerknes, R., Exponential growth. *Eur. J. Cancer,* 10:165 (1974).

34. Macdonald, P. D. M., The mathematical theory of exponentially-growing cell populations, in *Mathematical Models in Cell Kinetics* (A-j. Valleron, ed.), European Press Medikon, Ghent, p. 15 (1975).

35. Looney, W. B., Trefil, J. S., Schaffner, J. C., Kovacs, C. J., and Hopkins, H. A., Solid tumor models for the assessment of different treatment modalities. I. Radiation-induced changes in growth rate characteristics of a solid tumor model. *Proc. Natl. Acad. Sci. USA,* 72:2662 (1975).

36. Looney, W. B., Trefil, J. S., Hopkins, H. A., Kovacs, C. J., Ritenour, R., and Schaffner, J. G., Solid tumor models for assessment of different treatment modalities: Therapeutic strategy for sequential chemotherapy with radiotherapy. *Proc. Natl. Acad. Sci. USA,* 74:1983 (1977).

37. Tomasovic, S. P., Roti Roti, J. L., and Dethlefsen, L. A., Matrix algebraic simulation of mitotic cell selection experiments. *Cell Tissue Kinet.,* 13:117 (1980).

38. Vaidya, V. G. and Alexandro, F. J., Jr., Evaluation of some mathematical models for tumor growth. *Int. J. Bio-Medical Computing,* 13:19 (1982).

39. Coldman, A. J. and Goldie, J. H., A model for the resistance of tumor cells to cancer chemotherapeutic agents. *Math. Biosci.,* 65:291 (1983).

40. Takekawa, A., Kitamura, S., Mori, H., and Yamaguchi, N., Modelling and evaluation of the clinical states of acute leukemia, in *MEDINFO-83* (J. H. van Bemmel, M. J. Ball, and O. Wigertz, eds.), IFIP-IMIA, North-Holland, Amsterdam, p. 875 (1983).

41. Mendelsohn, M. L., The growth fraction: a new concept applied to tumors. *Science,* 132:1496 (1960).

42. Mendelsohn, M. L., Autoradiographic analysis of cell proliferation in spontaneous breast cancer of C3H mouse. II. Growth and survival of cells labelled with tritiated thymidine. *JNCI,* 25:485 (1960).

43. Rashevsky, N., Outline of a mathematical approach to the cancer problem. *Bull. Math. Biophys.,* 7:69 (1945).

44. Rashevsky, N., *Mathematical Biophysics,* Univ. of Chicago Press, Chicago (1948).

45. Verhulst, P. F., *Correspondence Mathématique et Physique 10.* Reprinted in *Readings in Ecology* (E. J. Kormondy, ed.), Prentice-Hall, Englewood Cliffs, N.J. (1965).

46. Pearl, R. and Reed, L. J., On the rate of growth of the popu-
     lation of the United States since 1790 and its mathematical
     representation. *Proc. Natl. Acad. Sci. USA, 6:*275 (1920).

47. Pearl, R., *Studies in Human Biology,* Williams and Wilkins,
     New York (1924).

48. Gause, G. F., *The Struggle for Existence,* Williams and Wilkins,
     New York (1934). Reprinted by Dover, New York (1971).

49. Swan, G. W., Cancer chemotherapy; optimal control using the
     Verhulst-Pearl equation. *Bull. Math. Biol., 48:*381 (1986).

50. Verhagen, A. M. W., Growth curves and their functional form.
     *Aust. J. Statistics, 2:*122 (1960).

51. Emanuel, N. M., *Kinetics of Experimental Tumour Processes,*
     Pergamon Press, Oxford (1982).

52. Schmid, F. A., Cappuccino, J. G., Merker, P. C., Tarnowski,
     G. S., and Stock, C. C., Chemotherapy studies in an animal
     tumor spectrum. I. Biologic characteristics of the tumors.
     *Cancer Res. Suppl., 26:*173 (1966).

53. Harding, H. R., Rosen, F., and Nichol, C. A., Depression of
     alanine transaminase activity in the liver of rats bearing Walker
     carcinoma 256. *Cancer Res., 24:*1318 (1964).

54. Swan, G. W., *Optimization of Human Cancer Radiotherapy,*
     Springer-Verlag, New York (1981).

55. Swan, G. W., *Some Current Mathematical Topics in Cancer Re-
     search,* Published for the Society for Mathematical Biology,
     University Microfilms International, Ann Arbor, Mich. (1977).

56. Skellam, J. G., Random dispersal in theoretical populations.
     *Biometrika, 38:*196 (1951).

57. Lefever, R. and Erneaux, T., On the growth of cellular tissues
     under constant and fluctuating environmental conditions, in
     Nonlinear Electrodynamics in Biological Systems (W. R. Adey
     and A.F. Lawrence, eds.), Plenum, New York, p. 287 (1984).

58. Gompertz, B., On the nature of the function expressive of the
     law of human mortality and on a new model of determining life
     contingencies. *Phil. Trans. Roy. Soc. (Lond.), 115:*513
     (1825).

59. Lloyd, H. H., Estimation of tumor cell kill from Gompertz growth
     curves. *Cancer Chem. Rept. Part 1, 59:*267 (1975).

60. Zotin, A. I., *Thermodynamic Aspects of Development Biology,*
     S. Karger, Basle (1972).

61. Winsor, P. C., The Gompertz curve as a growth curve. *Proc. Natl. Acad. Sci. USA*, *18*:1 (1932).

62. Gocka, E. F. and Reed, L. J., A method of fitting non-symmetric Gompertz functions for characterising malignant growth. *Int. J. Bio-Medical Computing*, *8*:247 (1977).

63. Brunton, G. F. and Wheldon, T. E., Prediction of the complete growth pattern of human multiple myeloma from restricted initial measurements. *Cell Tissue Kinet.*, *10*:591 (1977).

64. Sullivan, P. W. and Salmon, S. E., Kinetics of tumor growth and regression in IgG multiple myeloma. *J. Clinic Invest.*, *51*: 1697 (1972).

65. Swan, G. W. and Vincent, T. L., Optimal control analysis in the chemotherapy of IgG multiple myeloma. *Bull. Math. Biol.*, *39*:317 (1977).

66. Brunton, G. F. and Wheldon, T. E., Characteristic species dependent growth patterns of mammalian neoplasms. *Cell Tissue Kinet.*, *11*:161 (1978).

67. Brunton, G. F. and Wheldon, T. E., The Gompertz equation and the construction of tumor growth curves. *Cell Tissue Kinet.*, *13*:455 (1980).

68. Demicheli, R., Growth of testicular neoplasm lung metastases: Tumor-specific relation between two Gompertzian parameters. *Eur. J. Cancer*, *16*:1603 (1980).

69. Steel, G. G., Species-dependent growth patterns for mammalian neoplasms. *Cell Tissue Kinet.*, *13*:451 (1980).

70. Casey, A. E., The experimental alteration of malignancy with an homologous mammalian tumor material. I. *Am. J. Cancer*, *21*: 760 (1934).

71. Laird, A. K., Dynamics of tumour growth. *Br. J. Cancer*, *18*: 490 (1964).

72. Laird, A. K., Dynamics of growth in tumors and in normal tissues, in *Human Tumor Cell Kinetics*, Monograph 30, National Cancer Institute, Washington, D.C., p. 15 (1969).

73. McCredie, J. A., Inch, W. R., Kruuv, J., and Watson, T. A., The rate of tumor growth in animals. *Growth*, *29*:331 (1965).

74. Durbin, P. W., Jeung, N., Williams, M. H., and Arnold, J. S., Construction of growth curve for mammary tumors. *Cancer Res.*, *27*:1341 (1967).

75. Schabel, F. M., Jr. The use of tumor growth kinetics in planning "curative" chemotherapy of advanced solid tumors. *Cancer Res.*, *29*:2384 (1969).

76. Simpson-Herren, L. and Lloyd, H. H., Kinetic parameter and growth curves for experimental tumor systems. *Cancer Chem. Rept. Part 1*, *54*:143 (1970).

77. Norton, L., Simon, R., Brereton, H. D., and Bogden, A. E., Predicting the course of Gompertzian growth. *Nature*, *264*:542 (1976).

78. Norton, L. and R. Simon, Growth curve of an experimental solid tumor following radiotherapy. *JNCI*, *58*:1735 (1977).

79. Norton, L. and Simon, R., Tumor size, sensitivity to therapy, and design of treatment schedules. *Cancer Treat. Rep.*, *61*: 1307 (1977).

80. Wheldon, T. E. and Brunton, G. E., Tumor growth kinetics, therapeutic differentials, and design of treatment schedules. *Cancer Treat. Rept.*, *62*:845 (1978).

81. Norton, L. and Simon, R., Authors' response. *Cancer Treat. Rept.*, *62*:846 (1978).

82. Martinez, A. O. and Grieco, R. J., Growth dynamics of multi-cell spheroids from three murine tumors. *Growth*, *44*:112 (1980).

83. Skehan, P. and Friedman, S. J., Deceleratory growth by a rat glial tumor line in culture. *Cancer Res.*, *42*:1636 (1982).

84. Akanuma, A., Parameter analysis of Gompertzian function growth model in clinical tumors. *Eur. J. Cancer*, *14*:681 (1978).

85. von Eyben, F. E., Trope, C., Ljungberg, O., Alm, P., Wennerberg, J., and Gulberg, B., Histologic pattern and growth in two human testis cancers before and after transplantation to nude mice. *Cancer*, *50*:2845 (1982).

86. Swan, G. W., Optimal control in some cancer chemotherapy problems. *Int. J. Syst. Sci.*, *11*:223 (1980).

87. Swan, G. W., *Applications of Optimal Control Theory in Biomedicine*, Marcel Dekker, New York (1984).

88. Swan, G. W., Optimal control applications in the chemotherapy of multiple myeloma. *IMA Jl. Mathematics Applied in Medicine and Biology*, *2*:139 (1985).

89. Rofstad, E. K., Fodstat, Ø., and Lindmo, T., Growth characteristics of human melanoma xenografts. *Cell Tissue Kinet.*, *15*: 545 (1982).

90. Walter, R. and Lamprecht, I., Modern theories concerning the growth equations, in *Thermodynamics and Kinetics of Biological Processes* (I. Lamprecht and A. I. Zotin, eds.), de Gruyter, New York, p. 143 (1978).

91. Mendelsohn, M. L., Cell proliferation and tumour growth, in *Cell Proliferation* (L. F. Lamerton and R. J. M. Fry, eds.), Blackwell, Oxford, p. 190 (1963).

92. Mendelsohn, M. L. and Dethlefsen, L. A., Tumor growth and cellular kinetics, in *The Proliferation and Spread of Neoplastic Cells*, Williams and Wilkins, Baltimore, p. 197 (1968).

93. Dethlefsen, L. A., Prewitt, J. M. S., and Mendelsohn, M. L., Analysis of tumor growth curves. *JNCI, 40,* 389 (1968).

94. Goel, N. S., Maitra, S. C., and Montroll, E. W., *On the Volterra and Other Nonlinear Models of Interacting Populations,* Academic Press, New York. (The material in this book originally was printed in *Rev. Mod. Phys., 43*:231 (1971).)

95. Montroll, E. W., On coupled rate equations with quadratic non-linearities. *Proc. Natl. Acad. Sci. USA, 69*:2532 (1972).

96. Salzer, H. E., Toward a Gibbsian approach to the problems of growth and cancer. *Acta Biotheor. Series A, 12*:135 (1957).

97. Smith, C. J., Problems with entropy in biology. *Bio Systems,* 7:259 (1975).

98. Jones, D. D., Entropic models in biology: The next scientific revolution? *Perspectives in Biol. Med., 20*:285 (1977).

99. Lamprecht, I. and Zotin, A. I., eds., *Thermodynamics of Biological Processes,* de Gruyter, New York, (1978).

100. Lamprecht, I. and Zotin, A. I., eds., *Thermodynamics and Kinetics of Biological Processes,* de Gruyter, New York (1983).

101. Lamprecht, I. and Zotin, A. I., eds., *Thermodynamics and Regulation of Biological Processes,* de Gruyter, New York (1985).

102. von Bertalanffy, L., Principles and theory of growth, in *Fundamental Aspects of Normal and Malignant Growth* (W. W. Nowinsky, ed.), Elsevier, Amsterdam, p. 137 (1960).

103. Faybens, A. J., Properties and fitting of the von Bertalanffy growth curve. *Growth, 29*:265 (1965).

104. Savageau, M. A., Growth of complex systems can be related to the properties of their underlying determinants. *Proc. Natl. Acad. Sci. USA, 76*:5413 (1979).

105. Savageau, M. A., Allometric morphogenesis of complex systems: Derivation of the basic equations from first principles. *Proc. Natl. Acad. Sci. USA, 76*:6023 (1979).

106. Savageau, M. A., Growth equations: A general equation and a survey of special cases. *Math. Biosci., 48*:267 (1980).

107. Kendal, W. S., Gompertzian growth as a consequence of tumor heterogeneity. *Math. Biosci., 72*:1 (1984).

108. Heppner, G. H. and Miller, B. E., Tumor heterogeneity: Biological Implications and therapeutic consequences. *Cancer Metastasis Rev., 2*:5 (1983).

109. Fischer, J. J., Mathematical simulation of radiation therapy of solid tumors. I. Calculations. *Acta Radiol. Ther. Phys. Biol., 10*:73 (1971).

110. Marietta, M. G. and Swan, G. W., A Lagrangian formulation for continuous media. *Int. J. Non-Linear Mech., 12*:49 (1977).

111. Hore, P. and Koh, S. L., A continuum theory of growth processes of biological materials, in *Advances in Bioengineering* (R. E. Mates and C. R. Smith, eds.), American Society of Mechanical Engineers, New York, p. 40 (1976).

112. Hore, P. and Koh, S. L., A continuum theory of growth processes of biological materials; Report, Solid Mechanics and Materials Lab., Purdue Univ., West Lafayette, Ind. (1977).

113. Howard, A. and Pelc, S. R., Synthesis of deoxyribonucleic acid in normal and irradiated cells and its relation to chromosome breakage. *Heredity (Suppl.), 6*:261 (1953).

114. Verley, W. G. and Hunebell, G., Preparation of T-labeled thymidine. *Bull. Soc. Chim. Belg., 66*:640 (1957).

115. Taylor, J. H., Woods, P. S., and Hughes, W. L., The organization and duplication of chromosomes as revealed by autoradiographic studies using tritium-labeled thymidine. *Proc. Natl. Acad. Sci. USA, 43*:122 (1957).

116. Quastler, H. and Sherman, F. G., Cell population kinetics in the intestinal epithelium of the mouse. *Exp. Cell Res., 17*:420 (1959).

117. Kamentsky, L. A., Melamed, H. R., and Derman, H., Spectrophotometer: New instrument for ultrarapid cell analysis. *Science, 150*:630 (1965).

118. van Dilla, M. A., Trujillo, T. T., Mullaney, P. F., and Coulter, J. R. Cell microfluorometry: A method for rapid fluorescence measurement. *Science, 163*:1213 (1969).

119. Baserga, R., The relation of the cell cycle to tumor growth and control of cell division: A review. *Cancer Res.*, *25*:581 (1965).

120. Lajtha, L. G., On the concept of the cell cycle. *J. Cell Comp. Physiol. Suppl. 1, 62*:143 (1963).

121. Quastler, H., The analysis of cell population kinetics, in *Cell Proliferation* (L. G. Lamerton, and R. J. M. Fry, eds.), Blackwell Scientific, Oxford, p. 18 (1963).

122. Baserga, R., ed., *The Cell Cycle and Cancer*, Marcel Dekker, New York (1971).

123. Baserga, R., The cell cycle in cancer chemotherapy, in *Recent Results in Cancer Research*, Vol. 52, *The Ambivalence of Cytostatic Therapy* (E. Grundmann and R. Gross, eds.), Springer-Verlag, New York, p. 149 (1975).

124. Baserga, R., *Multiplication and Division in Mammalian Cells*, Marcel Dekker, New York (1976).

125. Mitchison, J. M., *The Cell Cycle*, Cambridge University Press, Cambridge (1971).

126. Lamerton, L. F., Tumor cell kinetics. *Brit. Med. Bull.*, *29*: 23 (1973).

127. Aroesty, J., Lincoln, T., Shapiro, N., and Boccia, G., Tumor growth and chemotherapy: Mathematical methods, computer simulations, and experimental foundations. *Math. Biosci.*, *17*: 243 (1973).

128. Fried, J., A mathematical model of proliferating cell populations: Further development and consideration of the resting state. *Math. Biosci.*, *18*:397 (1973).

129. Jansson, B., Mathematical models in cell cycle kinetics, in *Mathematical Models in Biology and Medicine* (N. T. J. Bailey, Bl. Sendov, and R. Tsanev, eds.), North-Holland, Amsterdam, p. 21 (1974).

130. Mazia, D., The cell cycle. *Scientific American 230* (Jan.): 54 (1974).

131. Bertuzzi, A., Gandolfi, A., and Giovenco, M. A., Mathematical models of the cell cycle with a view to tumor studies. *Math. Biosci.*, *53*:159 (1981).

132. Denekamp, J., *Cell Kinetics and Cancer Therapy*, Charles C. Thomas, Springfield, Ill., 1982.

133. Baserga, R., *The Biology of Cell Reproduction*, Harvard University Press, Cambridge (1985).

134. Barrett, J. C., A mathematical model of the mitotic cycle and its application to the interpretation of percentage labeled mitoses data. *JNCI, 37:*443 (1966).

135. Takahashi, M., Theoretical basis for cell cycle analysis, I. Labelled mitosis wave method. *J. Theor. Biol., 13:*202 (1966).

136. Takahashi, M., Theoretical basis for cell cycle analysis. II. Further studies on labelled mitosis wave method. *J. Theor. Biol., 18:*195 (1968).

137. Steel, G. G. and Hanes, S., The techniques of labeled mitoses: Analysis by automatic curve fitting. *Cell Tissue Kinet., 4:* 93 (1971).

138. Takahashi, M., Hogg, J. D. Jr., and Mendelsohn, M. L., The automatic analysis of FLM curves. *Cell Tissue Kinet., 4:*505 (1971).

139. Valleron, A-j. and Frindel, E., Computer simulation of growing cell populations. *Cell Tissue Kinet., 6:*69 (1973).

140. A-j. Valleron, ed., *Mathematical Models in Cell Kinetics,* European Press Medikon, Ghent (1975).

141. Simpson-Herren, L., Springer, T. A., and Lloyd, H. H., Ambiguity of the thymidine index. *Cancer Res., 36:*4705 (1976).

142. Hudson, H. M. and Hahn, G. M., The labelled mitosis curve for a population consisting of fast and slowly cycling cells. *J. Theor. Biol., 66:*63 (1977).

143. Shackney, S. E., Ford, S. S., and Wittig, A. B., The effects of counting threshold and emulsion exposure duration on the percent labelled mitoses curve and their implications for cell cycle analysis. *Cancer Res., 33:*2726 (1973).

144. Gray, J. W., Pallavicini, M. G., George, Y. S., Groppi, V., Look, M., and Dean, P. N., Rates of incorporation of radioactive molecules during the cell cycle. *J. Cell Physiol., 108:* 135 (1981).

145. Maurer, H. R., Potential pitfalls of [^{3}H]thymidine techniques to measure cell proliferation. *Cell Tissue Kinet. 14:*111 (1981).

146. Lang, W., Herrmann, H., and Georgii, A., Evaluation of continuous labelling data by a practical mathematical method with application to a virus-induced sarcoma of the rat. *Z. Krebsforsch, 92:*137 (1978).

147. Gray, J. W., Carver, J. H., George, Y. S., and Mendelsohn, M. L., Rapid cell cycle analysis by measurement of the

radioactivity per cell in a narrow window in S phase (RCS_i). *Cell Tissue Kinet.*, *10*:97 (1977).

148. Gray, J. W., Bogart, E., Gavel, D. T., George, Y. S., and Moore, D. H., II, Rapid Cell Analysis. II. Phase durations and dispersions for computer analysis of RC curves. *Cell Tissue Kinet.*, *16*:457 (1983).

149. *Cytometry*, *6*:499 (1985).

150. Van Dilla, M. A., Steinmetz, L. L., Davis, D. T., Calvert, R. N., and Gray, J. W., High-speed cell analysis and sorting with flow systems: biological applications and new approaches. *IEEE Nucl. Sci.*, *NS-21*:714 (1974).

151. Gray, J. W., Cell cycle analysis from computer synthesis of deoxyribonucleic acid histograms. *J. Histochem. Cytochem.*, *22*:642 (1974).

152. Gray, J. W., Carrano, A. V., Moore, D. H., II, Steinmetz, L. L., Minkler, J., Mayall, B. H., Mendelsohn, M. L., and Van Dilla, M. A., High-speed quantitative karyotyping by flow microfluorometry. *Clin. Chem.*, *21*:1258 (1975).

153. Gray, J. W., Carrano, A. V., Steinmetz, L. L., Van Dilla, M. A., Moore, D. H. II, Mayall, B. H., and Mendelsohn, M. L., Chromosome measurement and sorting by flow systems. *Proc. Natl. Acad. Sci. USA*, *72*:1231 (1975).

154. Gray, J. W., Cell cycle analysis of perturbed cell populations: Computer simulation of sequential DNA distributions. *Cell Tissue Kinet.*, *9*:499 (1976).

155. Melamed, M., Mullaney, P., and Mendelsohn, M., eds., *Flow Cytometry and Sorting*, John Wiley, New York (1979).

156. Zietz, S. and Nicolini, C., Flow microfluorometry and cell kinetics: A review, in *Biomathematics and Cell Kinetics* (A-j. Valleron and P. D. M. Macdonald, eds.), Elsevier, New York, p. 357 (1978).

157. Zietz, S., Desaive, C., Macri, N., Grattarola, M., and Nicolini, C., Deterministic mathematical models to obtain optimized drug metabolism and cell kinetic parameters as function of dosage from both autoradiographic and flow microfluoro-metric analysis, in *Biomathematics and Cell Kinetics* (A.-j. Valleron and P. D. M. Macdonald, eds.), Elsevier, New York, p. 431 (1978).

158. Baisch, H., Beck, H.-P., Christensen, I. J., et al. A comparison of mathematical models for the analysis of DNA histograms obtained by flow cytometry. *Cell Tissue Kinet.*, *15*:235 (1982).

159. Eisen, M., *Mathematical Models in Cell Biology and Cancer Chemotherapy*, Springer-Verlag, New York (1979).

160. Gray, J. W. and Dean. P. N., Display and analysis of flow cytometric data. *Ann. Rev. Biophys. Bioeng.*, *9*: 509 (1980).

161. Muirhead, K. A., Horan, P. K., and Poste, G., Flow cytometry: Present and future. *Bio/Technology*, *3*: 337 (1985).

162. Cox, E. B., Woodbury, M. A., and Meyers, L. E., A new model for tumor growth analysis based on a postulated inhibitory substance. *Comp. Biomed. Res.*, *13*: 437 (1980).

163. Bellman, R. and Cooke, K. L., *Differential Difference Equations*, Academic Press, New York (1963).

164. El'sgol'ts, L. E., *Introduction to the Theory of Differential Equations with Deviating Arguments*, Holden-Day, San Francisco, (1966).

165. Oğuztöreli, M. N., *Time-Lag Control Systems*, Academic Press, New York (1966).

166. Smith, J. A., and Martin, L., Do cells cycle? *Proc. Natl. Acad. Sci. USA*, *70*: 1263 (1973).

167. De Maertelaer, V. and Galand, P., Some properties of a "G_0"-model of the cell cycle. I. Investigation on the possible existence of natural constraints on the theoretical model in steady-state conditions. *Cell Tissue Kinet.*, *8*: 11 (1975).

168. De Maertelaer, V. and Galand, P., Some properties of a "G_0"-model of the cell cycle. II. Natural constraints on the theoretical model in exponential growth conditions. *Cell Tissue Kinet.*, *10*: 35 (1977).

169. Svetina, S., An extended transition probability model of the variability of cell generation times. *Cell Tissue Kinet.*, *10*: 575 (1977).

170. Svetina, S. and Zekš, B., Transition probability models of the cell cycle exhibiting the age distribution for cells in the indeterministic state of the cell cycle, in *Biomathematics and Cell Kinetics* (A-j. Valleron and P. D. M. Macdonald, eds.), Elsevier, New York, p. 71 (1978).

171. Piantadosi, S., A model of growth with first-order birth and death rates. *Comp. Biomed. Res.*, *18*: 220 (1985).

172. Jansson, B., A compartmental model including cell differentiation—Stability problems and a matrix notation, in *Mathematical Models in Cell Kinetics* (A-j. Valleron, ed.), European Press Medikon, Ghent, p. 32 (1975).

173. Jansson, B., Simulation of cell-cycle kinetics based on a multi-compartmental model. *Simulation*, 25:99 (1975).

174. Jansson, B., Mathematical models of cell kinetics—Tools for designing optimal protocols for treatment, in *Proceedings of the 29th Annual Symposium of Fundamental Cancer Research* (B. Drewinko and R. M. Humphrey, eds.), Williams and Wilkins, Baltimore, pp. 379–390 (1976).

175. Sandberg, I. W., On the mathematical foundations of compartmental analysis in biology, medicine, and ecology. *IEEE Trans. Circuits Syst.*, *CAS-25*:273 (1978). See same issue. p. 379.

176. Brown R. F., Compartmental system analysis: State of the art. *IEEE Trans. Biomed. Eng.*, *BME-27*:1 (1980).

177. Jacquez, J. A., *Compartmental Analysis in Biology and Medicine* 2nd ed., University of Michigan Press, Ann Arbor (1985).

178. DiStefano, J. J. III and Landaw, E. M., Multiexponential, multicompartmental, and noncompartmental modeling. I. Methodological limitations and physiological interpretations. *Am. J. Physiol. (Regulatory Integrative Comp. Physiol. 15)*, *246*:R651 (1984).

179. Landaw, E. and DiStefano, J. J. III., Multiexponential, multi-compartmental, and noncompartmental modeling. II. Data analysis and statistical considerations. *Am. J. Physiol. (Regulatory Integrative Comp. Physiol. 15)*, *246*:R665 (1984).

180. Mendelsohn, M. L., The kinetics of tumor cell proliferation, in *Cellular Radiation Biology*, Williams and Wilkins, Baltimore, p. 498 (1965).

181. Tannock, I., Cell kinetics and chemotherapy: A critical review. *Cancer Treat. Rept.*, *62*:1117 (1978).

182. Tannock, I., Cell kinetics—Where to now? *Cell Tissue Kinet.*, *13*:571 (1980).

183. Stryckmans, P., Cronkite, E. P., Fache, J., Fliedner, T. M., and Ramos, J. Deoxyribonucleic acid synthesis time of erythropoietic granulopoietic cells in human beings. *Nature*, *211*:717 (1966).

184. Todo, A., Proliferation and differentiation of hematopoietic cells in hematologic disorders. In vivo radioautographic study of leukemia including erythroleukemia. *Acta Haematol. Japan*, *31*:947 (1968).

185. Evert, C. F., CELLDYN—A digital program for modeling the dynamics of cells. *Simulation*, *24*:55 (1975).

186. Evert, C. F. and Palusiński, O. A., Application of discrete computer modeling to the dynamics of cell populations. *Acta Haematol. Pol.*, *6*:175 (1975).

187. Donaghey, C. E. and Drewinko, B., A computer simulation program for the study of cellular growth kinetics and its application to the analysis of human lymphoma cells in vitro. *Comp. Biomed. Res.*, *8*:118 (1975).

188. Donaghey, C. E., Computer simulation of cell kinetics models, in *Growth Kinetics and Biochemical Regulation of Normal and Malignant Cells* (B. Drewinko and R. M. Humphrey, eds.), Williams and Wilkins, Baltimore, p. 157 (1977).

189. Düchting, W., A cell kinetic study on the cancer problem based on the automatic control theory using digital simulation. *J. Cybernetics*, *6*:139 (1976).

190. Düchting, W., Some aspects of analysis cancer problems by means of control theory, in *Applied General Systems Research. Recent Developments and Trends* (G. J. Klir, ed.) Plenum Press, New York, p. 601 (1978).

191. Düchting, W. and Dehl, G., Computer studies of the spatial structure and temporal growth of tumor cells. *J. Biomed. Engng.*, *2*:167 (1980).

192. Düchting, W. and Vogelsaenger, Th., Aspects of modelling and simulating tumor growth and treatment. *J. Cancer Res. Clin. Oncol.*, *105*:1 (1983).

193. Düchting, W. and Vogelsaenger, Th., Modeling and simulation of growing spheroids. *Recent Results in Cancer Research*, *95*: 168 (1984).

194. Düchting, W. and Vogelsaenger, Th., Recent progress in modelling and simulation of three-dimensional tumor growth and treatment. *Bio. Systems*, *18*:79 (1985).

195. DeVita, V. T., Cell kinetics and the chemotherapy of cancer. *Cancer Chem. Rept. Part 3*, *2*:23 (1971).

196. Valeriote, F. A. and Edelstein, M. B., The role of cell kinetics in cancer chemotherapy. *Seminars in Oncol.*, *4*:217 (1977).

197. Hill, B. T., Cancer chemotherapy. The relevance of certain concepts of cell cycle kinetics. *Biochim. Biophys. Acta, 516*: 389 (1978).

198. Bingham, C. A., The cell cycle and cancer chemotherapy. *Am. J. Nursing*, *78*:1201 (1978).

199. van Putten, L. M., Cell kinetics, a guide for chemotherapy? in *Controversies in Cancer* (H. J. Tagnon and M. J. Staquet, eds.), Masson, New York, p. 117 (1979).

200. Walker, P. B. M., The mitotic index and interphase processes. *J. Expt. Biol.*, *31*:8 (1954).

201. Scherbaum, O. and Rasch, G., Cell size distribution and single cell growth in Tetrahymena Pyriformis GL. *Acta Pathol. Microbial. Scand.*, *41*:161 (1957).

202. von Foerster, H., Some remarks on changing populations, in *The Kinetics of Cellular Proliferation* (F. Stohlman Jr., ed.), Grune and Stratton, New York, p. 382 (1959).

203. Trucco, E., Mathematical models for cellular systems. The von Foerster equation. Part 1. *Bull. Math. Biophys.*, *27*: 285 (1965).

204. Trucco, E., Mathematical models for cellular systems. The von Foerster equation. Part 2. *Bull. Math. Biophys.*, *27*: 449 (1965).

205. Harris, T. E., A mathematical model for multiplication by binary fission, *The Kinetics of Cellular Proliferation* (F. Stohlman Jr., ed.), Grune and Stratton, New York, p. 368 (1959).

206. Rubinow, S. I., A maturity-time representation for cell populations. *Biophys. J.*, *8*:1055 (1968).

207. Haddow, A., David A. Karnofsky Memorial Lecture: Thoughts on chemical therapy. *Cancer*, *26*:737 (1970).

208. Burchenal, J. H., The historical development of cancer chemotherapy. *Seminars Oncol.*, *4*:135 (1977).

209. Goodman, L. S., Wintrobe, M. M., Dameshek, W., Goodman, M. J., Sternberg, S., and McLenan, M. T., Nitrogen mustard therapy. *JAMA*, *132*:126 (1946).

210. Farber, S., Diamond, L. K., Mercer, R. D., Sylvester, R. J. Jr., and Wolff, J. A., Temporary remissions in acute leukemia in children produced by folic acid antagonist 4-aminopteroyl-glutamic acid (aminopterin). *N. Eng. J. Med.*, *238*:787 (1948).

211. Frei, E. III., Curative cancer chemotherapy. *Cancer Res.*, *45*: 6523 (1985).

212. Tobey, R. A., Different drugs arrest cells at distinct stages in G_2. *Nature*, *254*:245 (1975).

213. Dibrov, B. R., Zhabotinsky, A. M., Neyfakh, A. Yu.,
     Orlova, M. P., and Churikova, L. I., Optimal scheduling for
     cell synchronization by cycle-phase-specific blockers. *Math.
     Biosci.*, *66*:167 (1983).

214. Skipper, H. E., Schabel, F. M., Jr., and Wilcox, W. S.,
     Experimental evaluation of potential anti-cancer agents. XIII.
     On the criteria and kinetics associated with "curability" of
     experimental leukemia. *Cancer Chem. Rept.*, *35*:1 (1964).

215. Chuang, S.-N. and Lloyd, H. H., Mathematical analysis of
     cancer chemotherapy. *Bull. Math. Biol.*, *37*:147 (1975).

216. Cooley, J. W. and Tukey, J. S., An algorithm for the
     machine calculation of complex Fourier series. *Math. Comput.*,
     19:297 (1965).

217. Simon, R. M., Stroot, M. T., and Weiss, G. H., Numerical
     inversion of Laplace transforms with application to percentage
     labelled mitoses experiments. *Comp. Biomedic. Res.*, *5*:596
     (1972).

218. Chuang, S.-N., Mathematic models for cancer chemotherapy:
     Pharmacokinetic and cell kinetic considerations. *Cancer Chem.
     Rept. Part 1*, *59*:827 (1975).

219. Shackney, S. E., A computer model for tumor growth and
     chemotherapy and its application to L1210 leukemia treated
     with cytosine arabinoside (NSC-63878). *Cancer Chem. Rept.
     Part 1*, *54*:399 (1970).

220. Chuang, S.-N. and Soong, T. T., Mathematical analysis of
     cancer chemotherapy: The effects of chemotherapeutic agents
     on the cell cycle traverse. *Bull. Math. Biol.*, *40*:499 (1978).

221. Cline, M. J., *The White Cell*, Harvard University Press,
     Cambridge (1975).

222. Clarkson, B. and Rubinow, S. I., Growth kinetics in human
     leukemia, in *Growth Kinetics and Biochemical Regulation of
     Normal and Malignant Cells* (B. Drewinko and R. M. Humphrey,
     eds.), Williams and Wilkins, Baltimore, p. 591 (1977).

223. Rubinow, S. I. and Lebowitz, J. L., A mathematical model of
     neutrophil production and control in normal man. *J. Math.
     Biol.*, *1*:187 (1975).

224. Rubinow, S. I. and Lebowitz, J. L., A mathematical model of
     the acute myeloblastic leukemic state in man. *Biophys. J.*, *16*:
     897 (1976).

225. Rubinow, S. I. and Lebowitz, J. L., A mathematical model of the chemotherapeutic treatment of acute myeloblastic leukemia. *Biophys. J.*, *16*:1257 (1976).

226. Rubinow, S. I., The dynamic two-state model of the kinetic behavior of cell populations, in *Differentiation of Normal and Neoplastic Hematopoietic Cells*, Cold Spring Harbor Laboratory, p. 93 (1978).

227. Kitamura, S., Takekawa, A., Mori, H., and Yamaguchi, N., A discrete-time model for acute leukemic process, its parameter estimation and clinical applications, in *Proceedings of IFAC*, Budapest, p. 75 (1984).

228. Athans, M. and Falb, P. L., *Optimal Control*, McGraw-Hill, New York (1966).

229. Swan, G. W., Some strategies for harvesting a single species. *Bull. Math. Biol.*, *37*:659 (1975).

230. Swan, G. W., Optimal control applications in biomedical engineering—a survey. *Optim. Control Appl. Methods*, *2*:311 (1981).

231. Swan, G. W. and Alexandro, F. J., Optimization of CNS methotrexate therapy, unpublished report to the National Cancer Institute (1979).

232. Swan, G. W. and Alexandro, F. J., Modeling methotrexate therapy for treatment of brain tumors, in *Proceedings of the 11th Pittsburgh Conference on Modeling and Simulation*, Instrument Society of America, Pittsburgh, p. 289 (1980).

233. Swan, G. W., An optimal control model of diabetes mellitus. *Bull. Math. Biol.*, *44*:793 (1982).

234. Swan, G. W., Optimal control in chemotherapy, *Biomed. Measure. Inform. Control*, *1*:3 (1986).

235. Swan, G. W., Optimal control analysis of a cancer chemotherapy problem, *IMA Jl. Mathematics Applied in Medicine and Biology*, to appear.

236. Holford, N. H. G. and Sheiner, L. B., Pharmacokinetic and pharmacodynamic modeling in vivo. *CRC Crit. Revs. Bioeng.*, *5*:273 (1981).

237. Brook, J., Bateman, J. R., Gocka, E. F., Nakamura, E., and Steinfeld, J. L., Long-term low dose melphalan treatment of multiple myeloma. *Arch. Intern. Med.*, *131*:545 (1973).

238. Farhangi, M. and Osserman, E. F., The treatment of multiple myeloma. *Semin. Haemat.*, *10*:149 (1973).

239. Buckles, R. G., New horizons in drug delivery. *CA-Cancer Jl. Clin.*, 28:343 (1978).

240. Dorr, R. T., Trinca, C. E., Griffith, K., Dombrowsky, P. L., and Salmon, S. E., Limitations of a portable infusion pump in ambulatory patients receiving continuous infusions of anticancer drugs. *Cancer Treat. Rept.*, 63:211 (1979).

241. McKinstry, D. W., Implanted drug delivery system for regional cancer chemotherapy. *Research Resources Reporter*, 5:1 (1981).

242. Cohen, A. M., Greenfield, A., and Wood, W. C., Treatment of hepatic artery chemotherapy using an implanted drug pump. *Cancer*, 51:2013 (1983).

243. Weiss, G. R., Garnick, M. B., Osteen, R. T., et al., Long-term hepatic arterial infusion of 5-fluorodeoxyuridine for liver metastases using an implantable infusion pump. *J. Clin. Oncol.*, 1:337 (1983).

244. Shepard, K. V., Levin, B., Karl, R. C., Faintuch, J., DuBrow, R. A., Hagle, M., Cooper, R. M., Beschorner, J., and Stablein, D., Therapy for metastatic colorectal cancer with hepatic artery infusion chemotherapy using a subcutaneous implanted pump. *J. Clin. Oncol.*, 3:161 (1985).

245. Kreis, W., Chaudhri, F., Chan. K., et al., Pharmacokinetics of low-dose 1-β-D-arabinofuranosylcytosine given by continuous intravenous infusion over twenty-one days. *Cancer Res.*, 45:6498 (1985).

246. Degos, L., Castaigne, S., Tilly, H., Sigaux, F., and Daniel, M. T., Treatment of leukemia with low-dose ara-C: A study of 160 cases. *Seminars Oncol.*, 12 No. 2 Suppl. 3:196 (1985).

247. Swan, G. W., On-line control of chemotherapy—Fact or fiction? presented at the conference New Concepts in Patient Care: Sensors, Pharmacokinetics, Adaptive Control, and Drug Delivery Systems, University of Washington, Seattle, Oct. 24, 1985.

248. Giraldo, G., Beth, E., Castello, G., Giordano, G. G., and Zarrilli, D., eds., *From Oncogenes to Tumor Antigens*, Elsevier, Amsterdam (1985).

249. Schumitzky, A., Stochastic control of pharmacokinetic systems, Technical Report: 85-2, University of Southern California School of Medicine, Laboratory of Applied Pharmacokinetics (1985).

250. *Seminars in Oncology*, Sept. 1985.

251. Bischoff, K. B., Dedrick, R. L., Zaharko, D. S., and Long-streth, J. A., Methotrexate pharmacokinetics. *J. Pharm. Sci.*, *60*:1128 (1971).

252. Reich, S. D., Application of advanced modelling techniques to anticancer drug pharmacokinetics, in *Pharmacokinetics of Anticancer Agents in Humans* (M. M. Ames, G. Powis, and J. S. Kovach, eds.), Elsevier, Amsterdam, p. 29 (1983).

252. Kuzma, J. W., Valand, I., and Bateman, J., A tumor cell model for the determination of drug schedules and drug effect in tumor reduction. *Bull. Math. Biophys.*, *31*:637 (1969).

254. Oğuztöreli, M. N., Tsokos, C. P., and Akabutu, J., A kinetic study of chemotherapy. *Appl. Math. Comp.*, *12*:255 (1983).

255. *Models for Biomedical Research. A New Prospective.* National Academy Press, Washington, D. C., p. 155 (1985).

257. Meyer, J. S., Growth and cell kinetic measurements in human tumors. *Path. Ann.*, *16*:53 (1982).

258. Meyer, J. S., Cell kinetic measurements of human tumors. *Human Path.*, *13*:874 (1982).

259. Gray, J. W., Quantitative cytokinetics: cellular response to cell cycle specific agents. *Pharmac. Ther.*, *22*:163 (1983).

260. Dibrov, B. F., Zhabotinsky, A. M., Neyfakh, Yu. A., Orlova, M. P., Churikova, L. I., Mathematical model of cancer chemotherapy. Periodic schedules of phase-specific cytotoxic-agent administration increasing the selectivity of therapy. *Math. Biosci.*, *73*:1 (1985).

261. Frenzen, C. L. and Murray, J. D., A cell kinetics justification for Gompertz' equation. *SIAM J. Appl. Math.*, *46*:614 (1986).

262. *Bull. Math. Biol.*, *48*:239 (1986).

263. Norton, L., Tumor growth kinetics. *The Mt. Sinai J. Med.*, *52*:March (1985).

4
Cell Population Models with Continuous Structure Variables

SUSAN L. TUCKER   *Department of Biomathematics, M.D. Anderson Hospital and Tumor Institute, The University of Texas System Cancer Center, Houston, Texas*

I. INTRODUCTION

The precise mechanism by which cancer kills an organism is not yet known, but it is clear that the "severity" of cancer is in some way related to the number of cancer cells present. For this reason, a wealth of mathematical models for tumor growth involving cell number has appeared in the literature.

The simplest models are those in which total cell number is expressed as a function of time, without distinguishing among cells on the basis of biochemical or physiological differences. The best-known and most frequently used model of this sort is the exponential model.

$$\frac{dN}{dt} = \gamma N \quad \text{or} \quad N(t) = N_0 e^{\gamma t} \tag{1}$$

where N_0 is the initial population size, $N(t)$ is the population size at time t, and the constant γ is the population growth rate. Two other well-known models involving total cell number are the logistic model

$$\frac{dN}{dt} = (\gamma_1 - \gamma_2 N)N \tag{2}$$

and the Gompertz model

$$\frac{dN}{dt} = \gamma_1 \, N \, \ln \left(\frac{\gamma_2}{N} \right) \tag{3}$$

where γ_1 and γ_2 are constants in each case. Whereas the exponential model assumes a constant population growth rate and, therefore, allows the population to become arbitrarily large, the logistic and Gompertz models assume that the growth rate depends on the population size. In particular, the growth rate tends to zero as the population approaches a limiting size. These models and others for total population size as a function of the single variable time are discussed in more detail by Swan [1].

As useful as population size models are for describing and analyzing tumor growth, they have in common a serious limitation. It is now well known that the cells making up a tumor are heterogeneous with respect to proliferative capacity, nutritional status, oxygen content, and other factors influencing their response to radiation and chemotherapeutic agents. Moreover, even cells in an otherwise homogeneous population will respond differently to drugs and radiation, depending on their relative positions in the cell cycle. Therefore, realistic models of cell populations and, ultimately, models of tumor treatment must include some mechanism for distinguishing among individual cells on the basis of one or more factors.

This chapter concerns cell population models containing continuous structure variables. A structure variable is some characteristic, such as age, volume, or DNA content, that might distinguish one cell from another; continuous structure variables are those that can assume a continuum of distinct values. These models could be contrasted, for example, with compartmental models in which each cell, at each time, is assumed to occupy one of only a finite number of discrete states. (For a discussion of compartmental models, see [2].)

Where possible, the ability of each model to reproduce observed cell population behavior will be discussed. In this connection, two characteristics of cell populations are worth mentioning at the outset. In a population of proliferating cells, each cell must double its DNA content during its lifetime in order to pass on a copy of its genetic material to each of two daughter cells at mitosis. In 1953, Howard and Pelc [3] showed that DNA synthesis occurs only during a portion of the cell cycle, or cell lifetime. This portion of the cell cycle was dubbed "S phase." After the birth of a cell, before onset of DNA synthesis, an intermitotic gap called G_1 occurs, and between the end of S phase and the beginning of mitosis (M), there is a second gap, G_2. Although DNA synthesis does not take place during G_1 or G_2, other biochemical events, such as RNA synthesis, occur then.

A fundamental characteristic of every otherwise apparently homogeneous cell population is that there is considerable variation in the generation times, or cell cycle times, of individual cells. Most of the variation, both under constant and varying environmental conditions, occurs in the length of G_1; the duration of $S + G_2 + M$ tends to be fairly constant for cells of any particular type. Experiments in which cells are synchronized at some point in the cell cycle show that synchrony is lost quite rapidly. That the variation in generation times is not due simply to inherent cell heterogeneity has been demonstrated by the same loss of synchrony in populations derived from single cells [4].

A second important characteristic of cells grown in batch culture is that before crowding sets in, the population quickly attains a state that is variously known as asynchronous, balanced, or steady-state exponential growth, in which the total population size grows exponentially with an intrinsic growth rate γ, but the proportion of cells in the population with any particular characteristic (e.g., age, volume, or DNA content) remains constant. This feature of cell populations has been used to investigate the underlying population dynamics (e.g., [5]). That is, by assuming a population to have *reached* a state of balanced exponential growth, we can estimate the rate of change of some structure variable (such as cell volume) from an experimentally determined distribution of cells with respect to that structure variable. This procedure requires a structured population model. An important consideration for any such model, therefore, is whether it is able to reproduce the phenomenon of balanced exponential growth for the population as a whole while allowing variation in the generation times of individual cells.

The variety of different structure variables included in published cell population models reflects ongoing disagreement concerning the factors responsible for regulation of mitosis and the source or sources of variation in cell cycle times. An attempt has been made here to discuss representatives of most of the major types of structured cell cycle models, but given the vastness of the literature, this survey is by no means exhaustive.

II. AGE-STRUCTURED MODELS

A. Models with Random Cycle Lengths

The earliest structured models that were applied to the description of cell populations were age-structured models. For such models, the structure variable is chronological age—i.e., the time elapsed since the birth of the cell from division of its mother cell.

Let a denote cell age, and let $n(a, t)$ be the population density function at time t. Since n is a density, the number of cells in the population at time t whose ages lie between a_1 and a_2 $(a_1 \leqslant a_2)$ is given by the integral

$$\int_{a_1}^{a_2} n(a, t) \, da$$

Scherbaum and Rasch [6] introduced the following model for the dynamics of an age-structured population:

$$\frac{\partial n}{\partial t}(a, t) + \frac{\partial n}{\partial a}(a, t) = 0 \tag{4}$$

A more general form for (4), one that does not require a priori that the solution n have partial derivatives, is

$$D_{(1,1)} n(a, t) = 0 \tag{5}$$

where

$$D_{(1,1)} n(a, t) \overset{\text{def}}{=} \lim_{h \to 0^+} \frac{n(a + h, t + h) - n(a, t)}{h} \tag{6}$$

is the directional derivative of n in the direction of the vector $(1, 1)$. Scherbaum and Rasch assumed the cycle time T to be equal for all cells. Thus their model is augmented by the boundary condition

$$n(0, t) = 2n(T, t) \tag{7}$$

and the initial condition

$$n(a, 0) = n_0(t) \tag{8}$$

representing the age distribution of the population at time $t = 0$.

The major drawback to the model of Scherbaum and Rasch is that it does not take into account the known existence of variation in cell cycle times, nor does it allow for the possible loss of cells from the population due to cell death or other causes. These limitations were corrected by von Foerster [7], who considered the model

$$\frac{\partial n}{\partial t}(a, t) + \frac{\partial n}{\partial a}(a, t) = -\lambda(a) \, n(a, t) \tag{9}$$

where $\lambda(a)$ is a loss term representing the probability per unit time that a cell of age a is lost from the population. The loss term is the sum of two components: $\lambda = \lambda_m + \lambda_d$, where λ_m is the "loss" rate due to mitosis—i.e., due to division of cells of age a into two daughters of age zero—and λ_d is the loss rate due to cell death or disappearance from all other causes. The boundary condition (7) is replaced by

$$n(0, t) = 2 \int_0^\infty \lambda_m(a)n(a, t) \, da \tag{10}$$

In other words, the number of new cells per unit time (at time t) is the sum, over all ages, of the expected number of daughters produced, in total, by cells of age a.

Formally, von Foerster's model is identical to the older McKendrick model [8] of age-structured growth for arbitrary populations which was used, for example, in demography. In the McKendrick model, the mitotic term $2\lambda_m(a)$ in (10) is replaced by the more general birth modulus $\beta(a)$, the average number of offspring produced per unit time by an individual of age a.

An expression for the solution to the McKendrick model is obtained by integrating along the characteristic curves t = a + constant:

$$n(a, t) = \begin{cases} n(0, t - a) \exp\left[-\int_0^a \lambda(\alpha) \, d\alpha\right] & \text{for } a < t \\[3em] n_0(a - t) \exp\left[-\int_{a-t}^a \lambda(\alpha) \, d\alpha\right] & \text{for } a \geqslant t \end{cases} \tag{11}$$

Letting B(t) denote the quantity n(0, t) and substituting (11) into the McKendrick version of the boundary condition (10) gives

$$B(t) = \int_0^t \beta(a) \, B(t - a) \exp\left[-\int_0^a \lambda(\alpha) \, d\alpha\right] da$$
$$+ \int_t^\infty \beta(a) \, n_0(a - t) \exp\left[-\int_{a-t}^a \lambda(\alpha) \, d\alpha\right] da \tag{12}$$

Thus, a solution n(a, t) to the population model can be reduced to a solution B(t) of the integral equation (12). The reduction of the problem to an integral equation is typical in the study of structured population models.

By definition, a balanced, stationary, or steady-state age distribution for the von Foerster model is a solution of the form n(a, t) = N(a)h(t). That is, the total population size may vary with time, but the proportion of the population in any age bracket remains constant.

Substituting the expression for a stationary age distribution into the population balance law (9) yields the condition

$$\frac{dN/da}{N(a)} + \lambda(a) = -\frac{dh/dt}{h(t)} \tag{13}$$

Since the left side of (13) is a function of age alone, whereas the right side is a function of time, the expression on each side must be constant. In particular, h(t) is proportional to $e^{\gamma t}$ for some constant γ (the intrinsic growth rate), so balanced population growth cannot occur unless the population as a whole grows exponentially (though possibly with growth rate $\gamma=0$). It then follows from integrating (13) that the age distribution N(a) has the form

$$N(a) = N(0) \exp\left[-\gamma a - \int_0^a \lambda(\alpha)\, d\alpha\right] \tag{14}$$

If N(0) = 0, then the steady-state solution n(a, t) = $N(a)e^{\gamma t}$ is identically zero. Otherwise, the birth condition (10) together with (14) implies that γ is a solution to the characteristic equation

$$1 = 2\int_0^\infty \lambda_m(a) \exp\left[-\gamma a - \int_0^a \lambda(\alpha)\, d\alpha\right] da \tag{15}$$

and for such γ, (14) determines a balanced age distribution for every choice of N(0). Under appropriate assumptions on the loss functions λ_m and λ_d, it can be shown that (15) has a unique solution γ. For example, if the mitotic rate λ_m is independent of age and if $\lambda_d = 0$, then $\gamma = \lambda_m$ is the unique solution to (15).

Feller [9] considered the time-dependent behavior of solutions to the McKendrick model. Under appropriate hypotheses on the birth and loss rates, Feller showed that solutions to the McKendrick model and, consequently, to the von Foerster model, exhibit the property of asynchronous exponential growth that is observed experimentally in cell populations in the absence of such limiting factors as cell crowding or nutritional deprivation. That is, every initial cell distribution evolves toward the unique stationary age distribution. More precisely, if n(a, t) is the solution to the von Foerster model corresponding to the initial distribution $n_0(a)$ and if γ is the unique solution to equation (15), then

$$\lim_{t \to \infty} \left| e^{-\gamma t} n(a, t) - N(a) \right| = 0 \tag{16}$$

uniformly on bounded subsets of age a, where $N(a)$ is defined by (14), and the constant $N(0)$ in (14) depends only on the initial age distribution $n_0(a)$.

In the von Foerster model of cell population dynamics, the variability in cell cycle times among individual cells is attributed entirely to a single random event, namely the probabilistic entry of a cell into mitosis governed by the term λ_m. A similar idea was proposed by Burns and Tannock [10], and later by Smith and Martin [11], who presented a model of the cell cycle that has come to be known as the *transition probability* model. In that model, the cell cycle is regarded as consisting of two distinct phases—a random phase and a deterministic phase, called A state and B phase, respectively. After division of a mother cell, both daughters are assumed to enter the random A state, where they are not actively progressing toward division and may remain for an indefinite length of time. Cells leave A state with some constant probability p per unit time (the transition probability) and enter B phase, which is assumed to have constant duration t_B. A cell divides when it completes B phase, and its daughters again enter A state. The deterministic B phase is regarded as representing that portion of the cell cycle of relatively constant duration, i.e., $S + G_2 + M$, and possibly some part of G_1 that might be essential for onset of DNA synthesis. The random A state represents G_1, or part of G_1, and therefore the transition probability model incorporates the observation that essentially all of the variation in cell cycle times occurs in G_1. Although the transition probability model was not presented explicitly as an age-structured model, it is included here in part because of its influence in the cell kinetic literature. Moreover, the model can be formulated in terms of the population balance law (9) by suppressing the distinction between A state and B phase, and using for the age-dependent rate of cell division the function

$$\lambda_m(a) \overset{\text{def}}{=} \begin{cases} 0 & \text{for } 0 \leqslant a \leqslant t_B \\ p & \text{for } a > t_B \end{cases} \tag{17}$$

The transition probability model and the von Foerster model are similar in that each attributes the variability in cycle lengths to the occurrence of a single random event, but the two models differ in

their views of when in the cell cycle the random event occurs (i.e.,
before or after DNA synthesis). Consequently, nonlinear versions
of the models involving regulation mechanisms for the transition
probability p would necessarily differ because of the differences in
timing of the random event.

Smith and Martin introduced a concept called the α-curve [11],
which illustrates the fit of the transition probability model to experimental data and is now widely used in the cell kinetic literature.
The function $\alpha(t)$ is defined to be the proportion of cells in the
population with generation times greater than or equal to t. Note
that $\alpha(t)$ is not well defined unless balanced exponential population
growth has been attained. The transition probability model predicts
the following expression for $\alpha(t)$:

$$\alpha(t) = \begin{cases} 1 & \text{for } 0 \leqslant t \leqslant t_B \\ \exp[-p(t - t_B)] & \text{for } t > t_B \end{cases} \tag{18}$$

In general, the model fits experimental data reasonably well, except
that in semilogarithmic coordinates the data are usually better described by a smooth curve near $t = t_B$ than by the piecewise linear
curve predicted by (18). This indicates that there is some variation
in the length of B phase as well as in the length of A state.

The transition probability model also provides an explanation for
the observed correlation between the generation times of sibling cells,
and also for the differences between the cycle times of sister cells.
This was noted by Minor and Smith [12], who defined the function
$\beta(t)$ to be the proportion of sibling pairs in which the two sister
cells have cycle times differing by at least t. According to the
transition probability model,

$$\beta(t) = e^{-pt} \tag{19}$$

so that although sister cells are expected to have different cycle
lengths, they are more likely to have cycle times differing by a
small amount than by a large amount. Equation (19) provides a good
fit to experimental data [12]. Note that the transition probability
model predicts the terminal slope of the α-curve, in semilogarithmic
coordinates, to be equal to the slope of the β-curve, which is, in
fact, usually observed in experimental data.

Burns and Tannock [10] emphasize that an advantage of the
transition probability model, compared with certain other cell population models, is that this model does not require a distinction between
the G_0 and G_1 phases of the cell cycle. The existence of a distinct
G_0 state was postulated by Lajtha [13] to explain the ability of
tissues such as liver to regenerate after injury. In a normal liver,

the proportion of cells undergoing DNA synthesis or mitosis at any time is quite small. However, after depletion of liver cells, e.g., via irradiation or surgical removal of part of the tissue, the proportion of actively proliferating cells increases dramatically. Lajtha suggested that under normal conditions, the majority of the cells are in a quiescent, or G_0 state, separate from the $G_1 + S + G_2 + M$ cell cycle. After injury, however, these G_0 cells could be recruited back into active proliferation.

Burns and Tannock point out that a large, apparently quiescent subpopulation could be explained on the basis of a very small transition probability from A state to B phase; increased recruitment into cycle could result simply from an increase in transition probability after tissue injury. The suggestion that there is no true quiescent phase is supported by data from cells exposed to radioactive thymidine. Thymidine is incorporated into the DNA of cells during S phase, and if exposure is brief, only those cells in S phase at the time of exposure will be radioactively labeled. However, experiments with slowly proliferating cell populations [10,14] have shown that all cells ultimately become labeled after prolonged thymidine exposure, indicating that all cells are in cycle. Data showing that the transition probability p can in fact be modified was presented by Smith and Martin [11]; for their data the value of p depended on culture conditions, although it is interesting to note that slight changes in the duration of B phase were also observed.

B. Inherited Cycle Length Models

1. The Model of Lebowitz and Rubinow

As an alternative to age-structured models in which variation in cell cycle times is attributed to occurrence of a random event, Lebowitz and Rubinow [15] proposed an age-structured model in which the generation time of each individual cell is determined at birth. In their model, variation in cell cycle times is due instead to a distribution in inherited generation times, and the model therefore includes a rule for determining the cycle length of a newborn cell. A major difference between the model of Lebowitz and Rubinow and that of von Foerster is that the concept of an inherited (i.e., predetermined) cycle time allows the possibility that the generation time of a cell depends at least in part on that of its mother. This is a matter of considerable debate: some investigators have found positive correlations between the cycle times of mother and daughter cells [16–18]; others have found negative correlations [19,20]; and still others have found no correlation at all [19,21].

The population density function in the model of Lebowitz and Rubinow has the form $n(a, t; \tau)$; the integral

$$\int_{a_1}^{a_2} \int_{\tau_1}^{\tau_2} n(a, t; \tau) \, d\tau \, da \qquad (a_1 \leqslant a_2; \ \tau_1 \leqslant \tau_2) \qquad (20)$$

represents the number of cells present at time t in the age bracket
$[a_1, a_2]$ whose cycle times lie between τ_1 and τ_2. Since each cell
divides when its age reaches its cycle time, $n(a, t; \tau) = 0$ for $a > \tau$.

For any particular cell, the value of the parameter τ does not
vary. Therefore, the population balance law is formally the same
as that for the von Foerster model of equation (9), namely

$$\frac{\partial n}{\partial t}(a, t; \tau) + \frac{\partial n}{\partial a}(a, t; \tau) = -\lambda(a)n(a, t; \tau) \qquad (21)$$

[More precisely, (21) is a parameterized family of balance laws, one
for each possible value of the cycle length τ.] Unlike the von
Foerster model, however, the loss term λ in (21) does not include
loss of cells of age a due to mitosis since (21) applies only for
$a < \tau$, i.e., for cell age less than the cell cycle length.

The boundary condition for the model is

$$n(0, t; \tau) = 2 \int_0^{\infty} K(\tau, \tau')n(\tau', t; \tau') \, d\tau' \qquad (22)$$

where the kernel $K(\tau, \tau')$, called the transition probability function
by Lebowitz and Rubinow, gives the probability that a dividing cell
of cycle length τ' produces a daughter cell with cycle length τ.
Since every cell must be assigned some cycle length at birth, K
satisfies the requirement

$$\int_0^{\infty} K(\tau, \tau') \, d\tau = 1 \qquad (23)$$

The factor 2 in (22) arises from the assumption that every dividing
cell produces two daughters. The choice of the transition kernel K
determines the degree of correlation between mother and daughter
cells. For example, if $K(\tau, \tau') = \delta(\tau - \tau')$, where δ denotes the
Dirac delta function, then every cell inherits the precise cycle
length of its mother. On the other hand, τ might be independent
of τ', the cycle time of the mother, in which case there is no
mother-daughter correlation and the Lebowitz-Rubinow model reduces
to that of von Foerster.

Since the balance law (21) is the same, for each τ, as (9), it follows from the discussion of the von Foerster model that a steady-state solution to the Lebowitz-Rubinow model must have the form

$$n(a, t; \tau) = \begin{cases} N(a; \tau)e^{\gamma t} & \text{for } 0 \leqslant a \leqslant \tau \\ 0 & \text{for } a > \tau \end{cases} \tag{24}$$

for some constant γ and for some distribution $N(a; \tau)$ of ages and cell cycle times. Integration of (21) shows that the steady-state distribution satisfies

$$N(a; \tau) = N(0; \tau)\exp\left[-\gamma a - \int_0^a \lambda(\alpha)\,d\alpha\right] \tag{25}$$

It then follows from the boundary condition (22) that the steady-state distribution $N(0; \tau)$ of generation times of newborn cells is required to satisfy the equation

$$N(0; \tau) = 2\int_0^\infty K(\tau, \tau')N(0; \tau')\exp\left[-\gamma\tau' - \int_0^{\tau'} \lambda(\alpha)\,d\alpha\right] d\tau' \tag{26}$$

Thus a necessary condition for the existence of a steady-state solution to the model of Lebowitz and Rubinow is that the integral equation (26) have a solution $N(0; \tau)$. It is evident that the existence of such a solution will depend on the transition kernel K. Consequently, one question of interest concerns properties of K that will guarantee the existence of a solution $N(0; \tau)$ to (26). If a solution to (26) exists for which

$$\int_0^\infty N(0; \tau)\,d\tau$$

is defined and nonzero, then integration of (26) with respect to τ implies that the growth rate γ is a solution to the equation

$$1 = 2\int_0^\infty g(\tau')\exp\left[-\gamma\tau' - \int_0^{\tau'} \lambda(\alpha)\,d\alpha\right] d\tau' \tag{27}$$

where $g(\tau')$ is the function

$$g(\tau') \overset{\text{def}}{=} \frac{N(0; \tau')}{\displaystyle\int_0^\infty N(0; \tau)\, d\tau} \tag{28}$$

When a solution to (26) does exist, however, it does not necessarily correspond to a solution of the cell population model representing balanced exponential growth. For example, Lebowitz and Rubinow
[15] note that if λ is constant and if there is perfect memory of
generation times—i.e., if $K(\tau, \tau') = \delta(\tau - \tau')$—then the model has
the infinite family of solutions $N(0; \tau) = \delta(\tau - \tau^*)$ for arbitrary τ^*,
with γ satisfying $1 = 2 \exp(-\gamma\tau^*)$. In this case, as observed
earlier by Rubinow [22], the population will rapidly be dominated by
cells having the shortest cycle length. Therefore, the population converges to one of infinitely many possible states, depending on the
initial data $n_0(a; \tau)$.

2. Results of Webb: Asynchronous Exponential Growth

Webb [23-24] has studied the time-dependent behavior of solutions
to the model of Lebowitz and Rubinow. In particular, he has considered conditions on the transition kernel K sufficient to guarantee
that solutions to the Lebowitz-Rubinow model converge asymptotically
to a state of balanced exponential growth.

   Webb's approach to the study of the Lebowitz-Rubinow model is
based on the theory of strongly continuous semigroups of bounded
linear operators. Certain of his results are applicable not only to
the inherited cycle length model but to linear structured population
models in general, and they will be outlined in this section.

   The use of operator theory in the study of population models requires that solutions to the model be contained in a Banach space
of functions. For example, in the model of Lebowitz and Rubinow,
suppose that time is normalized so that the cycle length of a cell lies
in the interval [0, 1]. At each time t, a solution to the Lebowitz-
Rubinow model is therefore a function defined on the triangle

$$T \overset{\text{def}}{=} \{(a, \tau): \ 0 \leqslant a \leqslant \tau \ \text{ and } \ 0 \leqslant \tau \leqslant 1\} \tag{29}$$

Let B be the space of continuous real-valued functions ϕ on T that
satisfy the condition

$$\phi(0, \tau) = 2\int_0^1 K(\tau, \tau')\phi(\tau', \tau')\, d\tau' \tag{30}$$

i.e., the functions in B satisfy the boundary condition (22). It can easily be verified that B forms a Banach space when equipped with the sup norm

$$\| \phi \| \overset{\text{def}}{=} \sup_{(a,\tau)\epsilon T} | \phi(a, \tau) | \tag{31}$$

Under appropriate conditions on the transition kernel K, Webb shows [23], by solving (21) along the characteristic curves t = a + constant, that for any initial distribution ϕ ε B of ages and cycle times, the model of Lebowitz and Rubinow has a unique solution n(a, t; τ) existing for all time. Moreover, one can show that n(a, t; τ) is continuous on T for each t, so the boundary condition (22) implies that the function n(a, t; τ) is in the Banach space B for each time t.

Since the population distribution n remains for all time in the Banach space B, provided the initial function ϕ is in B, it follows that one can define a family of operators {S(t): t ≥ 0} on B by

$$S(t)\phi(a,\tau) \overset{\text{def}}{=} n(a, t; \tau) \tag{32}$$

That is, for t ≥ 0, S(t) is the operator that transforms an initial distribution ϕ(a, τ) into the corresponding solution n(a, t; τ) of the Lebowitz-Rubinow model at time t.

Webb [25] shows that the collection of mappings {S(t): t ≥ 0} from the Banach space B into itself forms a *strongly continuous semigroup* of bounded linear operations. In other words, the mappings S(t) satisfy the following properties:

1. For each t ε [0, ∞), S(t) is a bounded linear operator on B. (In particular, the solution n(a, t; τ) at time t on the Lebowitz-Rubinow model depends linearly and continuously on the initial distribution ϕ.)

2. S(0) = I, where I is the identity operator [i.e., n(a, 0; τ) = ϕ(a, τ)].

3. For s, t ε [0, ∞), S(t + s) = S(t)S(s), where the latter denotes the composition of S(t) with S(s). (That is, the solution n(a, t + s; τ) corresponding to initial data ϕ is the same as the solution, at time t + s, corresponding to initial data n(a, t; τ), provided n(a, t; τ) is the solution at time t corresponding to initial data ϕ; this property follows from the uniqueness of solutions to the Lebowitz-Rubinow model.

4. For every ϕ ε B, the mapping from [0, ∞) into B defined by t ⟼ S(t) is continuous. (This condition says that solutions n(a, t; τ) in the Banach space B evolve continuously with time.)

Webb [25] makes the following definition concerning the asymptotic behavior of solutions to a linear structured population model: the semigroup {S(t): t ≥ 0} is said to have the property of *asynchronous exponential growth* with intrinsic growth constant γ ε [0, ∞) provided there exists a nonzero finite rank projection operator P on the Banach space B such that for every initial function φ in B,

$$\lim_{t \to \infty} e^{-\gamma t} S(t)\phi = P\phi \qquad (33)$$

In other words, asynchronous exponential growth occurs if every solution to the model converges asymptotically to one of a finite number of states of balanced exponential growth. Webb's use of the phrase "asynchronous exponential growth" differs somewhat from that of many other authors, who use it to describe a population that has already *reached* a state of balanced exponential growth.

For many population models, the rank of the projection operator P is equal to 1. In that case, there is a unique distribution φ*, characteristic of the population, such that every solution to the model converges to a multiple of the function $\phi^* e^{\gamma t}$. In particular, the proportion of the population with structure values lying in a specified range approaches a constant as t → ∞. In practice, i.e., in experiments with cell populations growing in an unlimited environment, the steady-state distribution is approached very rapidly, usually within just a few cell generations.

Webb [25] has determined necessary and sufficient conditions for the existence of asynchronous exponential growth. Associated with any strongly continuous semigroup {S(t): t ≥ 0} of bounded linear operators is an operator A called the *infinitesimal generator* of the semigroup. It is defined by

$$A\phi = \lim_{t \to 0^+} \left(\frac{1}{t}\right)[S(t)\phi - \phi] \qquad (34)$$

with domain consisting of those functions φ in B for which this limit exists. Roughly, Webb's result says that the strongly continuous semigroup {S(t): t ≥ 0} with infinitesimal generator A has the property of asynchronous exponential growth with intrinsic growth constant γ ε R if and only if γ is a dominant eigenvalue of A, γ is a simple pole of $(\lambda I - A)^{-1}$, and γ is greater than a constant ω_1, called the *essential growth bound* of the semigroup {S(t): t ≥ 0} (see [25] for a precise definition of ω_1).

Webb's results can be applied to the inherited cycle length model of cell populations. Lebowitz and Rubinow suggest [15] that a possible form for the transition kernel K in their model might be the function

$$K(\tau, \tau') = \beta\delta(\tau - \tau') + (1 - \beta)k[\tau - \tau_0 - \rho(\tau' - \tau_0)] \tag{35}$$

where τ_0 is the minimum generation time, β and ρ are constants, β lies in the interval $[0, 1]$, and k is a nonnegative function whose integral over $[0, \infty)$ is 1. The size of the constant β determines the amount of correlation between mother and daughter cells. For a transition kernel K of the form given by (35), one can solve for k if the distribution $g(\tau)$ of generation times is known from experimental data.

In [23], Webb considers a form for the transition kernel similar to that suggested by Lebowitz and Rubinow, namely

$$K(\tau, \tau') = r(\tau) + c\delta(\tau - \tau') \tag{36}$$

where $c \in [0, 1]$ is constant and r is a nonnegative continuous function on $[0, 1]$. Condition (23) on K implies that r and c must satisfy

$$\int_0^1 r(\tau)\, d\tau + c = 1 \tag{37}$$

Webb shows (when the loss function λ is continuous) that for the case in which fewer than half of the cells inherit the precise cycle lengths of their mothers (i.e., for $c < 1/2$), solutions to the Lebowitz-Rubinow model in the Banach space B exist for all time and have the property of asynchronous exponential growth. In fact, the rank of the projection operator P is 1, and Webb gives an explicit formula for P.

The transition kernel K given by (36) admits only positive correlations between the cycle times of mother and daughter cells. Since there is experimental evidence for negative mother-daughter correlations in some cell populations [19, 20], Webb [24] later considers a more general form for the transition kernel that could allow either a positive or a negative correlation in the cycle times of mothers and daughters.

Suppose there exist lower and upper bounds, denoted by τ_1 and τ_2, respectively, for the generation time of a cell. Let $K(\tau, \tau')$ be a nonnegative continuous function on $[\tau_1, \tau_2] \times [\tau_1, \tau_2]$ that satisfies condition (23) and for which $K(\tau_1, \tau) = K(\tau_2, \tau) = 0$, for $\tau \in [\tau_1, \tau_2]$, and $K(\tau, \tau) > 0$ for $\tau_1 < \tau < \tau_2$. Under these assumptions on K (and again assuming that the loss function is continuous), Webb shows [24] that solutions to the model form a strongly continuous semigroup $\{S(t): t \geq 0\}$ of bounded linear operators on a Banach space B and that $\{S(t): t \geq 0\}$ has the property of asynchronous exponential growth with a rank 1 projection operator. In this case, the appropriate Banach space B is the space of continuous functions $\phi(a, \tau)$ on the region

$$
T \overset{\text{def}}{=} \{(a, \tau) : 0 \leqslant a \leqslant \tau, \ \tau_1 \leqslant \tau \leqslant \tau_2\} \tag{38}
$$

such that ϕ satisfies (30) and $\phi(a, \tau_i) = 0$ for all $a \in [0, \tau_i]$, $i = 1, 2$.

III. MODELS WITH PHYSIOLOGICAL STRUCTURE VARIABLES

A. The Maturity-Time Model

A unique characteristic of any structure variable a proportional to chronological age is that da/dt is constant. Rubinow [22] proposed a model, called the maturity-time model, in which age is replaced by a structure variable μ representing some physiological measure of cell maturity that might have nonconstant rate of change $v = d\mu/dt$. For example, Rubinow suggested that μ could represent cell volume or DNA content. He postulated that all cells are born with the same level of maturity $\mu = \mu_1$ and undergo mitosis when they reach full maturity $\mu = \mu_2$. Variation in the cycle times of distinct cells would be explained by cell-to-cell differences in maturation velocity.

Let $n(\mu, t)$ represent the population density at time t with respect to the structure variable μ. The population balance law for the model of Rubinow has the form

$$
\frac{\partial n}{\partial t} + \frac{\partial}{\partial \mu} (vn) = -\lambda n \tag{39}
$$

where $\lambda(\mu)$ is the maturity-dependent proportion of cells lost per unit time due to causes other than mitosis. The maturation velocity v could depend on μ or on additional parameters such as culture conditions. Rubinow also suggested the possibility of a nonlinear model in which v depends on the population density n. Equation (39) can be derived [27,28] by regarding the cell population as an incompressible fluid moving in one dimension (maturity); then (39) is the equation for conservation of mass from fluid dynamics. The population balance law can also be made more general by writing it in the form

$$
D_{(1,v)} n = - \left(\lambda + \frac{\partial v}{\partial \mu} \right) n \tag{40}
$$

where D again denotes the directional derivative. In this formulation, a solution $n(\mu, t)$ is required a priori to be differentiable only in the direction of the (variable) vector (1, v).

If the range of possible maturity states $[\mu_1, \mu_2]$ is normalized to the interval $[0, 1]$, then the boundary condition for Rubinow's model, when maturation velocity depends on μ alone, is

$$n(0, t)v(0) = 2n(1, t)v(1) \tag{41}$$

The model also includes an initial maturity distribution

$$n(\mu, 0) = n_0(\mu) \tag{42}$$

The version of the maturity-time model just described does not explicitly include variability in the maturation velocity. If all cells have the same maturation rate $v(\mu)$, then Rubinow's model reduces to an age-structured model in which all cells divide at the same age. This is seen by applying the change of variables

$$\alpha = h(\mu) \overset{def}{=} \int_0^\mu \frac{du}{v(u)} \tag{43}$$

The integral in (43) is convergent because $v(\mu)$ is never zero; otherwise cells would never reach full maturity. Under this change of variables, equations (39) and (41) become, respectively,

$$\frac{\partial n}{\partial t} + \frac{\partial n}{\partial \alpha} = -\left(\lambda + \frac{\partial v}{\partial \mu}\right)n \tag{44}$$

and

$$n(0, t) = 2 \int_0^\infty \frac{v(\alpha)}{v(0)} \delta(\alpha - \alpha_1)n(\alpha, t)\, d\alpha \tag{45}$$

where α_1 is given by (43) with $\mu = 1$. Thus the model is like that of Scherbaum and Rasch [6], with the addition of a cell loss term. Webb [25] has investigated this model in terms of a strongly continuous semigroup $\{S(t): t \geq 0\}$ of bounded linear operators, and has shown, by demonstrating that the infinitesimal generator of $\{S(t)\}$ has no dominant eigenvalue, that solutions to Rubinow's model, when all cells have the same maturation function, do not exhibit the property of asynchronous exponential growth.

When the cell population is instead assumed to consist of subpopulations with different maturation velocities, then the maturity-time model is equivalent to the age-structured model of Lebowitz and Rubinow with transition kernal $K(\tau, \tau') = \delta(\tau - \tau')$, since the change of variables given by (43) can be applied to each subpopulation. Rubinow [22] found that this model provided a better fit than the von Foerster model to experimental data from a cell population in which cells were synchronized initially and then observed over several generations. However, since the model cannot reproduce the phenomenon of asychronous exponential growth, the good agreement to experimental data cannot persist indefinitely as the cell population approaches a stable distribution.

If the maturity variable μ in Rubinow's model represents DNA content, then it is reasonable to assume, as Rubinow does, that all cells are born at the same maturity level μ_1 and divide at the same maturity level μ_2. However, DNA content is not a suitable measure of maturity for those cells that do not synthesize DNA throughout their lifespans. Therefore, Rubinow also suggested that "maturity" could represent some physical characteristic of cells such as length, weight, or volume. In this case, however, the Rubinow model fails to take into account the fact that there is a distribution in the physical characteristics of newly formed cells, i.e., cells are not all born with the same weight or volume. Moreover, the total biomass of two new daughter cells must clearly equal that of the mother cell immediately before division. Thus, if μ represents some physical quantity, then there must be a conservation law relating the total maturity level of a pair of newborn sibling cells to the maturity of the mother. A number of cell cycle models have been proposed that include such a conservation law at mitosis. Models of this sort are discussed in the next section.

B. Structure Variables Satisfying a Conservation Law

1. Size Distributions in Models with Random Cycle Length

It is obvious that cells must increase in size before dividing, or else the average cell size would get progressively smaller with each generation. However, it is not yet known to what extent size is involved in the regulation of cell division. There is experimental evidence suggesting that cells cannot initiate DNA synthesis before a critical size is attained [29], in which case cell size would play a role in determining the length of the cell cycle. On the other hand, it has also been shown that cell growth and the division process can be dissociated [30,31]. It could be the case, to some extent, that cell growth simply occurs in parallel with the processes that do govern the division cycle. Baserga [32] has recently reviewed the evidence for and against the dependence of cell division on cell size.

Hannsgen, Tyson, and Watson [33] consider a model in which the cell cycle time is a random variable T with distribution function

$$\Pr\{T > t\} = \alpha(t) = \int_t^\infty f(s)\,ds \tag{46}$$

where the density f(s) is nonnegative and piecewise continuous.
Thus, they regard cell size x as an observable characteristic that
is independent of the mechanisms governing the dynamics of the
cell population. Individual cells are assumed to increase in size
according to a deterministic growth law $dx/dt = g(x)$, and Hannsgen
et al. [33] investigate whether various growth laws for individual
cells are consistent with the existence of a steady-state size distribution in a population of cells whose total number increases exponentially
with time. The structure variable x, called "size" for conveinence,
could equally well represent some other physical cell characteristics
such as RNA content.

Assuming that the cell population has already *reached* a state
of balanced exponential growth with respect to the structure variable x, Hannsgen et al. [33] consider the function $\phi(x)$, the proportion of *dividing* cells with size greater than x. Clearly $\phi(x)$
would not be well defined if the population size distribution were
not assumed constant. It is important to note that there are different ways to characterize a stationary size distribution. One could
instead consider the proportion of *newly formed* cells with size
greater than x or the proportion of *all* cells (of all ages) with size
greater than x; in general, these three functions will be different.

The physical interpretation of ϕ imposes several restrictions on
the function $\phi(x)$. In particular, ϕ must be nonincreasing in x,
with $\phi(0) = 1$ and $\lim_{x \to \infty} \phi(x) = 0$; i.e., cells cannot be arbitrarily
large. Hannsgen et al. also show [33] that a necessary condition
for the existence of balanced exponential growth, in the absence
of cell loss, is that the (negative) derivative $\psi(x) = -d\phi/dx$ satisfy
the equation

$$\psi(x) = 4 \int_0^\infty e^{-\gamma s} \psi[2m(-s, x)] \frac{\partial m}{\partial x} (-s, x) f(s) \, ds \tag{47}$$

where the constant γ is the population growth rate and $m(t, x)$ is
the size of a cell that grows to size x in time t. The function m
is determined by the growth law $g(x)$, and γ must satisfy the
characteristic equation

$$1 = 2 \int_0^\infty e^{-\gamma s} f(s) \, ds \tag{48}$$

(cf. (15), where $f(s) = \lambda_m(s) \exp[-\int_0^s \lambda_m(\alpha) \, d\alpha]$ when $\lambda_d = 0$).
Built into equation (47) is the assumption that each cell at mitosis

divides precisely in half to produce two daughters of equal size. (Actually, Hannsgen et al. [33] present the somewhat more general case that each dividing cell produces r daughters of equal size.)

A solution to the model of Hannsgen et al. is an integrable function ψ on $[0,\infty)$ such that $\psi(x) \geqslant 0$ almost everywhere,

$$\int_0^\infty \psi(x) \ dx = 1$$

and ψ satisfies (47) with γ determined by (48). For such ψ, the function

$$\phi(x) \overset{\text{def}}{=} \int_x^\infty \psi(y) \ dy \tag{49}$$

satisfies the requirements for a steady-state size distribution of mitotic cells; i.e., $\phi(0) = 1$, etc. Hannsgen et al. prove that if there is some $t_1 \geqslant 0$ such that the probability density function $f(t)$ of cell generation times is strictly greater than zero for $t \geqslant t_1$, then the model has at most one solution. Thus, the cell population cannot possess more than one steady-state distribution of cell sizes.

When the growth of individual cells is exponential, i.e., if $g(x) = kx$ for some constant k, so that $x(t) = x(0)e^{kt}$, then Hannsgen et al. [33] prove that the population model has no steady-state solution. (This was also noted by Bell and Anderson [5].) A more general result was proved by Trucco and Bell [34], who showed that if the size of individual cells is given by any function of the form $x(t) = x(0)h(t)$, with h positive and $h(0) = 1$, then there is no stationary distribution $\phi(x)$ of cell sizes at division. In fact, they showed that the variance of the time-dependent distribution $\phi(x,t)$ increases without bound as $t \to \infty$. For exponential cell growth, Hannsgen et al. [33] illustrate, by numerical simulations, the continual broadening of the cell size distribution of a population in which cell division is governed by the transition probability model.

On the other hand, if cell growth is linear, i.e., if $x(t) = x(0) + ct$ for some constant c, then steady-state solutions to the model of Hannsgen et al. are possible for at least certain choices of the cycle time density function $f(t)$. Hannsgen et al. obtain an explicit expression for the unique solution to the model for each of two specific functions $f(t)$; one of these is the density corresponding to the transition probability model of Smith and Martin [11]. They also find, for linear cell growth, the surprising result that the predicted coefficient of variation of cell age at division is approximately twice as large as that for cell size at division. This phenomenon has been observed experimentally [35] and could be interpreted to mean that cell division is more closely controlled by size than by age. The results of Hannsgen and co-workers [33] show that this interpretation of the data is not necessary, because in their model cell size plays no role at all in controlling division.

The time-dependent behavior of the cell size distribution in models with random cycle length was further investigated by Hannsgen and Tyson [36]. They assumed specific forms for the cell growth law g(x) and the cell cycle time density function f(t). The density f(t) is that of the transition probability model with duration t_B of B phase equal to 1:

$$
f(t) \overset{\text{def}}{=}
\begin{cases}
0 & \text{for } 0 \leqslant t \leqslant 1 \\
pe^{-p(t-1)} & \text{for } t > 1
\end{cases}
\tag{50}
$$

where p is the transition probability. Cell growth is assumed to be linear, and for simplicity the constant growth rate is chosen to be 1; i.e., $x(t) = x(0) + t$. These assumptions imply that $x = 1$ is the minimum cell size required for division. As in the model of Hannsgen et al. [33], cells are assumed to divide precisely in half.

Hannsgen and Tyson [36] consider the function $\hat{n}(x,t)$ [not the usual population density $n(x, t)$], where

$$
\int_{x_1}^{x_2} \hat{n}(x, t) \, dx
$$

represents the rate of division, at time t, of cells having size in the interval $[x_1, x_2]$. Then ϕ is defined to be the relation function $\phi(x, t) = -e^{-\gamma t}\hat{n}(x, t)$, where γ is the solution to the characteristic equation (48) with density function f(t) given by (50). In particular, γ is the solution to

$$
p + \gamma = 2pe^{-\gamma}
\tag{51}
$$

The function $\phi(x, t)$ must satisfy, among other requirements, the partial differential equation

$$
\frac{\partial \phi}{\partial t}(x, t) + \frac{\partial \phi}{\partial x}(x, t) = (p + \gamma)[-\phi(x, t) + 2\phi\{2(x - 1), t - 1\}]
\tag{52}
$$

for $x \in [1, \infty)$, $t \in (0, \infty)$. Under appropriate hypotheses, Hannsgen and Tyson prove [36] that their model has a unique solution $\phi(x, t)$. Moreover, $\phi(x, t)$ converges, in the following sense, to the unique stationary distribution $\phi_0(x)$ of cell sizes at division whose existence was proved by Hannsgen et al. [33]:

$$\lim_{t \to \infty} \int_1^\infty [e^{-\gamma t} \hat{n}(x, t) - c\phi_0(x)] \, dx \tag{53}$$

where c is a constant that depends on the initial conditions.

Webb and Grabosch [37] also considered the asymptotic behavior of time-dependent distributions of cell sizes at division in models in which cycle length depends only on time and in which each dividing cell produces two daughters of equal size. They consider a more general form for the probability density f(t) of cell cycle times, although they require f to be continuous, so the transition probability model (50) is excluded from their treatment. They also consider a more general growth law g(x) for individual cells. One of the assumptions on the growth law is that the quantity 2g(x) − g(2x) be positive and bounded away from zero. This condition excludes the possibility of exponential growth for individual cells and says that two daughter cells increase in total size more rapidly than the undivided mother cell would have.

Webb and Grabosch [37] define n(x,t) so that

$$\int_{x_1}^{x_2} n(x,t) \, dx$$

is the number of dividing cells at time t having size in the interval $[x_1, x_2]$. They derive the following equation for n:

$$n(x, t) = \begin{cases} 4 \int_1^{T(x)} n(2m(s, x), t - s) \dfrac{\partial m}{\partial x}(s, x)f(s) \, ds \\ \qquad\qquad\qquad \text{for } t \geq 0, \ x > M \\ 0 \qquad\qquad\quad \text{for } t \geq 0, \ x \in [0, M] \\ h(x,t) \qquad\quad \text{for } t < 0, \ x \geq 0 \end{cases} \tag{54}$$

where m is defined as it is for the model of Hannsgen et al., T(x) is the time required for a cell to grow from size 0 to size x, M is the minimum division size, and h(x, t) is historical data describing the size distribution of dividing cells before time 0. Webb and Grabosch define a Banach space B, whose elements represent cell size distributions at division, and prove under appropriate hypotheses on the functions f, g, and h that there is a unique solution γ to the characteristic equation (48), a unique steady-state division size distribution ϕ_0 in B, and a unique solution n(x, t) to (54) for which n($\cdot$, t) is in B for each t $\geqslant$ 0. The time-dependent size distributions n(x, t) converge to the steady-state distribution; specifically,

$$\lim_{t \to \infty} \| e^{-\gamma t} n(\cdot, t) - c\phi_0(\cdot) \|_B = 0 \tag{55}$$

where c is a constant depending only on the historical data h, and $\| \cdot \|_B$ denotes the Banach space norm. The results of Webb and Grabosch [37] are proved by the theory of strongly continuous semigroups of bounded linear operators, as described in Section I.B.2.

2. Cell Cycle Models with Size Control

In this section, cell cycle models are discussed in which "size" (representing any physical cell characteristic for which there is a conservation law) plays some role in determining the length of the cell cycle. Among the earliest models to include dependence of division on cell size was that of Bell and Anderson [5]. In their model, n(a, x, t) denotes the density of cells with respect to the structure variables a = age and x = size. That is,

$$\int_{a_1}^{a_2} \int_{x_1}^{x_2} n(a, x, t) \, dx \, da$$

is the number of cells in the population at time t with age in the interval [a_1, a_2] and size in the interval [x_1, x_2]. The population balance law for their model is analogous to that for the Rubinow model [22], namely,

$$\frac{\partial n}{\partial t} + \frac{\partial n}{\partial a} + \frac{\partial}{\partial x}(gn) = -(\lambda_m + \lambda_d)n \tag{56}$$

where g(a, x) = dx/dt is the rate at which cells of age a and size x increase in size, and λ_m(a, x) and λ_d(a, x) are the probabilities, per unit time, that a cell of age a and size x divides or disappears from the population, respectively.

Bell and Anderson assume that each cell divides precisely into two daughters of equal size, so the boundary condition for their model is

$$n(0, x, t) = 4 \int_0^\infty \lambda_m(a, 2x)n(a, 2x, t) \, da \qquad (57)$$

The factor 4 is due to two separate sources of doubling in the density function. One results from the assumption that two daughters are produced at each cell division. The other arises from the fact that cells in the size interval $[2x_1, 2x_2]$ divide to produce cells with sizes between x_1 and x_2.

Although the general model of Bell and Anderson admits the possibility that λ_m and λ_d might depend on cell age as well as on size, they primarily consider the age-independent version of (56) obtained by integrating with respect to age. Letting

$$N(x, t) \overset{\text{def}}{=} \int_0^\infty n(a, x, t) \, da \qquad (58)$$

and defining G, Λ_m, and Λ_d, respectively, by

$$G(x, t)N(x, t) = \int_0^\infty g(a, x)n(a, x, t) \, da$$

$$\Lambda_m(x, t)N(x, t) = \int_0^\infty \lambda_m(a, x)n(a, x, t) \, da \qquad (59)$$

$$\Lambda_d(x, t)N(x, t) = \int_0^\infty \lambda_d(a, x)n(a, x, t) \, da$$

we obtain, from (56) and (57), the balance law for N:

$$\frac{\partial N}{\partial t}(x, t) + \frac{\partial}{\partial x}(GN)(x, t) = -[\Lambda_m(x, t) + \Lambda_d(x, t)]N(x, t)$$
$$+ 4\Lambda_m(2x, t)N(2x, t) \qquad (60)$$

The first two terms on the right describe changes in the density $N(x, t)$ due to loss of cells of size x from death and mitosis; the last term represents changes in N due to cell birth. Models like (60), in which the probability of division per unit time depends on cell size but not on cell age and in which $\Lambda_m(x)$ is not a delta function (i.e., cells do not all divide at precisely the same size), have been called "sloppy size control" models [38,41].

If the population governed by (60) has achieved a state of balanced exponential growth, then the density $N(x, t)$ has the form $N^*(x)e^{\gamma t}$ for some constant γ. Bell and Anderson [5] observe that γ must satisfy (15), where $\lambda_m(a)$ and $\lambda(a)$ represent, in this case, integrals with respect to x of the rates $\lambda_m(a, x)$ and $\lambda(a, x) = \lambda_m(a, x) + \lambda_d(a, x)$ of mitosis and cell loss, respectively. Also, $G(x, t) = G^*(x)$, and similarly for Λ_m and Λ_d. Consequently, it follows from (60) that the balance for a population in a state of asychronous exponential growth has the form

$$\gamma N^*(x) + \frac{\partial}{\partial x} [G^*(x)N^*(x)] = -[\Lambda_m^*(x) + \Lambda_d^*(x)]N^*(x) + 4\Lambda_m^*(2x)N^*(2x)$$

$$(61)$$

Bell and Anderson use (61) to analyze experimentally determined cell size distributions $N^*(x)$ from an exponentially growing population of cells. They observe that if the size distribution $\Lambda_m^*(x)$ of dividing cells is known, then, in the absence of cell loss due to other causes, one can solve for the cell growth rate $G^*(x)$, or vice versa, but not for Λ_m^* and G^* simultaneously. However, they show how information concerning the forms of Λ_m^* and G^* over certain size ranges can be used to draw conclusions about Λ_m^* and G^* over larger regions. Using such an approach, they conclude that the best fit to experimental data is obtained when the growth of individual cells is exponential. Linear cell growth is inconsistent with the observed data. The apparent contradiction between this conclusion and the impossibility of reconciling exponential cell growth with balanced exponential population growth [5] could be explained in one of at least two ways; either cell growth is not *precisely* exponential, or daughter cells do not each receive precisely half of the cell material from the mother at mitosis.

The time-dependent behavior of solutions to the model (60), in which cells are characterized by size alone, was investigated by Diekmann, Heijmans, and Thieme [39]. They assume that no cell can divide before it reaches a minimal size x_0, so cells of size less than $x_0/2$ cannot exist. The rates Λ_m and Λ_d of mitosis and cell loss are assumed to depend only on cell size (not on time), and additional hypotheses on Λ_m are imposed so that every cell is guaranteed to divide by the time it reaches some maximal size, normalized to $x = 1$. Diekmann et al. [39] also assume that $x_0 \geqslant 1/2$; there is biological evidence for this condition [40], which says that the maximal size of a newborn cell is smaller than the minimum size at which cell division can occur. This implies the existence of a minimum cell cycle time

$$t_{min} \overset{def}{=} \int_{1/2}^{x_0} \frac{dx}{g(x)} \tag{62}$$

where $g(x) = dx/dt$ is the growth rate of individual cells.

Equation (60) is reformulated by Diekmann et al. [39]. Instead of the (time-dependent) cell size density $N(x, t)$, they consider the multiple $n(x, t) = h(x)N(x, t)$, where $h(x)$ is a function determined by the cell growth rate $g(x)$ and by the rates $\Lambda_m(x)$ and $\Lambda_d(x)$ of mitosis and cell loss, respectively. By a solution to their model they mean a continuous mapping $t \longmapsto n(x, t)$ from $[0, \infty)$ into the Banach space B of continuous functions on $[x_0/2, 1]$ with value zero at $x = x_0/2$ such that $n(\cdot, t)$ satisfies the transformed version of (60). They show [39] that the problem has a unique solution $N(x, t)$ for each choice $N_0(x)$ of tme initial data in B and that the mappings $N_0(\cdot) \longmapsto N(\cdot, t)$ for $t \geqslant 0$ for a strongly continuous semigroup of bounded linear operators on B.

For strictly positive, continuous cell growth laws satisfying the condition $g(2x) < 2g(x)$ on the interval $[x_0/2, 1/2]$, Diekmann et al. show [39] that there exists a unique real constant γ and a unique function $n^*(x)$ in B such that every solution $n(x, t)$ to their model converges, as $t \to \infty$, to $Ce^{\gamma t}n^*(x)$, where C is a constant depending only on the initial data $N_0 \varepsilon B$. Their proof uses operator-theoretic techniques similar to those used later by Webb [25] (cf. Section II.B.2). Specifically, they show that the infinitesimal generator of the strongly continuous semigroup of bounded linear operators has a dominant real eigenvalue γ. The eigenfunction $n^*(x)$ corresponding to γ determines the unique steady-state solution $N^*(x)$.

The results of Diekmann et al. [39] remain true if $g(2x) > 2g(x)$ on the interval $[x_0/2, 1/2]$, although this condition on the growth law is not considered biologically relevant, as discussed earlier (Section II.B.1). They prove, however, that when $g(2x) = 2g(x)$ on $[x_0/2, 1/2]$, e.g., when individual cells grow exponentially in size, asynchronous exponential growth is not achieved. However, Diekmann et al. show by example [39] that there exist growth laws $g(x)$ with $2g(x) = g(2x)$ on a proper subset of $[x_0/2, 1/2]$ for which convergence of solutions to a unique steady-state distribution is guaranteed.

In the size-structured models discussed so far in this section, cell age has not played a role in determining the cycle length of a cell. One model in which both age and size influence cycle time is the *tandem* model [42,43]. This model is similar to the transition probability model in that the cell cycle includes a probabilistic A state from which cells exit with constant probability p per unit time to a deterministic B phase of constant duration. The difference is that a critical size, normalized to $x = 1$, is required for a cell to enter A state. A cell born with size less than 1 must first enter a third state, called C state, where it remains until it grows to size $x = 1$, at which time it enters A state.

Assuming an exponential growth rate for individual cells, i.e., $g(x) = kx$ for some constant k, and assuming the division of mother cells into two daughters of equal size, Tyson and Hannsgen [44] describe sufficient conditions for the existence of a unique steady-state distribution of cell sizes for newborn cells in the tandem model. The proof uses results of Lasota and Mackey [45] which are based on the evolution of size distributions of newborn cells from generation to generation, instead of on their evolution with respect to time.

For populations in a state of balanced exponential growth, Tyson and Hannsgen derive the equation for $\alpha(t)$, the proportion of cells with cycle time greater than t, predicted by the tandem model. They show that the theoretical form for $\alpha(t)$ provides a good fit to experimental data [44,46]. However, from their estimates of the correlation coefficients r predicted by the model for the generation times of sibling cells $(0 < r < 1/2)$ and for mother-daughter pairs $(r \sim -1/2)$, they conclude that the values obtained are, on average, less than the values observed experimentally

Gyllenberg and Heijmans [47] present another model in which the cell cycle is assumed to consist of two distinct phases, one of variable and one of fixed duration t_B. The duration of the variable A state is determined by cell size; cells leave A state to enter the phase of constant duration at a rate that depends on cell size. Letting $n(x, t)$ denote the population density, with respect to size, of cells in the variable phase of the cell cycle, we obtain the population balance law for the model of Gyllenberg and Heijmans:

$$\frac{\partial n}{\partial t}(x, t) + \frac{\partial}{\partial x}[g(x)n(x, t)] = -[\lambda_d(x) + \tau(x)]n(x, t)$$

$$+ \frac{2f[y^{-1}(x)]\tau[y^{-1}(x)]}{y'[y^{-1}(x)]}n[t - t_B, y^{-1}(x)] \qquad (63)$$

Here, $g(x)$ is the growth rate for individual cells, $\tau(x)$ is the rate at which cells enter the deterministic phase from the variable phase, $y(x)$ is the size of a newborn cell whose mother entered B phase at time $t - 1$ with size x, and $f(x)$ is the probability that a cell entering B phase with size x will survive to divide into two daughter cells. Clearly $y(x)$ is determined by the function $g(x)$, and $f(x)$ depends on both g and λ_d. Cells are again assumed to divide precisely into two daughter cells of equal size at mitosis.

Gyllenberg and Heijmans assume, as do Diekmann et al. [39], that there is a minimum cell size $x = x_0$ required for division, and that the size-dependent transit rate function $\tau(x)$ is such that all cells are guaranteed to divide with size $x \leqslant 1$. In fact, the model of Gyllenberg and Heijmans reduces to that of Diekmann et al. if the duration t_B of the constant B phase is taken to be zero. A condition on the growth rate is also assumed that reduces to the condition $g(2x) < 2g(x)$ when $t_B = 0$.

Gyllenberg and Heijmans [47] transform the balance law (63) by considering a particular multiple u(x, t) = h(x)n(x, t) of the population density u. They obtain the delay-differential equation

$$\frac{\partial u}{\partial t}(x,\ t) + g(x)\ \frac{\partial u}{\partial x}(x,\ t) = k(x)\ u[t - t_B,\ y^{-1}(x)] \qquad (64)$$

for some function k(x). Equation (64) is supplemented with boundary and initial conditions, and it is shown that for an appropriate Banach space B, there exists a unique solution u(·, t) to the model, remaining in B for all time, for arbitrary initial data in B. Moreover, the solutions form a strongly continuous semigroup of bounded linear operators whose infinitesimal generator has a dominant real eigenvalue γ. It then follows that there is a unique stationary size distribution n*(x) such that $e^{-\gamma t}$n(x, t) converges, as t → ∞, to cn*(x) for some constant c that depends on the initial size distribution.

A common assumption among size-structured cell cycle models—in fact, one that has been made in every model discussed so far—is that each dividing cell produces two daughters of equal size. As noted by Bell and Anderson [5] and others (e.g., Diekmann et al. [39]), it is this assumption that prevents solutions to most size-structured models from exhibiting the property of asynchronous exponential growth when the growth of individual cells is exponential. We conclude this section by discussing a model in which cells divide into two daughters of unequal size.

Heijmans [48] presents a model in which the ratio p of the size of a newborn cell to that of its mother is a random variable having smooth probability density function f(p). Since the two values of p must sum to 1 for a pair of sibling cells, f(p) is symmetric about 1/2. The distribution of values p is not assumed to depend on the size of the mother. Heijmans's model for the unequal birth sizes of sibling cells was first suggested by Koch and Schaechter [49].

For n(x, t) the density of cells of size x at time t, the population balance law for the model of Heijmans is

$$\frac{\partial n}{\partial t}(x,\ t) + \frac{\partial}{\partial x}[g(x)n(x,\ t)] = -[\lambda_d(x) + \lambda_m(x)]n(x,\ t)$$

$$+ 2\int_{1/2-x_1}^{1/2+x_1} \frac{f(\rho)}{\rho}\ \lambda_m\left(\frac{x}{\rho}\right) n\left(\frac{x}{\rho},\ t\right)\ d\rho$$

$$(65)$$

where g(x), as usual, is the growth law for individual cells, λ_d and λ_m are the size-dependent probabilities, per unit time, of cell loss and mitosis, and $x_1 \in (0, 1/2)$ is a constant such that f(p) is zero outside the interval $(1/2 - x_1, 1/2 + x_1)$.

Under appropriate hypotheses on $\lambda_m(x)$, etc., Heijmans shows [48] that there exist unique solutions to his model in an appropriate Banach space B, provided the initial data correspond to a function in B. Using the theory of strongly continuous semigroups of bounded linear operators, he proves that solutions to his model exhibit the property of asynchronous exponential growth; solutions converge to constant multiples of a unique cell size distribution. This result is obtained for arbitrary growth laws g(x) that are continuous and strictly positive. In particular, the case of exponential growth for individual cells is not excluded.

IV. CONCLUSION

A wide variety of structured models with continuous structure variables has been introduced to describe the dynamics of cell populations. A major question tackled by these models concerns the nature of the source or sources of variation in the cycle times of otherwise identical cells. To date, most of the effort in modeling cell populations has been directed at understanding the dynamics of cells living in an unlimited environment, i.e., in uncrowded culture conditions with a nondiminishing nutrient supply. Mathematically, this means that the models are linear.

In the study of tumor cell dynamics in vivo, it is more likely that the relevant structured models will be nonlinear. A few efforts in this direction have been made, although the analysis of nonlinear models is considerably more difficult, in general, than for linear models. Gurtin and MacCamy [50] have studied a nonlinear version of the age-structured McKendrick model [8] in demography. They assume that the age-dependent birth modulus β and loss function λ also depend on the total population size at each time t, and they consider conditions necessary for the existence of a stable equilibrium population density, i.e., one that does not change with time. (This could be regarded as a special case of balanced exponential growth in which the intrinsic growth rate of the population is zero.) Murphy [51] considers a version of maturity-time model of Rubinow [22] in which the maturation rate depends on total population size (e.g., via depletion of nutrients), and proves the existence of solutions to the model. A last example is the work of Heijmans [48], who considers a model in which cells grow exponentially in size with growth rate depending on the concentration S of nutrients in the culture. The model includes both a population balance law and an equation for the rate of change in the substrate concentration. Under appropriate assumptions, the existence of a globally stable equilibrium solution is proved.

In addition to cell crowding and nutrient limitation, there are likely to be other factors causing nonlinearities in structure models of cancer processes. Two that come to mind immediately are the interactions between distinct cell subpopulations via the production of growth factors and changes in population dynamics resulting from treatment. Clearly this is an area ripe for further study.

ACKNOWLEDGMENTS

The author gratefully acknowledges the skillful assistance of Ms. Connie Seifert and Ms. Vickie Struwe in the preparation of this manuscript. Thanks are also due to Dr. Stuart Zimmerman, who first introduced me to this interesting topic. This work was supported by Grants CA-11430 and CA-29026 from the National Cancer Institute, National Institutes of Health.

REFERENCES

1. Swan, G. W., Tumor growth models and chemotherapy, in *Cancer Modeling* (J. R. Thompson and B. W. Brown, eds.), Marcel Dekker, New York (1987).

2. Bertuzzi, A., Gandolfi, A., and Giovenco, M. A., Mathematical models of the cell cycle with a view to tumor studies. *Math. Biosci.*, 53:159 (1981).

3. Howard, A. and Pelc, S. R., Synthesis of desoxyribonucleic acid in normal and irradiated cells and its relation to chromosome breakage. *Heredity, 6* (suppl.):261 (1953).

4. Peterson, D. F. and E. C. Anderson, Quantity production of synchronized mammalian cells in suspension culture. *Nature,* 203:642 (1964).

5. Bell, G. I. and Anderson, E. C., Cell growth division. I. A mathematical model with applications to cell volume distributions in mammalian suspension cultures. *Biophys. J.*, 7:329 (1967).

6. Scherbaum, O. and Rasch, G., Cell size distribution and single cell growth, in Tegrahyeme Pyriformis GL, *Acta Pathol. Microbiol. Scand.*, 41:161 (1957).

7. von Foerster, H., Some remarks on changing populations, in *The Kinetics of Cellular Proliferation* (F. Stohlman, ed.), Grune & Stratton, New York (1959).

8. McKendrick, A. G., Applications of mathematics to medical problems. *Proc. Edin. Math. Soc.*, 44:98 (1926).

9. Feller, W., On the integral equation of renewal theory. *Ann. Math. Stat.*, *12*:243 (1941).

10. Burns, F. J. and Tannock, I. F., On the existence of a G_0-phase in the cell cycle. *Cell Tissue Kinet.*, *3*:321 (1970).

11. Smith, J. A. and Martin, L., Do cells cycle? *Proc. Nat. Acad. Sci. USA*, *70*:1263 (1973).

12. Minor, P. D. and Smith, J. A., Explanation of degree of correlation of sibling generation times in animal cells. *Nature*, *248*:241 (1974).

13. Lajtha, L. G., On the concept of the cell cycle. *J. Cell. Comp. Physiol.*, *60*(suppl.):143 (1963).

14. Rubin, H. and Steiner, R., Reversible alterations in the mitotic cycle of chick embryo cells in various states of growth regulation. *J. Cell. Physiol.*, *85*:261 (1975).

15. Lebowitz, J. L. and Rubinow, S. I., A theory for the age and generation time distribution of a microbial population. *J. Math. Biol.*, *1*:17 (1974).

16. Dawson, K. B., Madoc Jones, H., and Field, E. O., Variations in the generation times of a strain of rat sarcoma cells in culture. *Exp. Cell Res.*, *38*:75 (1965).

17. Miyamoto, H., Zeuthen, E., and Rasmussen, L., Clonal growth of mouse cells (strain L). *J. Cell Sci.*, *13*:879 (1973).

18. Collyn-D'Hooghe, M., Valleron, A. -J., and Malaise, E. P., Time-lapse cinematography studies of cell cycle and mitosis duration. *Exp. Cell Res.*, *106*:405 (1977).

19. Schaechter, M., Williamson, J. P., Hood, J. R., and Koch, A. L., Growth, cell and nuclear division in some bacteria. *J. Gen. Microbiol.*, *29*:421 (1962).

20. Powell, E. O. and Errington, F. P., Generation times of individual bacteria: Some corroborative measurements. *J. Gen. Microbiol.*, *31*:315 (1963).

21. Shields, R. and Smith, J. A., Cells regulate their proliferation through alterations in transition probability. *J. Cell Physiol.*, *91*:345 (1977).

22. Rubinow, S. I., A maturity-time representation for cell populations. *Biophys. J.*, *8*:1055 (1968).

23. Webb, G. F., A model of proliferating cell populations with inherited cycle length. *J. Math. Biol.*, *23*:269 (1986).

24. Webb, G. F., Dynamics of structured populations with inherited properties, to appear.

25. Webb, G. F., An operator-theoretic formulation of asynchronous exponential growth, to appear.

26. Webb, G. F., *Theory of Nonlinear Age-Dependent Population Dynamics*, Marcel Dekker, New York (1985).

27. White, R. A., A review of some mathematical models in cell kinetics, in *Biomathematics and Cell Kinetics* (M. Rotenberg, ed.), Elsevier/North-Holland Biomedical Press, New York (1981).

28. Zimmerman, S. and White, R. A., Generalizations of a fluid dynamic model for analyzing multiparameter flowcytometric data, in *Biomathematics and Cell Kinetics* (M. Rotenberg, ed.), Elsevier/North-Holland Biomedical Press, New York (1981).

29. Killander, D. and Zetterberg, A., Quantitative cytochemical studies on interphase growth. I. Determination of DNA, RNA, and mass content of age determined mouse fibroblasts in vitro and of intercellular variation in generation time. *Exp. Cell Res.*, *38*:272 (1965).

30. Zetterberg, A., Engstrom, W., and Larsson, O., Growth activation of resting cells: Induction of balanced and imbalanced growth. *Ann. N.Y. Acad. Sci.*, *397*:130 (1982).

31. Zetterberg, A. and Engstrom, W., Induction of DNA synthesis and mitosis in the absence of cellular enlargement. *Exp. Cell Res.*, *144*:199 (1983).

32. Baserga, R., Growth in size and cell DNA replication. *Exp. Cell Res.*, *151*:1 (1984).

33. Hannsgen, K. B., Tyson, J. J., and Watson, L. T., Steady-state size distributions in probabilistic models of the cell division cycle. *SIAM J. Appl. Math.*, *45*:523 (1985).

34. Trucco, E. and Bell, G. I., A Note on the dispersionless growth law for single cells. *Bull. Math. Biophys.*, *32*:475 (1970).

35. Miyata, H., Miyata, M., and Ito, M., The cell cycle in the fission yeast, *Schizosaccharomyces pombe*. I. Relationship between cell size and cycle times. *Cell Struct. Funct.*, *3*:39 (1978).

36. Hannsgen, K. B., and Tyson, J. J., Stability of the steady-state size distribution in a model of cell growth and division. *J. Math. Biol.*, *22*:293 (1985).

37. Webb, G. F. and Grabosch, A., Asynchronous exponential growth in transition probability models of the cell cycle, to appear.

38. Wheals, A. E., Size control models of *Saccharomyces cerevisiae* cell proliferation. *Molec. Cell Biol.*, 2:361 (1982).

39. Diekmann, O., Heijmans, H. J. A. M., and Thieme, H. R., On the stability of the cell size distribution. *J. Math. Biol. 19*: 227 (1984).

40. Powell, E. O., A note on Koch and Schaechter's hypothesis about growth and fission of bacteria. *J. Gen. Microbiol.*, 37: 231 (1964).

41. Tyson, J. J. and Diekmann, O., Sloppy size control of the division cycle. *J. Theor. Biol.*, in press.

42. Shilo, B., Shilo, V., and Simchen, G., Cell-cycle initiation in yeast follows first-order kinetics. *Nature, 264*:767 (1976).

43. Lord, P. G. and Wheals, A. E., Variability in individual cell cycles of *Saccharomyces cerevisiae*. *J. Cell Sci.*, 50:361 (1981).

44. Tyson, J. J. and Hannsgen, K. B., Cell growth and division: A deterministic/probabilistic model of the cell cycle. *J. Math. Biol.*, 23:231 (1986).

45. Lasota, A. and Mackey, M. C., Globally asymptotic properties of proliferating cell populations. *J. Math. Biol.*, 19:43 (1984).

46. Tyson, J. J. and Hannsgen, K. B., The distributions of cell size and generation time in a model of the cell cycle incorporating size control and random transitions. *J. Theor. Biol.*, 113: 29 (1985).

47. Gyllenberg, M. and Heijmans, H. J. A. M., An abstract delay-differential equation modelling size dependent cell growth and division, Report AM-R8508, Centre for Mathematics and Computer Science, Amsterdam (1985).

48. Heijmans, H. J. A. M., On the stable size distribution of populations reproducing by fission into two unequal parts. *Math. Biosci.*, 72:19 (1984).

49. Koch, A. L. and Schaechter, M., A model for statistics of the cell division process. *J. Gen. Microbiol.*, 29:435 (1962).

50. Gurtin, M. E. and MacCamy, Non-linear age-dependent population dynamics. *Arch. Rational Mech. Anal.*, 54:281 (1974).

51. Murphy, L., Density dependent cellular growth in an age structured colony. *Comp. Maths. with Appls.*, 9:383 (1983).

5

Metabolic Events in the Cell Cycle of Malignant and Normal Cells
A Mathematical Modeling Approach

MAREK KIMMEL *Investigative Cytology Laboratory, Memorial Sloan-Kettering Cancer Center, New York, N.Y.*

I. INTRODUCTION

Proliferation of living cells is a process that requires completing a series of biological transformations between two successive cell divisions. The mass of the cell must approximately double, and the genetic material coded in the cell DNA (genome) must be duplicated to be divided among the two daughter cells. The interdivision period can be divided into three disjoint subintervals (Prescott [1]). The last of them, the G_2M phase [Fig. 1(a)], is the period of immediate preparations for the mechanics of cell division, of the physical separation of the two copies of the genetic information, and, finally, of the division itself. The G_2M phase must be preceded by a time interval in which a replica of the genome is produced. This period is called the S phase and is considered the central, most vital part of cell life.

Since the S and G_2M phases are devoted to well-defined tasks, their duration is rather precisely determined, and the course of events inside these stages of cell life is faithfully repeated from one cell generation to another. In contrast, the events inside the period called the G_1 phase, which precedes S phase, are governed by rules, that are not so clear. Also, it is the dispersion in cell residence times in G_1 which contributes the most to the overal dispersion of the cell generation time [1].

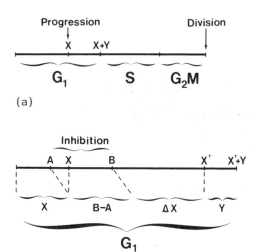

(a)

(b)

FIGURE 1   (a) Succession of events in the cell cycle: after division,
the cell enters the G_1 phase during which its RNA and protein contents are increased.   After completing these processes, the DNA
synthesis can begin and cell enters the S phase.   After concluding
the DNA replication, immediate preparations for division begin in the
G_2M phase.   Hypothetically, the G_1 phase is divided into (at least)
two parts by (at least) one "progression" point.   X and Y symbolize
the durations of the parts of G_1 before and after the progression
point.   Cell can pass a progression point only after completing necessary biochemical processes.   (b) Experiment demonstrating existence
of a progression point related to accumulating a threshold level of a
labile protein: if the synthesis of the protein is inhibited, in the
period from A to B (A < X), then X', the new time of threshold
accumulation is greater than just X + (B − A).   The difference ΔX
is the time required for resynthesizing the amount of labile protein
lost during the inhibition period.   Empirically, observing $\Delta X > 0$ is
considered a proof of existence of a progression point.   (In this
figure, for the sake of example, the interval ΔX is disproportionately
long.)

The more popular of the cell cycle models (e.g., Mitchison's [2] dependent pathway model and Smith and Martin's [3] A to B transition model) describe G_1 as the critical phase in which decisions occur as to whether (and when) a cell will synthesize DNA or enter a quiescent state. One of the recently recognized theories (Pledger et al. [4]) states that there exists a point (or points) in the G_1 phase which plays an important role in the progression of cells through G_1. Passing such a "progression" point in G_1 is possible only in the presence of certain growth factors in the surrounding medium. (Other names frequently used in the literature are "restriction" or "control" point. Without getting into too much detail, we use the term "progression" point generically throughout this chapter.) As postulated by Pledger et al. [4] for BALB/c-3T3 cells, the first of the "progression" points (called the competence point) is of special importance. Failure to pass it results in the cell sliding into quiescence.

The type of cell kinetic reasoning and experimental design aimed at demonstrating the existence of discrete progression points in the G_1 phase can be characterized as follows: suppose that the initiation of DNA synthesis requires accumulation of a threshold amount of a species of protein, a process which under normal conditions (i.e., enough nutrients and growth factors in the surrounding medium, absence of inhibitors), requires a time X [Fig. 1(a)]. (A substantial amount of this hypothetical protein may well have been inherited.) Then, after an additional delay Y, the cell automatically begins synthesizing DNA. In such cases it is considered that a progression point is located at X in the G_1 phase.

However, suppose that for a certain period of time [from A to B; cf. Fig. 1(b)], the cell is placed in an environment devoid of nutrients and/or growth factors and/or in the presence of agents inhibiting protein synthesis. If, moreover, the beginning of this period precedes the progression point (i.e., A < X), then, since the protein tends to decompose spontaneously and at the same time its synthesis is inhibited, its threshold level is reached with a delay greater than the duration (B − A) of the inhibition period. Denoting the new moment of reaching the threshold by X', we can write X' = X + (B − A) + ΔX. The new duration of G_1 is X' + Y. If the protein is labile (i.e., it decomposes quickly), then even a relatively short pulse of protein synthesis inhibitor will delay the exit from G_1 in an observable manner.

The experiments just described and the concept of a labile protein were introduced by Schneiderman, Dewey, and Highfield [5], who used the Chinese hamster ovary (CHO) cells, and applied by, among others, Rossow, Riddle, and Pardee [6] (cultured mouse fibroblasts). The latter paper (and the references therein) offers a simple mathematical model of this protein's kinetics.

If a mechanism described is responsible for triggering DNA synthesis, then it also seems reasonable to suppose that the processes
involved proceed at many sites in the cell simultaneously and have
a stochastic character; e.g., they are initiated by random encounters
of molecules of growth factors and specific receptor molecules on the
cell surface (Baserga [7]). In this context, it would then be natural
to suspect that the progression point(s) is (are) spread over an interval of G_1 rather than deterministically positioned. Such heterogeneity is suggested by Brooks [8], among others, who observed a
wide dispersal of exit times from G_1 under a constant, high concentration of inhibiting agent. Yen and Pardee [9] offer a mathematical
model to estimate the dispersion in the location of a progression
point (3T3 cells).

The primary aim of this paper is to consider the cell cycle
Recently, it has been argued that the chain of preparatory
events in the G_1 phase of the cell cycle is strictly coupled with the
expression of proto-oncogenes, units of genetic information which
supposedly code for growth factor-like proteins; conversely, such
growth factors can activate expression of certain proto-oncogenes
(Pardee et al. [10]). It appears that the oncogenes coding for successive growth factors are expressed one after another during the cell
cycle (cf. e.g., Thompson et al. [11]). Expression of any gene begins
from producing a string of mRNA, so the foregoing implies a connection
between kinetics of production of proteins and RNA during the cell
cycle, particularly in the G_1 phase.

The primary aim of this paper is to consider the cell cycle
effects predicted by specific assumptions on the metabolic events in
the cell's life. The case will be made for the heterogeneity of
kinetic characteristics in cell populations (among them progression
points). The impact of metabolic status on a cell's future will be
analyzed. Mathematical models will be presented, and their predictions will be discussed in the context of experimental evidence and
biological theories of the cell cycle. Our attention will be mostly
focused on the CHO cell line, which can be considered an experimental model of malignant cells. The CHO cells have certain characteristics of cancer cells (they form tumors in the nude mice), but they
retained some features of normal cells (they are anchorage dependent).
Secondary purposes of this chapter are to address the general question of the relevance of mathematical modeling in cell kinetics and to
provide the reader with a number of useful references.

The processes of RNA and protein synthesis are, in the exponentially growing cell cultures, tightly coupled to each other and to the
DNA synthesis process. However, it is possible to decouple them
by inhibiting synthesis of either proteins or RNA. By following the
effects of the resulting imbalance on cell cycle progression, one can
infer the kinetics of synthesis of basic cellular constituents.

First, in Section II, we will analyze the general kinetic relationships between production of protein, RNA, and DNA in the CHO

cells, under the action of inhibitors of RNA and protein synthesis. In the experiments performed (Traganos and Kimmel, in preparation), the CHO cells synchronized in mitosis or early G_1 phase were exposed to various concentrations of both agents. We show that the experimental results can be reproduced by an essentially continuous mechanism of cell cycle progression without introducing discrete progression points.

In Section III we consider a phenomenon of basic importance for the understanding of cell cycle kinetics: the unequal division during cytokinesis of metabolic cell constituents between two daughter cells and the mechanisms that control the length of the cell cycle. The analysis is carried out based on a mathematical model first described by Kimmel et al. [12]. This model offers an explanation for the origin of a considerable part of the variability of cell generation times in cell populations.

II. SYNTHESIS OF DNA, RNA, AND PROTEINS IN THE CYCLE OF CHO CELLS

The following material is based on the analysis of recent unpublished experimental data. Complete presentation of the experiments, including laboratory details, is beyond the scope of this chapter and is deferred to a separate publication (Traganos and Kimmel, in preparation).

A. Cell Kinetic Effects of Cycloheximide and Actinomycin D on CHO cells

Unperturbed (control) CHO cells, starting from a population synchronized in early G_1 by mitotic detachment and gradually producing the basic metabolic constituents, can be thought of as traversing, at a certain rate, a trajectory in RNA/DNA coordinates; these two coordinates are observable with the aid of the flow cytometric techniques we employ. The trajectory begins, at t = 0, at the point (1, 1) (i.e., both the RNA and the DNA contents are equal to 1) and ends, at t = T, at the point (2, 2) (a doubled content of RNA and DNA). The sigmoidal shape of the unperturbed trajectory (see Fig. 2) occurs because the RNA synthesis begins earlier and concludes later in the cell cycle than the DNA synthesis.

The notion of "trajectory" that is employed here concerns population averages; each cell follows its own trajectory (c.f. e.g., Kimmel et al. [12]). Also, the durations T_1 and T_2 of the G_1 and S phases, as well as the generation time T, vary from one cell to another, although for the CHO cells this variability is relatively small.

Two agents were employed to perturb the cell cycle kinetics: actinomycin D (AMD), which inhibits RNA synthesis, and

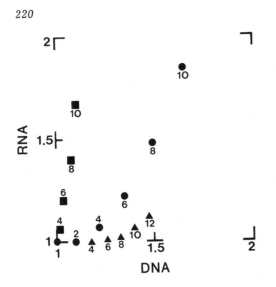

FIGURE 2   Cell cycle RNA/DNA trajectories of the CHO cells, initially synchronized at early G_1 by mitotic detachment. Model
simulations: control (circles); 0.1 µg/ml concentration of AMD
(inhibitor of RNA synthesis) at t = 0 (squares; and 0.1 µg/ml
concentration of CHX (inhibitor of protein synthesis) at t = 0
(triangles). Smaller numbers outside symbols are times in hours.

cycloheximide (CHX), which interferes with protein production. The
perturbations caused by the two agents differed considerably. Two
types of experiments were performed:

1. In the first type of experiment, various concentrations of
    either AMD or CHX were added to the culture immediately
    after synchronization in early G_1 phase.
    a. The result of the action of the AMD (cf. model simula-
        tions in Fig. 2) is, at the lowest dose, a sharp inhibition
        of RNA production, with the DNA production slowed
        down less markedly, so that the trajectory is almost
        vertical. At a larger dose, both RNA and DNA content
        are stagnant. The highest dose of the AMD causes a
        a gradual, slow decrease of the RNA content, with the
        DNA content unchanged.
    b. The result of the action of the CHX, an inhibitor of
        protein production (Fig. 2) is a gradual, dose-dependent
        slowdown of both the RNA and DNA production. How-
        ever, the DNA production is relatively more inhibited,
        so that the RNA/DNA trajectory is shifted downward.

2. In the second type of experiment, fixed doses of both
agents were added to the culture, after a time delay (t = 1,
2, or 3 hr) with respect to the initial synchronization.
   a. After the AMD is administered (Fig. 3) there is a short
      initial period of unperturbed growth and DNA synthesis
      slows down, whereas the amount of RNA decreases.
   b. The result of delayed administration of the CHX is
      qualitatively different (Fig. 3) from the result of experi-
      ment II.2. The RNA/DNA trajectory remains essentially
      unchanged, although the rate of cell progression is
      lower.

B. Mathematical Model of the Cell Cycle Events

We will employ a mathematical model of production of RNA, proteins,
and DNA during the cell cycle of an "average" cell. Idealized as it
is, this model will reproduce experimental data available to us.

Various species of RNA provide both templates and workshops
for production of cell proteins. Therefore, an increase in the RNA
quantity triggers a corresponding increase in the rate of protein

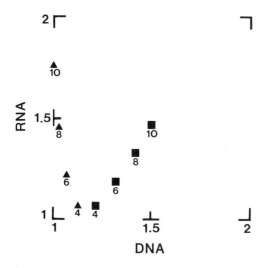

DNA

FIGURE 3   Cell cycle RNA/DNA trajectories of the CHO cells.
Model simulations: 0.1 μg/ml concentration of CHX (inhibitor of
protein synthesis) at t = 3 hr (squares); and 1 μg/ml concentration
of AMD (inhibitor of RNA synthesis) at t = 3 hr (triangles).   Smaller
numbers outside symbols are times in hours.

production. However, proteins (e.g., enzymes) are necessary for the transcription of genetic information from DNA into RNA, and thus the rate of RNA production may depend on the quantity of a specific cellular protein(s). Analogously, enzymes and histones are necessary for DNA synthesis.

It is convenient to think about these processes in terms of discrete portions of RNA, proteins, or DNA (not necessarily identical to individual chemical molecules). The relationships mentioned can then be uniformly symbolized by the acts of "promoting" the production of portions of a given species (e.g., protein) by the existence and activity of a portion of a different species (e.g., RNA). In this manner, it is possible to rewrite the general rules of the model as follows:

1. An "elementary" portion of the RNA promotes the event of production of an "elementary" portion of a protein.

2. A portion of protein promotes the event of production of a portion of the RNA.

3. A fraction of newly synthesized proteins may initiate the process which, after a time delay, increases the amount of DNA by a unit portion.

4. The portions of both RNA and proteins have finite life spans which are short in comparison to the length of the cell cycle.

There exist many sets of specific rules which can supplement the general scheme sketched here. Because we lack precise knowledge of the dynamics of the processes in question, we will use rules which yield very simple mathematical descriptions. Specifically, we assume that the mechanism of production of the RNA and the proteins is stochastic: in a time interval of length s, a portion of the RNA promotes synthesis of a portion of the protein with probability $a_{12}s + o(s)$ [where $o(s)$ is small compared to s; i.e., $o(s)/s$ tends to zero as s tends to zero]. Analogously, in a similar time interval, a portion of the protein promotes synthesis of a portion of the RNA with probability $a_{21}s + o(s)$. Decomposition of a portion of the RNA (protein) occurs, in a time interval of length s, with probability $a_{11}s + o(s)$ [respectively, $a_{22}s + o(s)$]. For probablistic background, see Rao [13].

The mechanism described here defines the production of the RNA and the proteins as a Markovian birth and death process with a very simple structure. Let R(t) denote the mean amount of RNA, and P(t) the mean amount of proteins in the cell at time t (time t = 0 corresponds to the beginning of the cell cycle, understood here as the moment immediately following cell division). Then the following differential equations are satisfied:

$$\dot{R}(t) = -a_{11}R(t) + a_{21}P(t) \tag{1}$$

$$\dot{P}(t) = a_{12}R(t) - a_{22}P(t) \tag{2}$$

Let us further suppose that a newly synthesized portion of protein promotes, in a short time interval of length s, with probability
bs + o(s), the event leading (after a delay T_1 corresponding to the
normal minimum duration of the G_1 phase of the cell cycle) to the
synthesis of a portion of DNA. Denoting by D(t) the mean amount
of DNA in the cell at time t, we obtain

$$\dot{D}(t) = \begin{cases} 0 & t < T_1 \\ b[P(t - T_1) - P(0)] & T_1 < t \leqslant T_1 + T_2 \\ 0 & T_1 + T_2 < t \leqslant T \end{cases} \tag{3}$$

where T_2 is the duration of the S phase of the cell cycle. The
amount of RNA, proteins, and DNA at t = 0 (i.e., at the beginning
of the cell cycle, inherited from the mother cell) will be set equal
to unity:

$$R(0) = P(0) = D(0) = 1 \tag{4}$$

Let T denote the duration of the cell cycle. Any solution of the system (1)-(3), corresponding to unperturbed cell growth, must satisfy

$$R(T) = P(T) = D(T_1 + T_2) = 2 \tag{5}$$

i.e., the RNA, proteins, and DNA duplicate during the intermitotic
period.

Equations (1)-(3) with initial conditions (4) can be explicitly
solved.

Inhibitory action of chemical agents on the production of RNA or
proteins can be modeled by manipulating the values of the coefficients
in the system (1)-(3). For instance, inhibition of the general protein synthesis is modeled by decreasing a_{12}, and inhibition of RNA
synthesis is modeled by decreasing a_{21}.

C. Experimental Results Versus Cell Cycle Model

For an initially synchronized cell population, the "averaged" RNA/
DNA trajectory leaves the level of DNA = 1, after a delay (T_1 = 2 hr)

approximately equal to the time spent in the G_1 by the fastest progressing cells, and the bulk of the cell cohort leaves G_1 later. (In our very simple model, no mechanism exists to explicitly account for the dispersion in the G_1 residence times.) We set $T_1 + T_2$ (joint duration of G_1 and S) to approximately 9 hr and the generation time T to approximately 12 hr.

The next step is to find a relationship between the remaining model coefficients such that condition (5) is satisfied (i.e., the cell RNA, proteins, and DNA are duplicated during the cell cycle), and thus the control experiment can be simulated by the model. As proved in the Appendix, all the versions of system (1), (2) with $R(0) = P(0) = 1$, $R(T) = P(T)$, satisfying

$$-a_{11} + a_{21} = -a_{22} + a_{12} = C \tag{6}$$

generate the same solutions $P(t)$, $R(t)$ for each given C. Thus to ensure that $P(T) = R(T) = 2$, it is enough for us to choose an appropriate C.

Attempts to reproduce the experimental RNA/DNA trajectories under drug action require extensive computer search in the space of coefficients a_{ij} and b, within the limits determined by equation (6). The coefficients are manipulated to obtain the simultaneously best least squares fit to the control trajectory and two trajectories perturbed by CHX and AMD (Fig. 2). The perturbed trajectories correspond to concentrations of 0.1 µg/ml of CHX and 0.1 µg/ml of AMD, which cause radical slowdowns in the DNA and RNA production, respectively (however, at this concentration of AMD a decrease in RNA content is not yet observed). These two perturbed trajectories are modeled under the assumption that the rate of synthesis of RNA or the synthesis of proteins (and thus of DNA) is reduced by the inhibitor to the level merely balancing the rate of spontaneous decomposition. Therefore, remembering condition (6) we have

for the unperturbed trajectory:

$$a_{11} = A_1 \qquad a_{21} = A_1 + C \qquad a_{12} = A_2 + C \qquad a_{22} = A_2$$

for the trajectory perturbed by AMD:

$$a_{11} = a_{21} = A_1 \qquad a_{12} = A_2 + C \qquad a_{22} = A_2$$

for the trajectory perturbed by the CHX:

$$a_{11} = A_1 \qquad a_{21} = A_1 + C \qquad a_{12} = a_{22} = A_2$$

Summarizing, we see that it is enough to search for the optimum
values of coefficients A_1, A_2, b, and C.
    The best fit provided by this search is $A_1 = 0.06$ hr^{-1}, $A_2 =$
0.04 hr^{-1}, b $= 0.40$, and C $= 0.05$ hr^{-1}. Resulting model trajectories are depicted in Fig. 2. The quality of this fit, to three
trajectories simultaneously, is characterized by a root-mean-square
error of approximately 10%.
    Further modeling results are presented in Fig. 3. The action
of CHX delayed by 3 hr is modeled with coefficients presented in
the foregoing. As is evident from examining Fig. 3, the RNA/DNA
trajectory is, in this case, very close to the control. Analogous
model simulations have performed for other delays in the action of
CHX (1 hr and 2 hr; not shown), with similar results.
    Action of a high dose, 1.0 μg/ml, of AMD was approximately
reproduced assuming $a_{21} = 0.03$ hr$^{-1} < a_{11}$, after a 3-hr delay
(Fig. 3). In this latter case, simulation reproduces the experiment
only qualitatively; modeling the action of higher concentrations of
cytostatic drugs is usually plagued by the fact that after a short
initial period the effects of the drug are propagated and affect all
the domains of cell metabolism (cf. Kimmel and Traganos [14]).
    Concluding, then, we see that a very simple mathematical model
reproduces quite satisfactorily the observed RNA/DNA trajectories
of the CHO cells perturbed by drug action. The model seems to be
the simplest possible: it is linear; it does not explicitly include any
threshold mechanisms or discrete progression points; and the underlying stochastic process is Markovian, etc.
    Further discussion of the simulation results follows in the last
section.

III. UNEQUAL DIVISION AND CELL CYCLE REGULATION

A. Background Information

It has long been suspected, based on observations of unicellular
organisms (mainly bacteria and yeasts), that asymmetric division of
cells and regulation of cell cycle duration are closely related. A
huge literature exists on this subject; basic sources can be found
in the references in Fantes [15]. The mechanism of regulation of
cell cycle duration is perhaps most explicitly presented in [15] for
the yeast *Schizosaccaromyces pombe*: yeast cells are cylindrical with
approximately hemispherical ends, and cell growth, between successive
divisions, occurs primarily by length extension. Fantes [15] notes
that cell length at birth determines the cell cycle duration: initially
long cells do not have to grow as long as the shorter cells to attain
a (hypothetical) threshold size which enables division. In most cells,
the size and cell cycle length regulation process requires only a

single cell generation. However, there exists a minimum cell cycle duration which is obligatory even for very long cells. For these cells the regulation requires a longer period.

It is known that in exponentially growing yeast populations the mean size and the variation around this mean are constant in time (Fantes [15]). In the presence of the regulatory mechanisms mentioned, this implies the existence of a mechanism which introduces variability into the population: either the size threshold for division is not precisely determined, or sibling cells are not of identical size (a combination of both factors is also possible).

Shields et al. [16] address the issue of cell size control in cultured mouse fibroblast cells. Mother cells have been sorted with respect to the cell size. Cells born of small mothers have longer generation times than those born of large mothers. Moreover, cell populations initially enriched in large (or small) cells return after a few cell divisions to the cell size distribution indistinguishable from that characteristic of the primary (unsorted) exponentially growing population.

Can cell size be the primary factor regulated during cell growth? It is conceivable that a more intrinsic quantity plays the primary role and that the cell size stabilization is a secondary effect of the regulation of this primary factor. An obvious candidate is cellular RNA, the amount of which continuously increases as a cell traverses the cell cycle. The experiments on cultured Chinese hamster lung cells published by Fujikawa-Yamamoto [17] demonstrate that cells overloaded with the RNA return after several cell cycles to normal content of this substance.

Further studies, performed mainly on CHO cells, illuminate the role of RNA production and unequal division in cell cycle regulation. In a study of RNA content and cell kinetics (Darzynkiewicz et al. [18]), CHO cells and lymphocytes stimulated to cycle by phytohemagglutinin were synchronized in G_1 phase, the former by mitotic detachment and the latter by treatment of 24-hr cultures with hydroxyurea. Since it was possible to follow both the cell cycle phase distribution and RNA content by flow cytometry, subpopulations with different RNA content could be identified and their rate of progression into and through S phase analyzed. This study shows that the rate of progression through S phase is directly related to the G_1 RNA content of cells (also, cf. Traganos et al. [19]). A later study confirmed that RNA content correlated with S phase transit times (Darzynkiewicz et al. [20]).

The most striking observation of the latter study is that the coefficients of variation (c.v.) of RNA and protein content are 15% greater in the immediately postmitotic part of the G_1 phase than in the mitotic cell population from which they arose. The interpretation of this small but highly reproducible difference is that both RNA and protein are unequally distributed among daughter cells as a result of asymmetric cytokinesis. It appears therefore that unequal cytokinesis may be responsible for generating intercellular hetero-geneity during the cell cycle. (The interesting fact is that cell progression through S phase is not associated with any significant increase in RNA or protein heterogeneity: on the contrary, short "windows" in the S phase have a 20-30% lower c.v. than postmitotic cells; cf. Discussion.) Another point of interest in Darzynkiewicz et al. [20] is that the c.v. of the distributions of the protein con-tent are higher than those of the RNA. This clearly suggests that RNA and not proteins (and thus not the cell size) is the primary regulating factor.

To what extent can the variability of the CHO cells generation times be caused by unequal division of the RNA? This question can be answered with the aid of mathematical modeling.

B. Model Assumptions and Basic Formulae

Two rules of RNA production and division are specified, based on results in Darzynkiewicz et al. [18,20]:

1. Cells which have more RNA in early G_1 phase (immediately after division) traverse the cell cycle faster than those that inherited less RNA.
2. RNA is divided unequally, in an apparently random way, be-tween the daughter cells.

Based on these assumptions, a mathematical model of the cell population kinetics was built by Kimmel et al. [12]. Unequal RNA division to daughter cells is the only source of randomness within the model.

The most important notions of the model are "instantaneous" RNA distributions at the end of mitosis and at the beginning of the G_1 phase. They are denoted by $m(t, x)$ and $n(t, x)$, respectively, and understood in the following way: $m(t, x)\, dt\, dx$ is equal to the number of cells with an RNA content between x and $x + dx$ which divided in the time interval from t to $t + dt$, and $n(x, t)\, dt\, dx$ is equal to the corresponding number of cells which entered the early G_1 phase. Both $m(t, x)$ and $n(t, x)$ are distribution densities with respect to x (RNA content) and rates of cell flow with respect to time t.

As mentioned, the only source of randomness in the model is the unequal division of RNA between two daughter cells. Suppose that the mitotic cell just before division has X units of RNA. The con-ditional probability density of a daughter size Y is denoted by $f(Y \mid X)$. Of course, $f(Y \mid X) = 0$ for $Y > X$ because no daughter cell can have more RNA than the original mother cell. The other daugh-ter cell with RNA content $X - Y$ must have the same conditional density; i.e., $f(X - Y | X) = f(Y | X)$, $0 \leqslant Y \leqslant X$, which is a symmetry requirement for $f(Y | X)$.

As a consequence of cell division, the number of cells doubles and the positions of the newly divided cells on the RNA scale change (due to unequality of division). In this quasi-probabilistic model the relation between $m(t, x)$ and $n(t, x)$ is

$$n(t, y) = 2 \int_0^\infty f(y | x) m(t,x) \, dx$$

as implied by the definition of conditional probability. Once the daughter cell has obtained its share (Y) of RNA, its fate is determined. Thus, the cell will spend $T = g(Y)$ units of time in the cycle. Cells with more RNA traverse the cell cycle faster, which implies that $g(\cdot)$ is a monotonic nonincreasing function. The amount X' of RNA at the end of the cycle (at the next division) is a function $X' = h(Y)$. It seems reasonable to assume that $h(\cdot)$ is a monotonic increasing function, i.e., cells richer in RNA at the outset of the cell cycle, conclude this cycle with a higher RNA content. These assumptions imply

$$m(t, x) = n\{t - g[h^{-1}(x)], \, h^{-1}(x)\}[h^{-1}(x)]'$$

and then, by elimination of $n(\cdot, \cdot)$, we obtain the equation which is the basis for the present analysis:

$$m(t, x) = 2[h^{-1}(x)]' \int_0^\infty f[h^{-1}(x) | u] m\{t - g[h^{-1}(x)], \, u\} \, du \qquad (7)$$

In the model, no limitations of cell growth are imposed, corresponding to experimental conditions in which cells are replated so that the population never becomes overcrowded or depleted of nutrients. Such cultures exhibit exponential growth for prolonged periods. The basic requirement for the model is to reproduce this phenomenon.

C. Properties of the Model

Analyses of the behavior of the unequal division model have been carried out by Kimmel et al. [12] and, in a more general setting, by Arino and Kimmel [21]. A basic property demonstrated rigorously in [21] is that under very broad hypotheses there exists a real positive constant b (the Malthusian parameter) and a distribution density $\overline{m}(x)$ such that the RNA distribution $m(t, x) \sim \exp(bt)\overline{m}(x)$ as t tends to infinity [cf. equation (7)]. This property, the existence of the exponential steady state (ESS), is obtained by using the theory of operator semigroups (see Discussion). Thus, the model reproduces the balanced exponential growth of the CHO cell cultures.

Using data from Darzynkiewicz et al. [18,20], one can demonstrate (Kimmel et al. [12]) that the model is capable of reproducing the ESS distribution of cell generation times with a c.v. of 8.4% (compared to values of about 12% observed by Prescott [1], Fig. 26, or of about 16%, estimated by Macdonald [22]). Thus, a slight (15% increase in c.v.) asymmetry of RNA division can be made responsible for at least a major part of kinetic variability. Another interesting prediction is the correlation coefficient of the generation times of sibling cells, close to the frequently reported value of 1/2.

IV. DISCUSSION

Recent discovery of relationships between proto-oncogenes, growth factors, and progression points in the cell cycle, has changed the understanding of the mechanisms of cell growth between divisions (Pardee et al. [10]). New experimental tools evolved from the techniques of molecular biology provide informaion on the details of metabolic pathways in individual cell development. In this new framework is there still a place for a traditional methodology of perturbing the cycling cell population with external agents and drawing inferences from the results? Contrary to views expressed by others (cf. Baserga [23]), it seems that the cell population kinetic approach has certain, even if limited, merits: a large number of cells are considered, and therefore the results are statistically unambiguous. Also, the behavior of cell population may be, in certain circumstances, not a simple sum of events observed in individual cells, isolated during the experiment. At least, examination of cell population kinetics provides clues about which of the metabolic events in the cell cycle might be of primary importance (as in the experiment of Pledger et al. [4]).

The role of mathematical modeling is to provide a quantitative link between outcomes of related experiments and to check the coherence of biological hypotheses regarding cell kinetics.

In this paper, we first consider if it was possible to describe, with a very simple (perhaps, the simplest possible) model, the kinetics of RNA and DNA production in CHO cells synchronized in early G_1 phase by mitotic detachment and subject to the action of two different cytostatic agents. Visual comparison of RNA/DNA trajectories for immediate (Fig. 2) and delayed (Fig. 3) administration may suggest that there exists a special protein which has to be synthesized in very early G_1 to promote preparation for DNA synthesis. Indeed, the RNA/DNA trajectory in the nondelayed case is shifted far to the bottom of the graph; in the delay case the

trajectory is identical with the control. Therefore, it is legitimate
to suspect that there exists a discrete, important protein synthesis
event (progression point?) in the early G_1 phase (less than 1 hr
after division), completion of which is necessary to trigger normal
DNA synthesis. Application of a protein synthesis inhibitor (here,
CHX) before this event would radically change the entire RNA/DNA
trajectory; this same inhibitor applied after a sufficient delay would
only slow down the progression along an essentially unchanged
trajectory.

Application of our method of analysis suggests that the discrete
progression point hypothesis is incorrect: translated into the
language of the mathematical model, the hypothesis would mean that
to reproduce the immediate CHX action it is necessary to decrease
coefficients a_{12} (rate of protein synthesis) and/or b (rate of DNA
synthesis), compared to their values employed to model the delayed
action. But, as is evident from Section III.C, both immediate and
delayed action of CHX can be modeled with the same values of these
coefficients.

To sum up, the principal result of the foregoing analysis is that
in the G_1 phase of CHO cells, the production of proteins and RNA
as well as expression of various growth factors is, viewed by kinetic
effects, a continuous process. Indeed, it has been hypothesized
(Pardee et al. [10]) that in cycling cells the progression event is
completed before the previous division. Only in cells arrested in
G_0 does the progression event have to be completed before cells
can enter the cycle. (Similar mechanism has been postulated previously as a unified theory for eukaryotic and prokaryotic cells [24,
25].) Another plausible explanation is that in tumorlike CHO cells
the cell cycle controls are relaxed, as opposed to the frequently
quoted 3T3 cells.

This latter point requires further discussion. The CHO cell line
used 15 years ago by Schneiderman et al. [5] had a G_1 residence
time of 7 hr and a generation time of 19 hr. Experiments performed
using this cell line indicated existence of a labile protein and a related progression point located at about 3.5 hr in G_1. For the CHO
line we use, the G_1 residence is never longer than 4 hr and the
generation time is close to 12 hr. Schneiderman's experiment has
been recently repeated using these cells (Traganos; unpublished
experimental data). The pulse of CHX, inhibiting protein synthesis
in interval (A, B) (see Fig. 1), was applied either from A = 0 hr
to B = 2 hr or from A = 1 hr to B = 3 hr or from A = 2 hr to B =
4 hr, after initial synchronization of cells, thus covering the entire
G_1 phase. In all three cases the "additional" delay ΔX (Fig. 1) was
identical: $\Delta X \cong 1$ hr. This suggests that either the progression
point location is different for individual cells or the progression
events spread over the entire G_1 (in accordance with the modeling
in this paper). Indeed, suppose that a discrete progression point

related to a labile protein is located in the first 2 hr of G_1 ($X < 2$ hr); then for the $(0, 2)$ hr-pulse of CHX, ΔX would be greater than zero, whereas for the $(2, 4)$-hr pulse, ΔX would be zero. If $2 < X < 4$, then the effect would be the opposite. This result, if confirmed, suggests that the cell cycle controls have evolved in the CHO line from those typical of normal cells to another pattern, perhaps more characteristic of malignant cells (cf. Riddle, Pardee, and Rossow [26] for related discussion).

The analysis in Section III indicates that a major portion of kinetic heterogeneity in the CHO cell population (including, perhaps, dispersed locations of progression events) can be attributed to variability in the metabolic status of cells in the population. Regulatory mechanisms keep the heterogeneity within limits that are stable with respect to perturbations.

As noted by Darzynkiewicz et al. [20] (cf. also Darzynkiewicz and Traganos [27]), the metabolic (RNA, protein) heterogeneity present in G_1 subpopulations is reduced during S phase. This suggests a negative stochastic dependence between durations of G_1 and S. Interestingly, such dependence is also suggested by cell kinetic analyses in Kimmel [28].

This chapter attempted to demonstrate examples of how mathematical modeling can help one understand the kinetics of cell populations. The examples chosen and methods applied reflect my own experience and preferences. It is necessary to acknowledge contributions by many investigators who have recently considered mathematical models of cell kinetics: Rigney [29] has investigated stochastic mechanisms which may produce the observed exponential tails of the distributions of cell generation times (so called alpha curves) and of the distributions of the differences of generation times of sibling cells (beta curves). Asymmetry of cell division, motivated by observations of yeast proliferation has been considered by Gyllenberg [30]. Conditions for the balanced exponential growth of cell populations under various assumptions regarding cell cycle controls have been reported by, among others, Tyson and Hannsgen [31], Diekmann, Heijmans, and Thieme [32], Lasota and Mackey [33], or recently by Webb and Grabosch [34].

Interestingly, the abstract theory of operator semigroups has become an important tool in analyzing cell kinetic models (Webb and Grabosch [34], Diekmann, Heijmans, and Thieme [32] and Arino and Kimmel [21]). Largely unexplored is the relationship of deterministic models based on differential, functional, and integral equations to stochastic models based on the theory of branching processes. For example, the process of cell proliferation with unequal division considered by Kimmel et al. [12] and by Arino and Kimmel [21] [described by Equation (7)] can be understood as a special case of a generalized continuous time branching process (see Mode [35], Chapter 7). In Mode's terminology, cells with different RNA content occupy different states in the process state space. Thus, equation (7) is an equation for the expected values of a branching process, analogous to Mode's [35] equation (7.7.2).

V. APPENDIX: A PROPERTY OF SYSTEMS OF LINEAR DIFFERENTIAL EQUATIONS

Let $x(t)$ denote a column vector function of dimension n, let A denote a square matrix of numbers, and let e denote a column vector composed of n 1's. The following property was used to reduce the number of numerical simulations necessary to investigate the model. (For background information on differential equations, cf. e.g., Hartmann [36]).

Proposition

Suppose that $x_i(t)$, i = 1, 2, $t \geqslant 0$, are solutions of systems of ordinary differential equations

$$\dot{x}_i(t) = A_i x_i(t) \tag{A1}$$

that

$$x_1(0) = x_2(0) = e \tag{A2}$$

and that

$$A_1 e = A_2 e = ve \tag{A3}$$

where v is a real number. Then $x_1(t) = x_2(t)$ for $t \geqslant 0$.

Proof: We show that $A_1^m e = A_2^m e$, $m \geqslant 0$. For m = 0 and 1, this is true. We proceed by induction: Suppose that the property holds for m. Then, based on (A3), $A_1^{m+1} e = A_1^m ve$, which, by the induction assumption, is equal to $A_2^m ve = A_2^{m+1} e$. Therefore, $[\exp(A_1 t)]e = [\exp(A_2 t)]e$. But, by (A2), this proves the Proposition.

For our system (1), (2), R(0) = P(0) = 1 [cf. equation (A2)]. Also,

$$-a_{11} + a_{21} = -a_{22} + a_{12} \tag{A4}$$

to ensure that R(T) = P(T). So, if two various sets of coefficients: $a_{ij}^{(k)}$, k = 1, 2, are used in system (1), (2) such that

$$-a_{11}^{(1)} + a_{21}^{(1)} = -a_{11}^{(2)} + a_{21}^{(2)}$$

[which, by (A4), also yields $-a_{22}^{(1)} + a_{12}^{(1)} = -a_{22}^{(2)} + a_{12}^{(2)}$],
then the corresponding solutions of system (1), (2) are identical.

ACKNOWLEDGMENTS

Writing this chapter would have been impossible without discussions and criticism of Frank Traganos, Ovide Arino, and Zbigniew Darzynkiewicz. The possibility of access to unpublished experimental data of Frank Traganos is gratefully acknowledged. Ms. Helen Gay provided excellent technical assistance. The author is a visiting investigator from the Institute of Automation, Silesian Technical University, Gliwice, Poland. This work was supported by the PHS grant CA 23296.

REFERENCES

1. Prescott, D. M., *Reproduction of Eukaryotic Cells*, Academic Press, New York (1976).

2. Mitchison, J. M., *The Biology of the Cell Cycle*, Cambridge University Press, Cambridge (1971).

3. Smith, J. A. and Martin, L., Do cells cycle? *Proc. Nat. Acad. Sci. USA*, *70*:1263 (1973).

4. Pledger, W. J., Stiles, C. D., Antoniades, H. N., and Scher, C. D., An ordered sequence of events is required before BALB/c-3T3 cells become committed to DNA synthesis. *Proc. Nat. Acad. Sci. USA*, *75*:2839 (1978).

5. Schneiderman, M. H., Dewey, W. C., and Highfield, D. P., Inhibition of DNA synthesis in synchronized Chinese Hamster cells treated with G_1 with cycloheximide. *Exp. Cell Res.*, *67*: 147 (1971).

6. Rossow, P. W., Riddle, V. G. H., and Pardee, A. B., Synthesis of labile serum-dependent protein in early G_1 controls animal cell growth. *Proc. Nat. Acad. Sci. USA*, *76*:4446 (1979).

7. Baserga, R., Growth in size and cell DNA replication. *Exp. Cell. Res.*, *151*:1 (1984).

8. Brooks, R. F., Continuous protein synthesis is required to maintain the probability of entry into S phase. *Cell*, *12*:311 (1977).

9. Yen, A. and Pardee, A. B., Exponential 3T3 cells escape in mid-G_1 from their high serum requirement. *Exp. Cell Res.*, *116*: 103 (1978).

10. Pardee, A. B., Campisi, J., Gray, H. E., Dean, M., and
     Sonenshein, G., Cellular oncogenes, growth factors, and cellu-
     lar growth control, in *Mediators in Cell Growth and Differentia-
     tion* (R. J. Ford and A. L. Maizel, eds.), Raven Press, New
     York, p. 21 (1984).

11. Thompson, C. B., Challoner, P. B., Neiman, P. E., and
     Groudine, M., Expression of the c-myb proto-oncogene during
     cellular proliferation. *Nature*, *319*:374 (1986).

12. Kimmel, M., Darzynkiewicz, Z., Arino, and Traganos, F.,
     Analysis of a model of cell cycle based on unequal division of
     mitotic constituents to daughter cells during cytokinesis. *J.
     Theor. Biol.*, *101*:637 (1984).

13. Rao, M. M., *Probability Theory with Applications*, Academic
     Press, New York (1984).

14. Kimmel, M. and Traganos, F., Kinetic analysis of drug-induced
     G_2 block in vitro. *Cell Tissue Kinet.*, *18*:81 (1985).

15. Fantes, P. A., Control of cell size and cycle time in *Schizo-
     saccaromyces Pombe*. *J. Cell. Sci.*, *24*:51 (1977).

16. Shields, R., Brooks, R. F., Riddle, P. N., Capellaro, D. F.,
     and Delia, D., Cell size, cell cycle and transition probability
     in mouse fibroblasts. *Cell 15*:469 (1978).

17. Fujikawa-Yamamoto, K., RNA dependence in the cell cycle of
     V-79 cells. *J. Cellular Physiol.*, *112*:60 (1982).

18. Darzynkiewicz, Z., Evenson, D. P., Staiano-Coico, L.,
     Sharpless, T. K., and Melamed, M. L., Correlation between
     cell cycle duration and RNA content. *J. Cell Physiol.*, *100*:425
     (1979).

19. Traganos, F., Darzynkiewicz, Z., and Melamed, M. R., The
     ratio of RNA to total nucleic acid content as a quantitative
     measure of unbalanced cell growth. *Cytometry*, *2*:212 (1982).

20. Darzynkiewicz, Z., Crissman, H., Traganos, F., and Steinkamp,
     J., Cell heterogeneity during the cell cycle. *J. Cell Physiol.*,
     113:465 (1982).

21. Arino, O. and Kimmel, M., Asymptotic analysis of a cell cycle
     model based on unequal division. *SIAM J. Appl. Math.*, *47*:128
     (1987).

22. Macdonald, P. D. M., Towards an exact analysis of stathmokinetic
     and continuous labeling experiments, in *Biomathematics and
     Cell Kinetics* (M. Rotenberg, ed.), Elsevier/North-Holland
     Biomedical Press, Amsterdam, p. 125 (1981).

23. Baserga, R., *The Biology of Cell Reproduction*. Harvard University Press, Cambridge (1985).

24. Cooper, S., A unifying model for the G_1 period in prokaryotes and eukaryotes. *Nature, 280*:17 (1979).

25. Kuczek, T., Stochastic modeling for the bacterial life cycle. *Math. Biosci., 69*:159 (1984).

26. Riddle, V. G. H., Pardee, A. B., and Rossow, P. W., Growth control of normal and transformed cells. *J. Supramolec. Structure, 11*:529 (1979).

27. Darzynkiewicz, Z. and Traganos, F., Multiparameter flow cytometry in studies of the cell cycle, in *Flow Cytometry and Sorting* (M. R. Melamed, M. L. Mendelsohn, and T. Lindmo, eds.), Alan R. Liss, New York, to appear.

28. Kimmel, M., Nonparametric analysis of stathmokinesis. *Math. Biosci., 74*:111 (1985).

29. Rigney, D. R., Multiple-transition cell cycle models that exhibit transition probability kinetics. *Cell Tissue Kinet., 19*:23 (1986).

30. Gyllenberg, M., The age structure of populations of cells reproducing by asymmetric division, in *Mathematics in Biology and Medicine* (V. Capasso, E. Grosso, and S. L. Paveri-Fontana, eds.), Lecture Notes in Biomathematics, Vol. 57, Springer, Berlin, p. 320 (1985).

31. Tyson, J. J. and Hannsgen, K. G., The distribution of cell size and generation time in a model of the cell cycle incorporating size control and random transitions. *J. Theor. Biol., 113*: 29 (1985).

32. Diekmann, O., Heijmans, H. J. A. M., and Thieme, H. R., On the stability of the cell size distributions. *J. Math. Biol., 19*: 227 (1984).

33. Lasota, A. and Mackey, M. C., Globally asymptotic properties of proliferating cell populations. *J. Math. Biol., 19*:43 (1984).

34. Webb, G. F. and Grabosch, A., Asynchronous exponential growth in transition probability models of the cell cycle, to appear.

35. Mode, Ch., Multitype branching processes, Elsevier, New York (1971).

36. Hartmann, Ph., *Ordinary Differential Equations*, Wiley, New York (1964).

6

A Modeling Approach
to Metastatic Progression of Cancer

ROBERT BARTOSZYŃSKI   *Department of Statistics, The Ohio State University, Columbus, Ohio*

I. INTRODUCTION

A metastasis is defined (see [1]) as "emergence of a new cancer at some distance from the original site of cancer as a result of the migration of cancer cells by way of blood vessels or lymphatic channels." Since a tumor (whether metastatic or not) cannot be detected until it reaches some appreciable size, the occurrence of a metastasis is not observable when it happens. On the other hand, the knowledge of the time of occurrence of metastases—even in a statistical sense, as an answer to the question whether metastases generally tend to occur at earlier or later stages of growth of the primary tumor—is of crucial importance for cancer research. Indeed, the motivation for the study of occurrence times of metastases is not only cognitive but also practical. If metastases tend to occur at early stages of primary tumors, long before the latter reach detectable sizes, the gain from introducing early detection methods (e.g., through costly screening programs) could be negligibly small. If this were the case, it might be wiser to allocate the funds to other areas of cancer research. If, on the other hand, metastases tend to occur at later stages of the life of the primary, then early detection is of paramount importance.

The impossibility of observing the metastatic process as it occurs poses challenging problems of creating new schemes of indirect inference. Such schemes must be based on some postulated mechanisms governing three interacting factors: growth of tumors, shedding metastases, and detection.   Problems of this type are primarily mathematical and belong to the domain of stochastic modeling.

This chapter presents some attempts to better understand the phenomenon of metastases; in particular, it attempts to answer the question of statistical characteristics of the time of its occurrence.

We start from showing (Section II) that the most commonly accepted ideas about tumor growth (fixed doubling time, hence exponential growth) and their propensity to metastasize (the larger the tumor, the more likely it is that it will shed a metastasis) are jointly incompatible with the data.   This forces us to examine the empirical validity of the two premises—at least one must be rejected.

Section III is devoted to testing the hypothesis of exponential growth.   We give theoretical results from [2] on estimating growth curves; we then give two sets of data and the empirical results. The latter indicate that for breast cancer, in the range of sizes typically seen at detection, the growth curve is indeed exponential (or at least empirically indistinguishable from it).

In Section IV we show some of the most important consequences of the fact that tumor growth is exponential.   One of them, perhaps the most remarkable, is the possibility of estimating the growth rate of a tumor on the basis of just one observation of its size, namely at the time of detection.

That growth is exponential necessitates, as explained, a revision of the second premise concerning the metastatic process.   The empirical data suggest that one must account for a fair number of metastases that occur early, when the primary tumor is still small. One possibility is explored in Section V, where we keep (see [3]) the assumption that metastatic rate is proportional to size of the primary, but we allow for the possibility of "systemic" tumors, that is, tumors that originate independently of the existence and size of the primary.

Finally, another possibility is presented in Section VI, which involves replacing the proportionality assumption in metastatic rate by an entirely new model of metastatic production (see [4]), where the latter is related to the randomly changing level of heterogeneity of the primary tumor.   This model is, thus far, theoretical only. However, at the end of the chapter we outline some possibilities for its empirical validation.

II.   WHERE IS THE FAULT?

The current thinking about the process of tumor growth and metastasis seems to be dominated by the following two ideas.   First, as regards growth, the concept commonly used by physicians is that of *doubling time*. Implicit in the use of this concept is the conviction that growth is unbounded, because for bounded growth, such as logistic, the tumor that reaches a certain size would continue growing but would never double.

Moreover, if doubling time is to serve as a useful measure of tumor growth, it should remain more or less the same—i.e., be independent of the actual size of the tumor. It is easy to show that the latter property is equivalent to the following hypothesis.

Hypothesis 1 (Exponential Growth). *Each tumor grows exponentially (with rates varying between patients).*

In other words, counting time from the (unobservable) moment t = 0 when the tumor originates, its size at time t is $ce^{t/\alpha}$, where c is the size (volume, mass, etc., depending on the chosen unit of measurement) of a single, and α is the (reciprocal of) the growth rate.

Clearly, $T_\alpha = \alpha \log 2$ is the doubling time of a tumor growing with rate α (so that smaller α correspond to faster growing tumors).

Next, as regards metastatic rate, the situation is somewhat less clear. Nevertheless, it is still possible to formulate a hypothesis which captures the most common convictions of the specialists. The source of information here lies in the typical doctor's pressure for an immediate surgery when an operable tumor becomes detected. The argument offered for avoiding any delay usually involves a reference to the risk of metastasis and to the fact that this risk is progressive: delay by two weeks (say) would more than double the risk connected with delaying the operation by one week. Such an argument is apparently motivated by the conviction that the larger is the tumor, the more likely it is to metastasize. The assumption of proportionality formulated next is only one possibility here, giving the exponential growth of risk. Incidentally, the exponential growth of tumors allows us to leave unresolved the question of whether metastases can be shed from the whole mass of the tumor or only from its surface: the latter changes as a power of the volume, which again gives exponential growth.

We formulate therefore the following hypothesis.

Hypothesis 2 (Metastatic Rate). *Suppose that at time t the size of the tumor is f(t). Then the probability that it will metastasize between t and t + h is $\mu f(t)h + o(h)$, where μ is some proportionality constant (metastatic force), and $o(h)/h \to 0$ as $h \to 0$.*

This hypothesis asserts simply that for short intervals of time, the chances of a metastasis are in direct proportion to the tumor size and the length of the interval.

As mentioned in the Introduction, Hypotheses 1 and 2 taken jointly are not compatible with the empirical data. Intuitive arguments (see [3] and [5]) involve the fact that under these hypotheses, most metastases would have to occur just prior to detection of the primary and, hence, would at that time be very small. Since it takes about 30 doubling times for a tumor to become detectable, most patients would be expected to enjoy an appreciably long cancer-free period (perhaps as much as two years or so). This, regretfully, is not true.

When this argument is made formal, it leads to the following two theorems. Suppose that a tumor with doubling time T is detected at some time t, and let p = p(t) be the probability that the tumor, if not removed, would metastasize during the first doubling time following t, i.e., at some time between t and t + T. We then have

Theorem 1. *The probability that the tumor will metastasize during the first k doubling periods following t, i.e., between t and t + kT, equals*

$$P(k) = 1 - (1 - p)^{2^k - 1}$$ (1)

Theorem 2. *The probability that the tumor has already metastasized during the last k doubling periods preceding t, i.e., between t − kT and t, equals*

$$Q(k) = 1 - (1 - p)^{1 - 2^{-k}}$$ (2)

Taking k = 2 in formula (1), we get $P(2) = 1 - (1 - p)^3 = 3p - 3p^2 + p^3$. For small p we have $P(2) \approx 3p$, so (under hypotheses 1 and 2) the risk of metastasis is indeed progressive: delaying the operation by two doubling periods about triples the chances of metastasis, as compared with the risk of delaying the operation by one doubling period.

On the other hand, letting k → ∞ in formula (2), we obtain the probability $Q(\infty) = p$ that the tumor has already metastasized. We may formulate it as follows.

Corollary. *Under Hypothesis 1 and 2, the chances that the tumor has already metastasized are always equal to the chances of a metastasis during the nearest doubling period.*

Now, $Q(k)/Q(\infty) = Q(k)/p$ is the probability that the tumor has metastasized during the last k doubling periods, if it has metastasized at all. It may be shown that $Q(1)/p$ exceeds 0.5 for all p, so that in over 50% of cases, the metastasis (if it occurred at all) happened during the most recent doubling period.

Similarly, $Q(6)/p$ exceeds 0.97 for all p, which means that in over 97% of all cases the metastasis occurs during the six doubling periods of the primary that precede its detection.

As already mentioned, if the statements above were true, then most patients would be expected to have a long cancer-free period following the detection of the primary. This is not the case, as may be seen from Fig. 1, which shows the changes of the proportion of patients free of metastases as a function of the time elapsing from the detection of the primary. These data (collected in Curie-Skłodowska Cancer Institute in Warsaw, Poland) concern breast cancer and include only Category 1 cases (i.e., least serious cases, when the lymph nodes are not affected, no mastectomy is performed, and no radiotherapy or chemotherapy is applied). Yet, as may be seen from Fig. 1, even in such cases, in about 8% of patients, a metastasis is detected within two years from detection of the primary. For other groups of patients the situation is much worse, and a

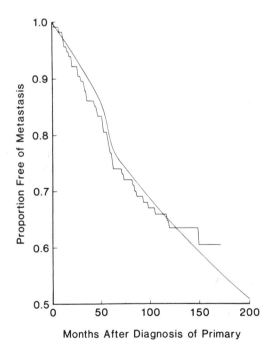

Months After Diagnosis of Primary

FIGURE 1   Kaplan-Meier estimate of time to metastasis and the fit obtained from the model of Section V.

substantial percentage of patients are metastatic (lymph nodes affected) already at detection of the primary.

These data, by being in direct contradiction to the consequences of Theorems 1 and 2, force us to reject at least one of the hypotheses underlying these theorems. We formulate this conclusion as the following logical dilemma:

Either the tumors do not grow exponentially, or, if they do, the rate of shedding metastases cannot be proportional to the tumor size.

III. ANALYSIS OF TUMOR GROWTH CURVES

This section contains two main parts: theoretical and empirical. In the first part we present the methods (introduced in [2]) which allow tumor growth curves to be determined, given the sample of tumor sizes as measured at the times of their detection. We also formulate some theorems concerning the properties of the introduced estimator of the growth curve.

In the empirical part we show the results of estimation, based on two sets of data (see [2,6,7]).

A. Growth Function Estimator

The question of the shape of the growth function of tumors has been a center of attention of cancer specialists in view of its relevance for assessing the risk of metastasis. The main competitors to exponential growth, as described by Hypothesis 1, are various forms of bounded or subexponential growth curves, such as logistic or Gompertzian.

The main trouble here is with empirical evidence. The obvious source of information is to take measurements of tumor sizes at several times—at least three for each tumor. This may be possible in animal studies, but for human cancer one faces an ethical problem: when a tumor is detected, it ought to be removed, and even if for some reasons it cannot be removed, the patient should receive treatment intended to inhibit the growth of the tumor. As a result, subsequent observations of tumor sizes, even if available, are confounded with treatment effects.

We are therefore left with a seemingly impossible task of estimating the growth curve, while being able to measure the size of each tumor only once, when it is detected.

We start from presenting the essential part of the results given in [2], which show that, contrary to intuitive expectations, the growth curve may indeed be estimated from such data. The key to the solution is that the size of the tumor at detection is random.

Since the inference about the growth curve is indirect, it has to be based on some theoretical relationships between appropriate features of the observable data and the growth curve. Such a relationship, in turn, must be derived from certain hypotheses—i.e., from a model of the phenomenon under study.

First, we must postulate that the object we are after—the common growth curve—does exist. Accordingly, we assume the following hypothesis.

Hypothesis 1a (Existence of Common Growth Curve). *Each tumor grows like f(t/α), where f is the common growth function, assumed to be strictly increasing and continuous, and α is the (reciprocal of) the growth rate, specific for a given tumor.*

In more picturesque language we may say that each patient has an "internal clock" set at some value α, and the tumor grows according to the function f, whose graph is traversed at the rate α (in Hypothesis 1 it was assumed that f was exponential).

Observe that we assume that the growth of each tumor is deterministic, so size variability at detection is due to randomness of the detection process. The latter is described by the following assumption.

Hypothesis 3 (Detection). *Suppose that the tumor has not been detected until time t, and its size is f(t/α). Then the probability that it will become detected between t and t + h equals bf(t/α)h + o(h), where h is some constant (detection rate) assumed to be independent of the patient.*

What this hypothesis asserts is that the factor responsible for detection of the tumor is its size: the larger the tumor, the more likely that it will be detected. The relation is linear. This hypothesis is of the same type as Hypothesis 2 (metastatic rate); thus, it is postulated that detection and shedding a metastasis are events governed by the same stochastic laws.

The tumors for which Hypothesis 3 might be closest to reality are those located on or near the surface of the body. One tumor is breast cancer, used in this chapter. Another natural possibility is skin cancer.

Finally, the last hypothesis is more technical.

Hypothesis 4 (Variability of Growth Rates). *The scaling factors α vary in the population of patients according to a gamma distribution.*

This assumption is not too restrictive, provided that the distribution of scaling factors is unimodal: the class of gamma-distributions is sufficiently rich to provide a fair approximation to most unimodal distributions.

To formulate the result, we need to introduce some notation. Firstly, we let X denote the size of the tumor at detection, and let

$$W(x) = P(X \leq x) \tag{3}$$

so that W(x) is estimated by the fraction of patients in the sample who had their tumor detected at size x or less.

Next, let $f(0) = c$, so c is the size of a single cell, and let $g(x)$ be the function inverse to the common growth function $f(t)$.

Finally, let a and r denote the scale and shape parameters of the gamma distribution of scaling factors α, so the mean scaling factor is r/a and the variance is r/a^2. We then have the following theorem (see [2]).

Theorem 3.   *Under Hypothesis 1a, 2, and 4 for all* $x \geq c$ *we* have

$$g(x) \;=\; \frac{a}{br} \int_{c}^{x} \frac{dW(u)}{u[1 - W(u)]^{1+1/r}} \equiv \frac{a}{br}\, h(x) \tag{4}$$

This theorem provides a relationship between the empirical data (distribution function W of tumor sizes at detection) and the function g (hence also the common growth function f, which is the inverse of g). To put it differently, this theorem shows that each hypothetical growth function is determined by the observable distribution of sizes at detection.

Consequently, we can use Theorem 3, replacing the cumulative distribution function W_N as follows. Suppose we have the data on sizes at detection (of tumors of some type) in a sample of N patients. sizes at detection (of tumors of some type) in a sample of N patients. Let the measurements, arranged in increasing order, be $u_1 \leq u_2 \leq \cdots \leq u_N$. Further, let

$$N(x) = \max\{j: \; u_j \leq x\} \tag{5}$$

so N(x) is the number of patients in the sample who had their tumors detected at size x or less. Then the empirical cumulative distribution function is $W_N(x) = N(x)/N$.

For x between u_1 and u_N define

$$h_N(x) \;=\; \sum_{j=1}^{N(x)} \frac{1}{u_j(N - j + 1)^{1+1/r}} \tag{6}$$

One may then show that $h_N(x)$ is an estimator of $A + Bg(x)$, where A and B are some constants, of which A, and possibly also B, are not estimable.

Two problems have to be resolved before we can use this fact for inference about the function $g(x)$, hence also about the growth function $f(t)$:

1. We need to know r in order to calculate the values of the function $h_N(x)$ from the data.
2. Even if r were known, the values $h_N(x)$ would provide estimates not of $g(x)$, which is the main object of our interest, but of $A + Bg(x)$, with unknown A and B.

The situation for problem 2 is relatively simple: we may get rid of constants A and B by observing that the ratios

$$\frac{h_N(x + y) - h_N(x)}{h_N(z + w) - h_N(z)} \tag{7}$$

are estimators of the corresponding ratios

$$\frac{g(x + y) - g(x)}{g(z + w) - g(z)} \tag{8}$$

Quantity (8) is the ratio of the time it takes a tumor to grow from size x to size $x + y$ to the time it takes the tumor to grow from size z to size $z + w$. This ratio is independent of the scaling factor α, no matter whether the growth is exponential (in which case $g(x) = \log x$) or not.

There remains the problem of estimating the parameter r. To do that, we need two or more samples of patients, characterized by different detection constants b (with the remaining parameters, r and a, and the growth function f being the same). Omitting the technical details, we may estimate r by using the fact that the function $g(x)$, estimated from both samples, must be the same. This gives the condition for r; the ratio

$$\frac{W_1'(x)}{W_2'(x)} \left\{ \frac{1 - W_2(x)}{1 - W_1(x)} \right\}^{1+1/r}$$

must have the same value for all x (here W_1 and W_2 are the distributions of tumor sizes in the two samples).

There is a natural set of questions connected with every estimator. They concern its bias, mean square error, exact or

asymptotic distribution, and so forth. Some answers are given in [8];
we shall briefly mention the most important.

First, as regards the bias and mean square error of the estimator
$h_N(x)$ of the function $h(x)$ defined in (4), we have the following
theorem.

Theorem 4. *Assume that* $1/r$ *is an integer, say* $1/r = m$. *Then
for every* x *such that* $W(x) < 1$ *we have*

$$Eh_N(x) = h(x) + \frac{m(m+1)}{2N} \left\{ \int_c^x \frac{dW(u)}{u[1 - W(u)]^{m+2}} \right.$$

$$\left. - \int_c^x \frac{dW(u)}{u[1 - W(u)]^{m+1}} \right\} + o\left(\frac{1}{N}\right) \tag{10}$$

and

$$Var[h_N(x)] = \left(\frac{1}{N}\right)\left\{ \int_c^x \frac{dW(u)}{u^2[1 - W(u)]^{2m+2}} \right.$$

$$+ 2m(m+1) \int_c^x \int_c^x \frac{dW(u)\, dW(v)}{uv[1 - W(u)]^{m+1}[1 - W(v)]^{m+2}}$$

$$\left. - m^2 \left[\int_c^x \frac{dW(u)}{u[1 - W(u)]^{m+1}} \right]^2 \right\} + o\left(\frac{1}{N}\right)$$

$$= \frac{c(x)}{N} + o\left(\frac{1}{N}\right) \tag{11}$$

Moreover, as $N \to \infty$ *the asymptotic distribution of*

$$\sqrt{N}[h_N(x) - Eh_N(x)] \tag{12}$$

is $N[0, c(x)]$, *where* $c(x)$ *is given in* (11).

Theorem 4 allows us to construct confidence intervals for $h(x)$
for any fixed value of x. Some other theorems proved in [8] extend this possibility to (12), regarded as a function of x, hence
to the situation when the result of estimation is treated as a sample
path of a certain stochastic process.

The assumption of Theorem 4, namely that $1/r$ is an integer,
is not too restrictive: as will be seen from analysis of the data
presented in the next section, the value of r is close to 1 (at least
for breast tumors).

B. Empirical Results

1. The Data

The following results are based on two sets of data, both concerning breast tumors. One set consists of some 4000 cases treated at M. D. Anderson Hospital and Tumor Institute in Houston between 1945 and 1981. In the sequel, we shall refer to this set as MDA data. The second set comprises 600 cases of breast cancer treated at The Ohio State University Hospital between 1948 and 1983; this set is called OSU data.

In the MDA data the tumor volumes were assessed from mammographs, where tumor length and width were recorded. The volume was calculated using the assumption that the tumor is a prolate ellipsoid whose axes are the measured length and width. When a tumor appeared as spheroid, only one measurement was recorded and the volume was calculated accordingly.

In the OSU data the sizes were assessed by palpation, and one (44% of cases), two (48% of cases), or three (8% of cases) dimensions were recorded. Again, the volume was calculated using the assumption that the tumor was ellipsoidal.

For estimating the shape parameter r of the gamma distribution of growth rates, we partitioned the MDA data into four equal subgroups according to the time of diagnosis. Subsequent partitioning of the OSU data according to the same time intervals did not lead to equal groups (see Table 1).

The OSU data partitioned into groups of about equal size are shown in Table 2. Patients in OSU data entered the study at a more or less uniform rate of approximately one per month. On the other hand, in the MDA data we note a scarcity of patients in the first 20 years. This may be due in part to a relatively low usage of mammography (on which MDA data are based) before the early 1960s (see [9]).

Note that in both sets of data, the median sizes, mean sizes, and maximum and minimum sizes tend to decrease. This indicates that there has been a systematic progress in detection methods during the last 30 years or so.

We also note that the median volume at detection appears to be significantly smaller (p < 0.0001 based on the median test) in the OSU data as compared with the MDA data. The same holds for means and standard deviations (however, as explained later, the latter statistics should not be used in this case).

One possible explanation may be that many tumors were not ellipsoidal but consisted of a solid nucleus surrounded by a more elastic outer shell. The sizes obtained by palpation are of the more solid core, whereas those sizes obtained by mammography include the more pliable outer layer. A second explanation could be that tumors, though oblong in shape, tend to be oriented with respect to the

TABLE 1   Comparison of MDA and OSU Data

Begin date	End date	No. cases		Median size		Mean size		Standard deviation	
		MDA	OSU	MDA	OSU	MDA	OSU	MDA	OSU
3/12/45	4/2/65	934	244	22.4	14.1	87.5	50.7	189.4	197.8
4/6/65	12/8/70	934	96	18.9	5.8	80.9	47.2	159.6	191.0
12/15/70	8/26/75	934	84	14.1	5.2	72.1	17.6	153.4	28.3
8/28/75	5/31/83[a]	934	172	14.1	4.2	51.3	12.6	128.5	24.4

[a]The final period for MDA data ends 2/12/81.

TABLE 2   Characteristics of OSU Data for Four Time Periods

No. Cases	Begin date	End date	Min. size (cm^3)	Max. size (cm^3)	Median size (cm^3)	Mean size (cm^3)	Standard deviation (cm^3)
150	7/18/48	8/4/59	0.188	2,827.4	68.7	14.1	248.1
147	9/12/59	5/2/68	0.335	1,767.2	40.8	6.3	158.5
149	7/1/68	3/15/77	0.131	205.3	17.1	5.2	29.1
150	3/29/77	5/31/83	0.079	150.8	11.3	4.2	19.7

mammary ducts and thus directed toward the nipple. On mammographs both the longer and shorter axes tend to be visible, whereas palpation may lead to the two shorter axes. A final explanation,
in view of the fact that all OSU measurement were made by the
same physician, might be a systematic underestimation of the actual
tumor sizes for those patients with moderate to large tumor masses.

2. Estimation of Growth Curve

It is not unreasonable to assume that the biological characteristics,
as expressed by the growth function f and variability of doubling
times in the population of patients (parameters r and a), remained
the same during the last 30 years or so. The only changes may be
(1) the overall incidence of breast cancer (which need not concern
us here) and (2) the detection rates b. Consequently, we may regard the four strata as four samples corresponding to different
values of the parameters b (in other words, we postulate here that
within the times that separate the subsamples, the detection rates
remained constant).

Without the technical details, the situation is as follows. The
estimate of r, based on formula (9) and using the four groups in
MDA data, is r = 0.53. With this r, the graphs of f (more precisely,
inverse to the function $h_N(x)$, drawn on a logarithmic scale) for the
four groups are shown on Fig. 2.

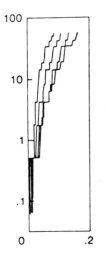

FIGURE 2   Estimates of growth curve based on $h_N(x)$ for r = 0.53
(MDA data). Horizontal axis: time in arbitrary units. Vertical
axis: log volume (cm³).

The apparent linearity of these estimates is good evidence that growth is indeed exponential, at least between about 0.1 cm^3 to 100 cm^3. If there is any flattening of the growth curve (as one may expect from considering physical or nutritional limitations on growth), then it occurs beyond the range of sizes typically observed at detection.

The time scale (horizontal axis on Fig. 2) is expressed in arbitrary units, because the data with one measurement per tumor cannot possibly carry any information about actual values of growth rates. We may only know how they vary with respect to one another: this is expressed through the parameter r, since $1/\sqrt{r}$ is the coefficient of variation of scaling factors (hence also of doubling times).

IV. SOME CONSEQUENCES OF EXPONENTIAL GROWTH

We have now identified the source of troubles encountered in Sections I and II: since tumor growth appears to be exponential (or close to it), the fault must lie with Hypothesis 2. Before analyzing certain alternatives to this hypothesis, let us explore some of the consequences of exponentiality of tumor growth.

First, we do not claim that tumor growth is in reality *exactly* exponential. The model of exponential growth is based on the crudest and most intellectually primitive assumptions, which are unlikely to hold in the analyzed situations. As soon as one takes into account any factor that must affect tumor growth (such as pressure from the surrounding tissue, nutritional effects, existence of "dormant" cells), one arrives at some form of bounded or subexponential growth, resulting typically from a solution of an appropriate system of differential equations (for a review of models of tumor growth, see [10]). The main point is, however, that all these models predict that initially the growth will be approximately exponential. Our findings indicate that tumor growth up to the size of about 80–100 cm^3 ought to be regarded as its "initial" phase, with the growth curve indistinguishable from an exponential curve.

In what follows, we simply accept Hypotheses 1 (exponential growth) 3 (detection), and 4 (variability of growth rates). We now have the following theorem.

Theorem 5. *The density of distribution of sizes X at detection is*

$$w(x) = \frac{rb}{a} \left[1 + \frac{b}{a}(x - c) \right]^{-(r+1)} \tag{13}$$

Consequently, the expectation of X exists only if $r > 1$, and
equals $E(X) = c + a/[b(r - 1)]$, and the variance exists only if
$r > 2$.

The importance of this theorem lies mainly (though not solely)
in the possibility of deriving maximum likelihood equations for estimating the parameter r and the ratios b/a for various groups of
patients (characterized, in different periods, by different detection
constants b).

The maximum likelihood estimates are probably more precise than
the estimate of r based on formula (9). This latter estimate was
obtained by a rather rough method of trial and error and visual
comparison of the resulting curve with a straight line.

Note, however, the logic underlying the process of testing the
hypothesis of exponentiality of growth: the estimate based on (9)
does not rely on the assumption tested, and because of that it was
justifiable to conclude from Fig. 2 that growth is (approximately)
exponential. It is only after this claim was accepted as an assumption that we could use the results of this section.

The maximum likelihood of r are 1.038 for MDA data and 1.17
for OSU data, with standard error of the latter estimate being about
0.23 (see [2] and [7]). This means that the distribution of doubling
times is close to exponential. It appears therefore that variability of
growth rates in the population of patients is higher than one might
have expected a priori.

With these values of r, the estimates of the growth function f
[i.e., estimates based on the function $h_N(x)$] were evaluated again.
The results (for MDA data) are shown in Fig. 3 (the graphs for
OSU data are analogous).

The observed values of r so close to 1 mean that the variance
of sizes X at detection is infinite, whereas the expectation $E(X)$,
even if finite, is probably very large (this is supported empirically
by occasional detection of very big tumors). The practical consequence of these facts may be summarized as a warning to avoid
using the sample mean and sample variance of tumor sizes, in view
of the likely instability of these measures between samples. Instead,
one should use measures such as the median, whose role in the
present context is stressed by the following theorem.

Theorem 6. The medians m_i in populations characterized by detection constants b_i satisfy the relation

$$m_i b_i = c + \frac{a}{b_i} (1^{1/r} - 1) \tag{14}$$

If c (size of a single cell) is neglected, this means that the
product $m_i b_i$ is constant. Consequently, progress in detection

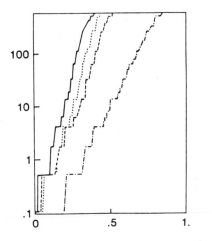

FIGURE 3   Estimates of growth curve based on $h_N(x)$ for r = 1.038 (MDA data). Horizontal axis: time in arbitrary units. Vertical axis: log volume (cm^3).

methods (as measured by the ratio b_1/b_2 in two periods) is reflected in the ratio m_2/m_1 of the corresponding median sizes at detection.

As the next consequence of exponential growth, let us mention the possibility of testing a generalization of Hypothesis 3. It is natural to suspect that the probability of detecting a tumor is proportional to some power of the tumor size; the obvious "candidates" for the exponent are 1/3, if the probability of detection depends linearly on the diameter of the tumor, or 2/3, if it depends on the two-dimensional cross section. If one assumes exponential growth, it is easy to derive the equations for maximum likelihood estimates of the exponent in the generalized Hypothesis 3. Such an estimation was carried out for MDA data [11] and for OSU data [7]. Again, the results are consistent: the MDA estimate of the exponent is 0.9, with the upper limit of the 95% confidence interval being 0.95, and the OSU data yield the exponent to be about 1, with the lower limit of the 95% confidence interval equal to 0.85. These findings constitute an argument in favor of the original version of Hypothesis 3, with exponent 1 (which means that the probability of detection is proportional to the tumor volume). It is worth mentioning that Hypothesis 3 with exponent close to 1 is acceptable only for primary tumors: in local recurrence (see [11]), this exponent was found to be about 0.44, an exponent giving values close to the diameter of the tumor.

Finally, the most far-reaching consequences of the fact that
tumor growth is exponential are contained in the following theorem
(see [2]).

Theorem 7. *The conditional distribution of growth rates given*
the size X a detection is gamma, with parameters $r + 1$ *and* $a +$
$b(X - c)$.

Consequently, the conditional expectation of growth rate given
the size X at detection is

$$E(\alpha \mid X) = \frac{r + 1}{a + b(X - c)} \tag{15}$$

Intuitively, this means that a tumor detected when it is large is
likely to be fast growing.

As already mentioned, the maximum likelihood estimates of the
ratio b/a are available; alternatively, one can use Theorem 6 and
estimate b/a (for a given period) as $m/2^{1/r} - 1$), where m is the
observed median size at detection in this period. Consequently, the
practical use of Theorem 7 depends on obtaining an estimate of a or,
equivalently, of the mean doubling time $(r/a)\log 2$.

Clearly, we need some data involving more than one observation
per tumor. As explained in the Introduction, such data are difficult
to obtain, since measurements of tumor sizes after detection (even
if available) would typically be confounded with treatment effects,
whereas before detection the tumor sizes are not observable.

The last part of the previous sentence looks like a logical
tautology; in reality, however, it is simply false, and this provides
us with an estimate of the mean doubling time for breast tumors.
In screening programs it is sometimes found that a tumor detected
at some screening was overlooked in the preceding screening or even
in several screenings (see [12]), thus giving a series of observations
of sizes of the same tumor at various times. The survey [13] suggests a mean doubling time for breast tumors of about 107 days,
which yields $a = 6.72 \times 10^{-3}$. Given an estimate of b/a, one may
find the value of b (for a given period, since b changes with the
progress of detection methods). For instance, for MDA data and
the most recent period b is about 5.04×10^{-4} (with time measured
in days). Using the estimated value of r, one may easily compute
the expected doubling time of a tumor detected at size X simply by
multiplying the value in formula (15) by $\log 2$.

In addition to the point estimate (15), Theorem 7 specifies the
posterior distribution of the rate α given the size X at detection,
and this allows us to construct confidence intervals.

Figure 4 shows the point estimate (middle curve) and the upper
and lower endpoints of a 95% confidence interval with symmetric

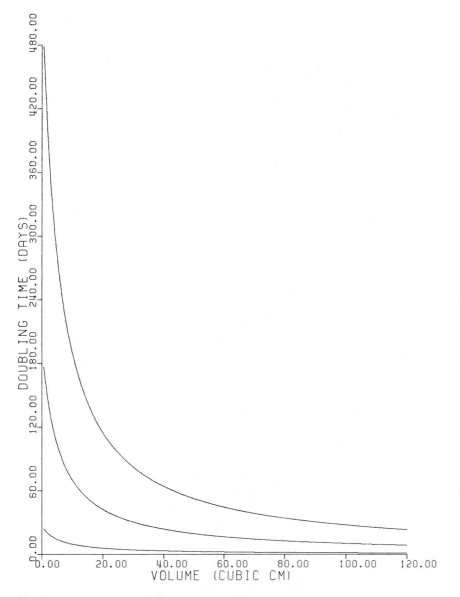

FIGURE 4   Point estimate (middle curve) and 95% confidence interval for doubling time of a tumor detected at a given size.

probabilities for the doubling time of a tumor just detected at size X (see [7]). We used here the mean doubling time of 107 days and the values of r and b from OSU data for the most recent period.

Notice that for small tumors the upper limit (which is a rapidly decreasing function of size) is so large that it provides little insight into the doubling time, but the lower limit gives a reasonable upper bound on growth. For example, if X is 1 cm^3, the doubling time is at least three weeks, whereas if X is 5 cm^3, the doubling time is at least two weeks, etc. On the other hand, for large tumors the upper bound for doubling time is rather low, thus giving a lower bound for growth. For example, if X = 100 cm^3, the doubling time is no more than four weeks.

The confidence intervals in Fig. 4 are rather wide. Since the underlying distribution is asymmetric, they could be somewhat shortened if one used the optimal allocation of probabilities to the two tails of the distribution. But even the shortest confidence intervals would be wide, which ought to be expected: after all, they are based on a *single* observation of tumor size, and one should rather marvel at the fact that such an observation allows *any* inference about the growth rate.

The foregoing estimator of the doubling time was used in [11] to shed some light on the following questions: Do all tumors of the same person grow with the same rate? If not, what is the relationship between rates of growth of the primary and metastatic tumors of the same person?

Observe that one of the difficulties here lies in the detection mechanism of secondary tumors, which may be quite different than that for the primary tumors. Even assuming the same basic mechanism, as described in Hypothesis 3, the detection constants for metastatic and primary tumors would certainly be different. Consequently, it is not possible to use estimator (15) for tumors other than the primary ones.

The analysis in [11] concerned local recurrences, i.e., tumors that result from an error in surgical operation of removal of the primary: some part of it is left and therefore allowed to develop into a new tumor.

Now, local recurrences are the only kind of tumors whose age at detection is known exactly. Consequently, knowing the final size, one can easily compute the growth rate, the only problem being that one does not know the initial number of cells. One can, however, estimate the mean initial number of cells and use it for assessing the growth rates of recurrent tumors. Combined with the knowledge of size of the primary (hence also an estimate of its growth rate), one gets bivariate data on growth rates of the primary and recurrence for the same person. It appears that (1) the mean initial size is about 60,000 cells, (2) the primary and recurrent tumors have the same doubling time of about 3.1 months,

and (3) the growth rates of the primary and recurrence are nearly
unrelated (for details, see [11]).

V. SYSTEMIC COMPONENT IN CANCER PROGRESSION

Figure 1 shows the data on time to metastasis for breast cancer
taken from Curie-Sklodowska Cancer Institute in Warsaw. As already argued, the relatively frequent occurrence of times to
metastasis below the limit of two years or so is incompatible with
Hypothesis 2. More precisely, Hypotheses 1 and 2 jointly imply
that *most metastases must occur shortly before detection of the
primary.* Consequently, if Hypotheses 1 and 2 are to be retained,
then it is necessary to find some additional factors to adequately
explain the frequent short waiting time for detecting a metastasis.

Now, the obvious factors that may (at least partially) account
for early detection of metastases are the following:

1. Different detection mechanism, or higher detection rate
    (with the same mechanism) for secondary tumors than for
    primary tumors.
2. Possible higher growth rates for metastatic tumors.
3. Metastatic tumors need not start from a single cell.

For a discussion of these issues and some empirical evidence, see
[5].

The role of factor 1 may be partially assessed by analyzing the
sizes of metastatic tumors at detection (though records of such sizes
are scarce). But even if metastatic tumors tend to be detected at
smaller sizes, the difference (in terms of number of doubling periods)
cannot be very large: there is a threshold, about 10^7 cells, below
which no tumor, primary or metastatic, is going to be detected, at
least for years.

Regarding 2, very little is known about growth rates of different tumors of the same person. Thus far we considered only primary tumors, and this problem did not arise; consequently, we
needed only an assumption about interpersonal variability of growth
rates. When the analysis concerns more than one tumor of the
same patient, the problem of intrapatient variability arises.

Some information here was obtained from recurrences, as mentioned at the end of the last section, and it appears that the growth
rates of primary and recurrence are largely unrelated. Whether the
same remains true for metastatic tumors is unknown, since we do
not have a good method of estimating the growth rate of a metastatic
tumor. (In [5], p. 273, the author assumes that "the net rate of
growth of the metastasis is somewhat larger than that of the primary,"
and comments that such an assumption is "not unreasonable."

However, no empirical evidence is mentioned, and the author may have been motivated to accept this assumption because it was needed to evaluate some formulas.)

Regarding the third factor, the size at which a metastatic tumor starts, not much is known, except that this size must be restricted by the size of blood vessels traversed. Some data (see [5]) suggest that tumor cells do not adhere well to one another, which would indicate that perhaps most metastases originate from a single cell.

Without trying to diminish the possible importance of factors 1–3, we follow the usual research strategy of isolating the research objective and (conceptually) disregarding all other factors. Consequently, we shall suppress the roles of 1–3 and explore two possibilities:

1. Retain Hypothesis 2 and allow for the possibility that some tumors are not metastases from the primary.
2. Abandon Hypothesis 2.

In this section we shall deal with the first possibility and see how much can be explained by assuming that there exists another source of secondary tumors (besides metastases).

The results of this section were, to a large extent, inspired by the discoveries reported in [14]. We had been conducting a preliminary statistical analysis of cancer data on waiting time of detection of a metastasis (see Fig. 1), treating the observed times of successive metastases as a nonhomogeneous Poisson process. The estimation of the (time-dependent) intensity of this process led to a somewhat puzzling result that this intensity is reasonably constant, instead, as had been expected, of increasing after about two years.

Consequently, in [3] we suggested a model combining two mechanisms for spread of tumors. The first represents the traditional metastatic mechanism, as specified in Hypothesis 2. The second mechanism, called "systemic," contributes a constant probability to new tumor occurrence that is independent of existing tumors.

Hypothesis 5 (Systemic Tumors). *The probability of a systemic occurrence of a new tumor in the time interval between t and t + h is $\lambda h + o(h)$ and is independent of the prior cancer history of the patient. Here λ is some constant (systemic rate), and $o(h) \to 0$ as $h \to 0$.*

In the sequel, tumors originating from the systemic source will be called *quasi-metastases*; the blanket term for both metastases and quasi-metastases will be *secondary tumors*.

The situation would be simple if one could always tell whether a given secondary tumor is a metastasis from the primary. Often it is not possible.

As in all stochastic models, to enable any inference, we must first deduce (from the hypotheses of the model) some logical consequences which describe the statistical properties of the observable events. In our case the events are those connected with the time T that elapses between the detection of the primary tumor and the detection of the first secondary tumor (the empirical distribution of T is shown in Fig. 1).

To enable derivation of such consequences and to keep the number of parameters under control, we make the following (likely counterfactual) assumptions:

Hypothesis 6 (Simplification). (1) *The detection rate is the same for all tumors, primary or secondary.* (2) *All tumors of the same patient grow with the same rate.* (3) *Every tumor starts its growth from a single cell.*

One can prove (under some additional technical assumptions that need not concern us here) the following theorem.

Theorem 8. *Let* $v(u)$ *be determined from the relation*

$$u = \int_0^v \frac{ds}{u + b + \frac{s}{\alpha} + \mu e^{-s}} \tag{16}$$

and let

$$k(s) = \lambda \left[\int_0^s e^{-v(u)} \, du - 1 \right] \tag{17}$$

The the probability of no secondary tumor for the time at least t *is*

$$P(T > t) = \frac{a^r b}{\Gamma(r)} \int_0^\infty \alpha^{r-1} e^{-a\alpha} \int_0^\infty \left\{ \exp \; k(t) + \frac{u}{\alpha} + \alpha \lambda v(t) \right.$$
$$- \alpha b (e^{u/\alpha} - 1) - \alpha \lambda \log[1 + e^{-u/\alpha}(e^{v(t)} - 1)]$$
$$\left. + \alpha \mu e^{u/\alpha}(e^{v(t)} - 1) \log[1 + (e^{-u/\alpha} - 1)e^{-v(t)}] \right\} \, du \, d\alpha \tag{18}$$

Formula (18) involves quadruple integration and contains five parameters: a, r, b, μ, and λ. To reduce computational complexity to a manageable level, we disregarded the variability of growth rates α: parameters a and r were then replaced by the common growth rate, say β, and the formulas involved only triple integration.

The sample comprised 116 women with localized breast cancer from Curie-Skłodowska Cancer Institute in Warsaw. To reasonably satisfy the assumptions of the model concerning the growth of metastatic and quasi-metastatic tumors, the sample contained only those patients whose primary tumor was classified as Category 1 (least serious). For such patients the primary tumor was removed, but no mastectomy was performed, lymph notes were not affected, and no chemotherapy or radiotherapy was applied. In short, at the time of removal of the primary tumor, no action was taken that would affect the growth of any secondary tumor existing at that time.

The maximum likelihood estimates of the parameters were as follows: metastatic rate, $\mu = 0.17 \times 10^{-9}$; detection rate, $b = 0.23 \times 10^{-8}$; mean growth rate, $\beta = 3.23$; and systemic rate, $\lambda = 0.0030$. Figure 1 presents the Kaplan-Meier estimates of the proportion free of discovered secondary tumors and the proportion from the model, with the above values of the parameters. The agreement of the model with the data appears quite satisfactory.

Some of the consequences of the obtained parameters are as follows. The mean doubling time is 2.2 months. The median time from primary origination to detection is 59.2 months, and at that time the tumor consists of $9.3 \times 10^{+7}$ cells. The mean time to quasi-metastasis due to systemic process is 27.7 years. The probability of a metastasis prior to detection of the primary is 0.069.

An attempt was made to fit the same model, without the systemic mechanism, to the data. The attempt failed: the fitting procedure tried to drive μ to 0 and β to ∞, and the likelihoods were much smaller than for the full model.

In Table 3 we examine the relative significance of the metastatic and systemic processes. For all times examined the cumulative risk of a systemic tumor exceeds that of a metastatic tumor.

With our present knowledge, it is easy to criticize the estimated values of parameters. The mean doubling period of 2.2 months appears too short (the current view, as mentioned in Section IV, puts this value at 107 days). This however, is not too serious, since the data allowing the mean doubling time to be estimated are scarce and not too precise.

What is more troublesome is the calculated median size at detection: $9.2 \times 10^{+7}$ cells is about 0.1 cm^3, which is two orders of magnitude below the actual value. Similarly, the obtained detection rate $b = 0.23 \times 10^{-8}$ (with time measured in months and size in number of cells) is about two orders of magnitude off the value $b = 5.04 \times 10^{-4}$ (units: days, cm^3) reported in preceding sections.

These discrepancies are not too essential, though: it suffices to realize that the estimates in this section were based on small sample (116 cases) and, moreover, they used only the information about the time to secondary tumor, not about the sizes at detection.

TABLE 3 Probability of One or More
Metastases from Two Mechanisms Before
Various Times from Primary Origination

Time (years)	Metastatic mechanism	Systemic mechanism
1	2.26×10^{-8}	0.0345
2	9.34×10^{-7}	0.0695
3	3.85×10^{-5}	0.102
4	1.57×10^{-3}	0.134
5	0.0423	0.165
6	0.0688	0.194
10	0.0688	0.302

The main conclusion, that the data cannot be explained if
Hypothesis 2 is retained unless we assume the existence of a systemic component, has been questioned by LeCam [5]. According to
him, the role of systemic component was overstressed, primarily due
to neglecting the variability of growth rates. However, private
communication from Brown and Thompson indicates that even when
variability of the growth rate is introduced into the model the systemic component is essential if Hypothesis 2 is to be retained.

VI. ABANDONING THE HYPOTHESIS OF METASTATIC RATE

In this section we consider some alternatives to Hypothesis 2. The
ultimate question that has to be answered in order to build any co-
herent theory of metastatic progression of cancer is, when do
metastases originate? Specifically, at which size is the primary
tumor most likely to shed a metastasis?

To put if formally, let $m(\alpha, u)$ stand for the metastatic intensity
of a tumor which grows with rate α (to be called simply α-tumor)
upon reaching size u. This means that the probability of shedding
a metastasis by an α-tumor between the times when it is of sizes u
and $u + h$ is $m(\alpha, u)h + o(h)$. The first issue one has to settle
is whether there exist observable events which could provide, however indirect, access to the function $m(\alpha, u)$.

The natural candidates for such events are those associated
with two variables: the size X of the primary at detection, and

the time T till the first secondary tumor is observed. The following
theorem, proved in [4], shows that the joint distribution of X and
T contains the desired information.

Theorem 9. *Assume that both the primary and metastasis grow
with the same rate* α, *satisfying Hypothesis 4, and their detections
occur according to Hypothesis 3, with constants b and b*. Then
the metastatic intensity* $m(\alpha,u)$ *satisfies the relation*

$$F(t, x) = P(T < t \mid X = x)$$

$$= \frac{[a + b(x - c)]^{r+1}}{\Gamma(r + 1)} \int_0^\infty \alpha^r e^{-\alpha[a+b(x-c)]}$$

$$\times \int_c^x \left\{ 1 - \exp\left[-\frac{\alpha}{u}b^*cx(e^{t/\alpha} - 1)\right] \right\} m(\alpha, u) \, du \, d\alpha \qquad (19)$$

The probability F(t, x) is estimated by the fraction of patients
who had their secondary tumor detected in time less than t after
detection of the primary, among those whose primary tumor was detected at size x.

This theorem gives us some qualitative information about the
risk $m(\alpha, u)$. We know namely that F(t, x) is not negligibly small
for small t, which means that for small t the inner integral cannot
be too close to zero. This, in turn, implies that $m(\alpha, u)$ must be
relatively large for small u. We have therefore, at least qualitatively,
what we suspected from the start: small, hence young, primary
tumors must be more prone to metastasize than large ones.

This argument and, more precisely, formula (19) are based on
the crucial assumption that the mechanisms of detection are the
same for primary and metastatic tumors, the only difference being
the values of the detection constants. Such an assumption for
metastatic tumors may at best be treated only as a crude approximation to reality. Indeed, detection of metastatic tumors typically
occurs during control visits, and therefore the distribution of time
T depends on the schedule of such visits. These problems are being investigated, and the results will be published elsewhere. In
their final form these results will provide a connection between the
metastatic rate $m(\alpha, u)$ and properties of some observable random
variables, a connection analogous to (19).

At any rate, the qualitative information contained in Theorem 8
suggests a search for explanatory hypotheses. One such possibility
has been analyzed in [4], and we give some of the main features of
the model.

The idea which we propose to explore is that (1) as the tumor grows it becomes gradually more heterogeneous, and (2) heterogeneity is inversely related to metastatic proneness.

The concept of heterogeneity is somewhat vague, and may be explicated in a number of ways, each conforming to the general intuition of "diversity," "internal variability," and the like. The way we suggest is to assume that each cell of a tumor belongs to one of a number of types. When a cell divides, it usually produces two daughter cells of the same type, but with some small probability a mutation to a new type may occur. Heterogeneity of the tumor is then defined as the number of types that are already present (regardless of the frequency of various types). The question of possible interpretation of the notion of type is left entirely open to creative imagination and factual knowledge of specialists.

Suppose that the total number of types is $R + 1$. Let us agree to say that the tumor is in state E_n if $R + 1 - n$ types are present in the tumor (i.e., n types are still missing). Thus, each tumor starts in state E_R, and the consecutive transitions are $E_R \to E_{R-1} \to \cdots \to E_0$. These transitions are governed by the following hypothesis.

Hypothesis 7 (Mutations). *If the state of the tumor at time t is E_n, then each of the existing cells has probability $\rho n h + o(h)$ of mutating to another type between t and $t + h$. When a mutation occurs, it always produces a cell of a type not yet present in the tumor.*

Next, Hypothesis 2 is replaced by the following hypothesis.

Hypothesis 8 (Heterogeneity and Metastases). *Suppose that an α-tumor is in state E_n at time t (and has not yet been detected). Then the probability that it will shed a metastasis between t and $t + h$ is $\mu n c e^{t/\alpha} h + o(h)$.*

According to Hypothesis 8, two factors contribute to proneness of metastasis: the size $c e^{t/\alpha}$ of the tumor, as in the original version of Hypothesis 2, and the degree n of homogeneity (number of missing types).

One can now prove the following theorem.

Theorem 10. *The distribution of the time V of shedding the first metastasis by an α-tumor is*

$$G(\alpha, t) = P_\alpha(V \leqslant t)$$

$$= 1 - \left(\frac{\rho}{\mu + \rho}\right)^R \left\{ 1 + \frac{\mu}{\rho} \exp[-\alpha c(\mu + \rho)(e^{t/\alpha} - 1)] \right\}^R \tag{20}$$

Observe that the metastatic risk at size u is then

$$m(\alpha, u) = \frac{\alpha}{u} G' \left[\alpha, \alpha \log \frac{u}{c} \right] \tag{21}$$

which can be used in Theorem 8.

The problem of testing this model (as well as related models, obtained by some modifications of Hypotheses 7 and 8), estimating the parameters, etc., are now under investigation, and the results will be published elsewhere.

The model leads to some interesting consequences about metastatic hazard rates (see Fig. 5) associated with density (20). The graphs show the hazard rates for some values of ρ and μ, and R = 5 (i.e., six cell types). As may be seen, tumors with large α (slow growing) are most dangerous at smaller sizes and become less dangerous (less metastatic prone). On the other hand, tumors with small α (fast growing) are less dangerous at smaller sizes, but their hazard function begins to dominate for larger sizes.

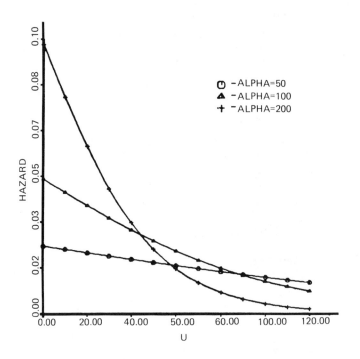

FIGURE 5   Metastatic hazard rate for three selected values of α.

VII. CONCLUSIONS

The aim of this chapter is twofold. The main objective was to present some specific results, both theoretical and empirical, which constitute the (admittedly rather meager) outcome of our attempts to understand the mechanisms of metastases. The second objective was to illustrate the role and importance of mathematics, especially modeling, in cancer research.

At this point it is necessary to stress the distinction between modeling and statistical research on cancer. The latter may provide basic information relating incidence, survival, etc., with different variables, of known or suspected partinence, such as age, type of diet, pollution, and so forth. The analysis here, by its nature, is always at the level of what is observable.

On the other hand, the attempts to explain the causes of various statistical phenomena related to cancer refer usually to statistical properties of events which are not observable. Such explanations (typically in the form of hypothetical "mechanisms" that generate unobservable events) require more or less extensive mathematical treatment, whose final product is one or more theorems connecting the properties of postulated mechanisms with the statistical characteristics of observable variables. Perhaps the best example here is our result on determining the shape of the growth curve from the data which involve only one observation per tumor—a small feast, totally impossible according to "common sense" logic. But it ought to be realized that only such theorems could provide us with an insight into the realm of unobservable events. They also allow us to test various hypothetical mechanisms and, eventually to discover the "laws of cancer."

It has been remarked (LeCam, personal communication) that, for any law of cancer that one may advance, it is always possible to find in the medical literature some cases that contradict it. This might indicate that the field is still too poor to look for regularities, and it is perhaps too early to attempt modeling.

The view advocated in this chapter is not so pessimistic. To be sure, the "freak" cases which contradict some of the current theories or beliefs do exist, and it would be a serious mistake to disregard them entirely. Actually, these freak cases constitute an enormously valuable source of information: it is the attempts to understand the causes behind any of these cases that often lead to inspiring conjectures, and it is quite possible that most of the progress in cancer research may ultimately be traced down to an analysis of such cases.

The latter, however, are, almost by definition, rare. The bulk of "typical" cases remains, for which we may hope that Nature follows some laws that can ultimately be discovered. It is here that mathematical modeling and statistics provide a meaningful and,

hopefully, valuable contribution to our understanding of the phenomenon of cancer.

REFERENCES

1. Encylopaedia Britannica, Vol. VI, p. 834 (1984).

2. Atkinson, E. N., Bartoszyński, R., Brown, B. W., and Thomp-
    son, J. R., On estimating the growth function of tumors. *Math.
    Biosci.*, *67*:145–166 (1983).

3. Bartoszyński, R., Brown, B. W., and Thompson, J. R.,
    Metastatic and systemic factors in neoplastic progression, in
    Probability Models and Cancer (L. LeCam and J. Neyman, eds.),
    North-Holland, Amsterdam, pp. 253–263 (1982).

4. Bartoszyński, R., Jones, B. F., and Klein, J. P., Some stochas-
    tic models of cancer metastasis. *Stochastic Models, 1(3)*:317–339
    (1985).

5. LeCam, L., On some mathematical models of tumor growth and
    metastasis, in *Probability Models and Cancer* (L. LeCam and
    J. Neyman, eds.), North-Holland, Amsterdam, pp. 265–283
    (1982).

6. Brown, B. W., Atkinson, E. N., Bartoszyński, R., Thompson,
    J. R., and Montague, E. D., Estimation of human tumor growth
    rate from distribution of tumor size at detection. *JNCI, 72*:
    31–38 (1984).

7. Klein, J. P., Bartoszyński, R., and James, A. G., Characteristic
    of growth rates and metastatic proneness of breast tumors,
    The Ohio State University, Dept. of Statistics Technical Re-
    port No. 339 (1986).

8. Bartoszyński, R. and Dynin, S. M., Asymptotic properties of
    the tumor growth curve estimator. *Journal of Statistical Planning
    and Inference* (in press).

9. Heshiki, A. and F. Osterman, The role of radiological examina-
    tions in the management of patients with suspected breast
    cancer, in *Current trends in the Management of Breast Cancer*
    (R. Baker, ed.), The Johns Hopkins University Press, Balti-
    more, pp. 66–76 (1977).

10. White, R. A., A review of some mathematical models in cell
    kinetics, in *Biomathematics and Cell Kinetics* (M. Rotenberg,
    ed.), Elsevier/North Holland, New York, pp. 243–261 (1981).

11. Brown, B. W., Atkinson, E. N., J. R. Thompson, and Montague, E. D., Lack of concordance of growth rates of primary and recurrent breast cancer, submitted.

12. Heuser, L., Spratt, J. S., and Polk, H. C., Growth rates of primary breast cancers, *Cancer*, *43(5)*:1888–1894 (1979).

13. Sasaki, T., Sato, Y., and Sakka, M., Cell population kinetics of human solid tumors: A statistical analysis in various histological types. *Gann*, *71*:520–529 (1980).

14. Bartoszyński, R., Brown, B. W., McBride, C. M., and Thompson, J. R., Some non-parametric techniques for estimating the intensity function of cancer-related nonstationary Poisson process. *Ann. Stat.* *9*:1050–1060 (1981).

7

Repair of Radiation Injury and the Time Factor in Radiotherapy

HOWARD D. THAMES, Jr. *Department of Biomathematics, University of Texas System Cancer Center, M.D. Anderson Hospital and Tumor Institute, Houston, Texas*

I. INTRODUCTION

Although the first radiotherapy treatments at the turn of the twentieth century were given as daily doses of low-dose-rate x-rays protracted over several days [1], technical advances in the design of x-ray tubes soon led to single-dose treatments [2]. It was recognized thereafter that the effectiveness of a given dose was greatly intensified when it was given a single, high-dose-rate shot rather than as multiple, daily exposures. Controversy over methods of treatment continued into the 1920s, when it became apparent that the successful treatment of deep-seated tumors required that the total radiation dose be broken up (or *fractionated*), into multiple small doses (or fractions) separated by time intervals sufficient for normal tissue recovery between doses [3].

The nature of this recovery was not understood, and it was defined in terms of the increase in dose required to elicit a given biological effect as treatment time (and usually, number of fractions) was increased. When the log of biologically isoeffective doses was plotted against the log of number of treatments [4,5] or log overall time [6], a straight line was obtained. The same was true when the log isoeffect dose was plotted against the log of exposure time, when radiation was given in a single shot at various dose rates. Many workers tried to link this behavior in a purely formal way to the

Schwarzschild law of photochemistry, which states that the effect
of a given exposure of light is proportional to the product of intensity (I) and time (T) raised to the power p, where p is less
than 1:

$$IT^p = constant \qquad (1)$$

Typical values of p for the dose-rate effect were in the range 0.8–
0.95. This relationship corresponded to a diminished effect with
decreasing dose rate (I), suggesting some type of "recovery"
process in the exposed material.

In his investigation of the time factor with fractionated radiation,
Strandqvist [6] found that log isoeffect dose was linear in log treatment time:

$$D = constant \times T^q \qquad (2)$$

where q = 0.22. He was taken by the mathematical symmetry between the Schwarzschild relationship (1) for dose-rate and fractionation effects, on the one hand, and the biological conception of low
dose rate as approximated by a series of many, small fractional doses.
Thus, in his discussion (pp. 232–233) on the significance of the
slope. Strandqvist pointed out that dose rate I equals dose divided
by time (D/T), so equation (1) could be rewritten $DT^{p-1} = constant.$
which is (2) with q = 1 − p.

Subsequently, the fractionation exponents for tumors were compared to those of normal tissues, notably, by Cohen [7]. It was
concluded that the q-value for skin was higher than that for skin
tumors, and therefore that normal tissues might recover to a greater
extent than tumors, the more radiation was fractionated. The
validity of Cohen's analysis [7,8] has since been questioned [9],
but the possibility of improving the results of radiotherapy by altering the pattern of dose delivery remains a lively topic [10].

Our purpose is to present mathematical models for recovery
processes after radiation-induced injury that involve repair. These
will be distinguished from recovery due to regeneration of survivors,
and experimental data will be set out, that typify the salient aspects
of repair. The most influential models of cellular survival after
radiation injury will be presented along with critical experimental
tests of the two main currents of thought on models of radiation
sensitivity. Finally, their extensions to fractionated and low-dose-
rate exposures will be described.

II. DATA

A. Dose-Survival, Repair, and Target Cells

The understanding of recovery from radiation injury was changed almost overnight after the publication of the first dose-survival curve for mammalian cells by Puck and Marcus [11] and the two-dose recovery curve of Elkind and Sutton [12]. The data of Puck and Marcus are shown in Fig. 1. A surviving cell is defined as one that retains the capability to divide indefinitely. The curve is characterized by the presence of an initial "shoulder" in the low-dose region; it terminates in an exponential with steeper slope than the initial slope, indicating an increased efficiency of killing at higher doses. The negative reciprocal of the terminal slope is called D_0, which defines the dose required to reduce survival by the factor $0.37 = 1/e$. The intercept on the dose axis of the terminal exponential is a dose called D_q, and is a measure of shoulder width. Extrapolation of the final exponential region to zero dose gives the extrapolation number n. These quantities are related by $D_q = D_0 \ln n$.

Elkind and Sutton [12] showed that when two sufficiently large radiation doses were given a few hours apart, the shoulder on the

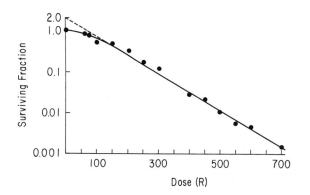

FIGURE 1   The first survival curve for mammalian (HeLa) cells. Cells were irradiated in vitro, and their viability was assayed as ability to form colonies in special culture medium. The curve has a "shoulder" preceding the exponential decrease in surviving fraction with increasing radiation dose (adapted from Ref. 11).

survival curve was reproduced in the second dose-survival curve
(Fig. 2). They interpreted the disappearance of memory of the
first dose as due to a repair process. Repair occurred approximately exponentially in time with a half-period of about 1 hr. It is
readily appreciated that if the shoulder of the survival curve is
always repeated between doses, then the response to multiple dose
fractions will be linear, with increasingly steeper slope as size of
dose per fraction increases. This was confirmed for 5 fractions
(Fig. 3) by Elkind and Sutton [13].

These developments introduced a new way of thinking about
radiation-induced injury to tissues, namely as a manifestation of
killing of target cells characterized by specific survival curves
[14−18]. Thus, the recovery effects observed in cell culture could
be used to predict tumor and normal tissue response to fractionated
radiotherapy. Also, a large component of the dose increase with
increasing time was seen to be due to repair, and, in fact, the
number (and size) of fractions, not time, might be the important
parameter.

B. Number of Fractions Versus Overall Time

In the developments described in the previous paragraphs, the
crucial assumption that varying the number of fractions for the
same total dose in the same overall time did not appreciably affect
the degree of reaction was rarely challenged. An exception was
Cohen's [19] suggestion that the recovery of mammary cancer was
dependent on number of fractions rather than overall time, when
these were large and separated by relatively long intervals (a suggestion that influenced subsequent clinical practice).

Fowler et al. [20] designed experiments on pigskin to distinguish
between two competing explanations of recovery: Elkind recovery,
and slow tissue repair (or repopulation). They knew that the effect
produced by 2000-rad x-rays given as a single dose was equal to
that produced by 3500 rad in 5 fractions over five days or by 5500
rad in 21 fractions over four weeks. The critical experiment was to
give 5 fractions distributed evenly over 28 days. If 3500 rad were
required for the same effect, the important factor would be the number of fractions, because the effect of slow repair and repopulation
would be relatively small, and the increase in dose with overall time
would be due to the effect of the smaller fractions. If, on the other
hand, 5500 rad were required to produce the same effect, then the
overall time of 28 days would be the important factor, and the number of fractions would be irrelevant, whether 5 or 21.

The results showed that 5 fractions over 28 days gave the same
skin effect with total doses of about 4200 rad, leading the authors
to conclude that overall time between 5 and 28 days was less important, and that the main effect determining the increase in dose

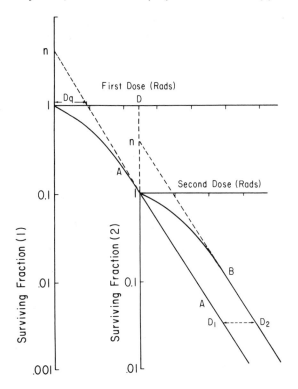

FIGURE 2 The effect of repair of sublethal injury on the survival of mammalian cells when a dose is delivered in two separate fractions. Curve A traces the single-dose response and curve B the response to a second dose given several hours after a first dose, D. If the single dose required to produce a certain surviving fraction is D_1, and the total dose required in two fractions to produce the same surviving fraction is D_2, then in the ideal case when all sublethal injury is repaired the slope of the second dose survival curve is the same as that for single doses (adapted from Ref. 12).

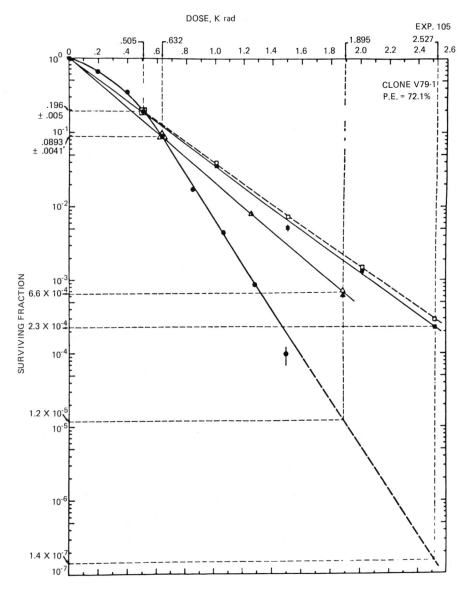

FIGURE 3 Response to fractionated doses with different sizes of dose per fraction. Single high dose-rate exposures of nongrowing cells (●) resulted in a shouldered survival curve. Complete recovery between doses of 5 (□) or 6.3 (△) Gy would be expected to lead to repetitions of the initial shoulder (cf. Fig. 2) and therefore to an exponential response to fractionated doses. Moreover, the response would be steeper, the larger the dose per fraction. The observed survival after doses of 5 (■) or 6.3 (▲) Gy separated by 22 hr confirmed this expectation (modified from Ref. 13).

with extended fractionation was the size and number of the individual fractions. The effect of overall time was, however, not negligible, because it contributed about one-third of the increase in total dose. The main conclusion was that the use of fewer and larger fractions required a reduction in total dose.

In the sequel we shall ignore the contribution of cellular proliferation to the response of tissues and cells to fractionated and low-dose-rate irradiation, and develop models of cell survival and fractionation effects that can describe significant components of the time factor in radiotherapy.

III. MODELS

Survival-curve models may be classified on the basis of their explanation of the shoulder. We shall label models that give an explanation based on the types of lesions induced by radiation "damage" models and those that ascribe the shoulder to repair processes will be labeled "repair" models.

A. Damage Models

1. Target Theory

Suppose that, as a result of the absorption of energy from the radiation beam, a density ξ of potentially damaging events exists, caused primarily by fast-moving electorns set into motion by Compton interactions between x rays and the biological material in the cell. Assume further that each member of the population presents a volume cross section σ for biologically damaging interaction; σ is the "target size" of the cell. If the total cell volume of the population is V, then

$$\rho \equiv \text{prob}\{a \text{ damaging event registers in a cell}\}$$

$$= \frac{\sigma\xi}{V\xi} = \frac{\sigma}{V}$$

ρ is know as the *hit probability* of a cell. Since $\sigma \leqslant$ volume of a single cell, ρ is quite small:

$$\rho \leqslant N^{-1} = O(10^{-5})$$

The probability that a cell will receive h "hits" from a total of $V\xi$ "tosses" is

$$\binom{V\xi}{h} \rho^h (1 - \rho)^{V\xi - h} = p(\rho, V\xi, h)$$

If a *single hit* suffices to kill the cell, then the surviving fraction is given by

$$p(\rho, V\xi, 0) = (1 - \rho)^{V\xi} \cong e^{-\rho V\xi}$$

which accounts for the pure exponential survival curve A shown in Fig. 4 (ξ is proportional to dose).

Now suppose that each cell has n targets, each with equal probability of being hit, and that a single hit is sufficient to inactivate each target. Carrying over the notation from above, we assume that

$$e^{-\rho V\xi} = \text{prob \{a target is not hit during } V\xi \text{ active events\}}$$

Then the probability that a cell survives with ν targets hit and $n - \nu$ targets missed is

$$P(\rho V\xi, n, \nu) = \binom{n}{\nu} (1 - e^{-\rho V\xi})^n (e^{-\rho V\xi})^{n-\nu} Q(\nu)$$

in which $Q(\nu) = \text{prob \{cell survives with } \nu \text{ targets hit\}}$. If inactivation of all n targets is required, then the surviving fraction is

$$\sum_{\nu=0}^{n-1} \binom{n}{\nu} (1 - e^{-\rho V\xi})^{\nu} (e^{-\rho V\xi})^{n-\nu} = 1 - (1 - e^{-\rho V\xi})^n$$

which is curve B in Fig. 4. This is known as the *multitarget single-hit* (sometimes simply multitarget) model.

The foregoing derivations have been simplified. More detail may be found in Elkind and Whitmore [22].

Curve C of Fig. 4 is the product of a curve of type A and a curve of type B. The rationale behind this form is that many radiation beams are heterogeneous in regard to the amount of energy deposited by secondary particles (electrons) along their tracks, defined by the LET (linear energy transfer) distribution for a particular energy in the spectrum of the radiation beam. X-rays and ^{60}Co γ-rays are usually termed low LET beams; neutrons give rise to tracks of high LET. Exponential killing (curve A) characterizes high LET beams, whereas curves with a "shoulder" like that of B are typical of low LET irradiation. It is natural to suppose that a beam with components of both types would lead to a curve of type C, where surviving fraction is given by

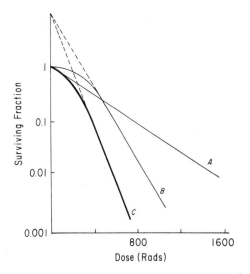

FIGURE 4   Diagram showing how the experimentally determined survival curve C can be reconstructed as the summation of two processes: single-hit inactivation, and killing from accumulation of sublethal injury (target inactivation). Curve A describes the dose-survival relationship for single-hit inactivation and is derived from measurements of cell survival at doses or dose rates low enough to exclude significant killing by accumulated sublethal injury. The curve for lethality from accumulated sublethal injury (B) is the multitarget, single-hit model derived in the text. It has zero initial slope; its extrapolation number coincides with that of the measured single-dose survival curve (C); and its terminal slope is the difference between the slope for single-hit inactivation (curve A) and the measured terminal slope of C. $s.f._C = s.f._A \times s.f._B$ and $slope_C = slope_A + slope_B$. (From Ref. 21 with permission.)

$$e^{-\rho'V\xi}[1 - (1 - e^{-\rho''V\xi})^n]$$

The primes are used to indicate the different target and dose-rate characteristics of the beam components. This model has been called the "two-component" model.

   Two features of the two-component model are noteworthy. First, the initial slope is nonzero, in agreement with almost all experimental observations of the response of mammalian cells. Second, the curve tends toward a linear asymptote as $\xi \to \infty$; this agrees with the wide results of the study of bacterial survival over an extremely wide range of doses (Fig. 5).

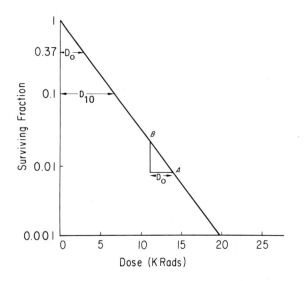

FIGURE 5   Survival curve for *E. Coli B.*   Survival is a simple exponential function of dose. D_0 is the mean lethal dose, i.e., the dose required to deliver an *average* of one lethal event per bacterial cell.   Because of the randomness of dose deposition, e^{-1} (or 37%) of cells survive a dose of D_0 rads, and the other 63% of cells receive one or more lethal events.   At any point on an exponential survival curve, a dose of D_0 rads reduces survival to 37% of its previous value, i.e., by one natural logarithm.   One of the important implications of an exponential survival curve is that, however great the dose, there is always a finite probability of a cell's surviving.   In the figure, $A = Be^{-1}$ (modified from Ref. 23).

2.   Linear-Quadratic (LQ) Models

Kellerer and Rossi [24] derived a quadratic dependence of lesion induction on dose based on microdosimetric considerations.   An analysis of the relative biological effectiveness (RBE) of various types of radiation as a function of absorbed dose led to the conclusion that cellular damage is proportional to the square of the specific energy, z, in the nucleus or in sensitive sites of the nucleus from about 1 to several micrometers diameter [24]:

$$\varepsilon(z) = kz^2$$

According to this relation, cellular damage results from the interaction of paris of radiation-induced sublesions. The quadratic dependence on specific energy leads to a LQ dependence on absorbed dose:

$$\varepsilon(D) = k(\zeta D + D^2) \qquad (3)$$

The linear term corresponds to that component of the damage due to lesions produced in one and the same particle track; ζ is the average increment of specific energy brought about by a single charged particle in the site. The quadratic term corresponds to the component of damage due to lesions produced by separate particles. Accordingly, one can state that the linear term represents the intratrack effect, and the quadratic term represents the intertrack effect.

Before the microdosimetric concepts had been developed which lead to (3), the LQ dose dependence had been deduced for the induction of dicentric chromosomes and centric rings. In this case $\varepsilon(D)$ represents the mean number of these aberrations per cell. Lea [25] gave an account of the reasoning, which, in essence, corresponds to the microdosimetric arguments. Kellerer and Rossi showed [24] that (3) reduced to

$$\varepsilon(D) = k\left(22.9 \, \frac{\bar{L}_D}{d^2} \, D + D^2\right)$$

where $\bar{L}_D$ is the dose average LET (keV/μm), d is the site diameter (μm), and D is the absorbed dose (rad). The relation expresses the fact that the chromosome aberrations are the result of two "single breaks"; the linear term represents the yield of aberrations resulting from the interaction of two breaks produced by the same particle track, and the quadratic term represents the yield due to interaction of breaks produced by different charged particles.

Chadwick and Leenhouts [26] arrived at the LQ model starting from molecular considerations. Thus, it was assumed that radiation-induced DNA double-strand breaks were the most critical lesions in cell reproductive death, chromosomal aberrations, and somatic mutations. Suppose α represents the average number per unit dose of double-strand breaks by induced by single radiation events, and β represents the average number per unit dose squared of double-strand breaks resulting from the combination of two unrepaired single-strand breaks. If p is the probability that a DNA double-strand break leads to cell reproductive death, then, by Poisson statistics, survival (S) is

$$S = \exp[-p(\alpha D + \beta D^2)] \qquad (4)$$

If q is the probability that a DNA double-strand break leads to a specific mutation, then the mutation frequency per surviving cell (M) can be described by

$$M = 1 - \exp[-q(\alpha D + \beta D^2)]$$

which, if $M \ll 1$, reduces to

$$M = q(\alpha D + \beta D^2) \tag{5}$$

This is a reasonable assumption, since doses that give an appreciable reduction in survival result in only one in a few thousands of mutations.

If a chromosome has a single DNA double-helix backbone (for references see Ref. 27), then a chromosome backbone break will be a DNA double-strand break. Chadwick and Leenhouts [26] proposed that one chromosome backbone break could lead to a visible chromosomal aberration and that the yield of chromsomal aberrations (Y) was therefore

$$Y = k(\alpha D + \beta D^2) \tag{6}$$

Using equations (4)–(6), they related cell survival to mutation frequency per surviving cell or chromosomal aberration yield

$$\ln S = -\left(\frac{p}{q}\right) M$$

or

$$\ln S = -\left(\frac{p}{k}\right) Y$$

These equations indicate that ln S is linearly related to mutation frequency per survivor or chromosome aberration yield, independent of the type of radiation, dose rate, or stage of the cell cycle, which affect only the coefficients α and β. The validity of these relations is illustrated in Fig. 6 for mutations induced by neutrons and γ-rays and for chromosomal aberrations induced at different stages of the cell cycle. Similar straight-line correlations have been found by others (for references see Ref. 27). These linear correlations between survival and mutation or chromsomal aberration indicate that the basic molecular lesions may be similar.

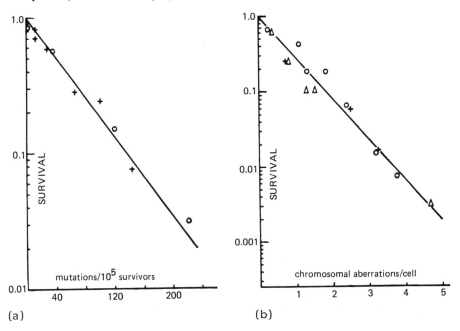

FIGURE 6   (a) The relationship between survival and mutation frequency for neutrons and gamma radiation: o = ^{60}Co, + = neutrons. (b) The relationship between survival and chromosomal aberrations for cells in different stages of the cell cycle: o = G1, + = M, Δ = S (modified from Ref. 27).

B. Exponential Repair Models

According to the damage models we have outlined, the survival-curve shoulder results from the accumulation and interaction of sublethal damage to produce lethal damage. Repair models have a radically different conceptual basis, distinguishing only between reparable lethal damage and irreparable lethal damage. In the absence of repair, survival curves would be exponential, and cells would therefore be considered to be essentially "single-hit detectors" [28]. The slope of the response in the absence of repair would be D_0, the terminal slope. If all reparable lesions were repaired, the slope would equal $_1D_0$, the initial slope; i.e., the exponential response in the absence of repair would swing upward to give a shallower exponential response reflecting complete repair. If there were no irreparable component of damage, there would be no cell killing when repair was complete .

Survival curves bend downward at higher doses, however, and repair models explain this in two distinct ways: by the saturation of repair, through depletion of a pool of substance(s) critical for repair that is replenished between doses or during a low-dose-rate exposure [23,28–30]; or by the fixation of damage by interaction of reparable lesions to produce irreparable lesions [31,32].

1. Pool Depletion

Laurie et al. [29] assumed that as repair occurred a pool of substances was consumed that was replenished much more slowly. The time scale for consumption was about the same as the time for dose delivery (e.g., minutes); the time scale for its replenishment was about the same as the time for Elkind repair (e.g., hours). The model is pictured in Fig. 7. Each increment in dose produces more B (potentially lethal damage); some of this is converted to C (lethal damage), and, depending on the amount of P (pool), some is repaired to the normal state A. However, as this repair proceeds, P is consumed, and as dose increases, repair becomes less efficient. The differential equations for the model are

$$\dot{B} = -kPB - KB$$

$$\dot{C} = KB$$

$$\dot{A} = kPB = -P \qquad\qquad P(0) = Po$$

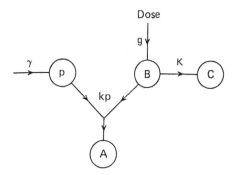

FIGURE 7   Model for the competition between development and repair of damage and the separation of the repair from recovery by consumption as opposed to replenishment of p. p = pool; g = production of B/rad; K = rate of production of C per unit B; k = rate of production of A per unit B and per unit p; γ = rate of production of p per unit deviation from initial value. Symbols represent quantities per cell where appropriate (modified from Ref. 29).

The total amount of B produced is gx, where x is dose. The solution is given by

$$x = \frac{1}{g}[-\ln f + P_0(1 - f^{\alpha})] \tag{7}$$

where $\alpha = k/K$ and f = surviving fraction = exp(-final value of C). Equation (7) may be solved numerically to give f as a function of dose x, and shouldered survival curves result.

2. Fixation (Misrepair)

The RMR (repair-misrepair) model of Tobias et al. [31] and the LPL (lethal–potentially lethal) model of Curtis [32] were founded on the concept that reparable lesions could interact to produce irreparable ones. This process was considered either as misrepair or fixation of damage, but since the lesions are unspecified there is no way of making a distinction. The formal aspects of the model are pictured in Fig. 8.

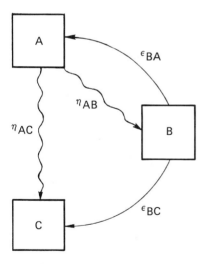

FIGURE 8   Basic schematic representation for the production, repair and misrepair of radiation lesions. η_{AB} and η_{AC} denote the rates of production (per unit absorbed dose) of reparable and irreparable damage, respectively. ε_{BA} and ε_{BC} denote the rates (per unit time) for enzymatic repair and misrepair, respectively (modified from Ref. 33).

The hypotheses on which the model is based are as follows [32]:

1. Long-lived (minutes) spatially separated lesions (B-lesions in Fig. 8) in the amount η_{AB} per unit dose are created in cell nuclei by (low LET) radiation. These lesions are repaired by a first-order enzymatic process, but may interact to produce irreparable lesions (C-lesions), one of which is sufficient to result in loss of cell reproductive capacity. Thus, the rate of the repair process will depend on the first power of the number of lesions, whereas their interaction and fixation will proceed at a rate dependent on its second power. The latter process may also be interpreted as "misrepair" [31]. Its probability is assumed to depend on the overall concentration of lesions, not on their initial proximity.

2. The lesions can interact with each other on a very short time scale (one second or less) to create an irreparable lesion, if they are created simultaneously and very close to each other (e.g., by a single charged particle). This is considered a C-lesion, created directly as a result of radiation, as shown in Fig. 8, in the amount η_{AC} per unit dose.

3. η_{AB} and η_{AC} are independent of dose.

The part of the model having to do with repair, of most interest for our purposes, is as follows. Let $N_B(t)$ = mean number of reparable lesions per cell at time t, and let $N_C(t)$ = mean number of irreparable lesions per cell at time t (Fig. 8). The differential equations describing the evolution of the concentrations are

$$\frac{dN_B}{dt} = -\varepsilon_{BA}N_B - \varepsilon_{BC}N_B^2 \qquad N_B(0) = \eta_{AB}x$$

$$\frac{dN_C}{dt} = \varepsilon_{BC}N_B^2 \qquad N_C(0) = \eta_{AC}x \qquad (8)$$

The solutions are

$$N_B = \frac{\eta_{AB}x\exp(-\varepsilon_{BA}t)}{1 + (\eta_{AB}x/\varepsilon)(1 - \exp(-\varepsilon_{BA}t))}$$

$$N_C = \frac{\eta_{AB}x(1 + \eta_{AB}x/\varepsilon)(1 - \exp(-\varepsilon_{BA}t))}{1 + (\eta_{AB}x/\varepsilon)(1 - \exp(-\varepsilon_{BA}t))}$$

$$-\varepsilon\ln[1 + (\eta_{AB}x/\varepsilon)(1 - \exp(-\varepsilon_{BA}t))] + \eta_{AC}x \qquad (9)$$

In (9) x is the radiation dose and $\varepsilon = \varepsilon_{BA}/\varepsilon_{BC}$.

To calculate survival, we make the following necessary assumption: (1) all lesions are lethal, some are reparable (B), and some are irreparable (C); (2) all B-lesions become irreparable if the repair process is halted by some experimental treatment (fixation of damage); and (3) the distribution of lesions per cell is random (Poisson).

Therefore the surviving fraction at time t, f(x, t) is

$$f(x, t) = \exp(-N_B - N_C)$$

which, upon combining (9) and substituting, becomes

$$f(x, t) = \exp[-(\eta_{AC} + \eta_{AB})x]\left[1 + \left(\frac{\eta_{AB}x}{\varepsilon}\right)(1 - \exp(-\varepsilon_{BA}t))\right]$$

(10)

Several remarks may be made in connection with the foregoing:

1. The initial conditions in (8) include all of the lesions of types B and C induced by radiation alone; thus this is a high-dose-rate setting in which induction of lesions by the radiation dose x is essentially instantaneous in comparison with repair processes.

2. Low-dose approximation of (10): when terms of order $(\eta_{AB}x)^3/\varepsilon^2$ may be neglected, i.e., at "low" doses, the logarithm may be expanded in a Taylor series to give log survival:

$$\ln f(x, t) = -[\eta_{AC} + \eta_{AB}\exp(-\varepsilon_{BA}t)]x$$

$$- \left(\frac{\eta_{AB}}{2\varepsilon}\right)^2 [1 - \exp(-\varepsilon_{BA}t)]^2 x^2$$

(11)

For long repair times after the dose x, (11) becomes

$$\ln f(x) = -\eta_{AC}x - \left(\frac{\eta_{AB}}{2\varepsilon}\right)^2 x^2$$

(12)

which is the LQ model with

$$\alpha = \eta_{AC} \qquad \beta = \frac{\eta_{AB}^2}{2\varepsilon}$$

(13)

IV. EXPERIMENTAL TESTS

The survival models presented in the foregoing may be generalized
to include the effects of fractionation and low dose rate, our ultimate purpose. It is instructive to consider first, however, whether
we may exclude some of the models on the basis of experimental
tests which have been designed to distinguish between them. We
will first describe experiments designed to decide whether damage
or repair models make more sense, and, second, we will describe
experiments designed to test the models on the basis of their predictions of the dose-rate effect.

A. Damage Versus Repair

The LQ model was based on the consideration of the relative roles
of one-track and two-track actions in the production of lesions and
the hypothesis of the need for interaction or accumulation of sublesions to produce lesions. These ideas are illustrated in Fig. 9,
where A and B are sublesions that interact to produce a lesion that
leads to an observable biological effect. Microdosimetric calculations
show that for sparsely ionizing radiation the average distance between tracks is of the order of micrometers. Therefore, since
dose-response curves are visibly curved for these radiations, the
interaction distance must be of the same order.

Goodhead et al. [34-37] tested this hypothesis directly by observing the effectiveness of radiations (ultrasoft x-rays) that produce only tracks much shorter than this interaction distance. On
average then, the probability of finding two sites of radiation

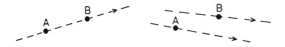

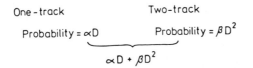

FIGURE 9   Schematic diagram of one-track and two-track hypotheses
of radiation action. It is often assumed that two sublesions (A and
B) must interact to form a lesion with a dose-dependent probability
of $\alpha D + \beta D^2$. It is assumed that the observable biological effect
can result from lesions but not sublesions (modified from Ref. 37).

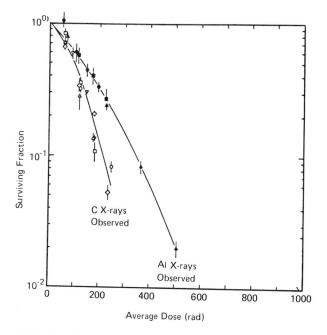

FIGURE 10   Observed inactivation and mutation induction of V79
Chinese hamster cells after irradiation with 1.5-keV aluminum ultrasoft x-rays (solid symbols) [40] and 0.3-keV carbon ultrasoft
x-rays (open symbols) (Goodhead et al. [36], compared with the
observed curves for γ-rays [40] (modified from Ref. 37).

damage at a distance of micrometers is close to zero for these radiations. By hypothesis they should be very inefficient in one-track
action; i.e., the survival curve should have zero initial slope. The
observed effect of these radiations (Fig. 10) was quite contrary to
this prediction of the dual-action theory [24,38]:   there was a pro-
nounced nonzero initial slope.

On the molecular theory [26], on the other hand, one would not
have expected curvature in the survival response to ultrasoft x-rays.
This theory assumes that two-track action occurs over distances of
6 nm, with the second track having a greatly enhanced effect over
the first [39].   The probability of two-tracks occurring this close
together in a nucleus at a small dose is very much less than 10^{-6},
so no curvature would be expected, contrary to what was observed
(Fig. 10).

Further disagreement with the sublesion hypothesis arises from
the fact that a shoulder on the dose-response curve is not a general

characteristic of mammalian cells [40]. For established cells, its presence varies through the cell cycle, but for asynchronous early-passage human diploid fibroblasts there is no visible shoulder under conventional in vitro growth conditions (Fig. 11). If the absence of a shoulder is explained by lack of susceptibility to interaction of sublethal damage, then these early-passage cells should be more resistant than established cell lines to low LET radiation; but they are observed not to be more resistant. If instead, it is suggested that

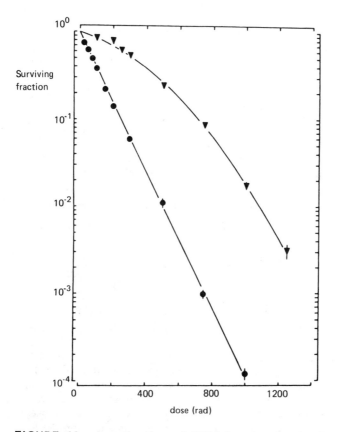

FIGURE 11   Inactivation of HF19 human diploid fibroblasts after low-LET irradiation (250-kV x-rays) compared with that of an established cell line (V79 Chinese hamster cells; γ-rays) (Cox et al. [40]). • = HF19 human; ▼ = V79 Chinese hamster (modified from Ref. 37).

they are so sensitive that they are inactivated by what would be individual sublethal lesions for other cell types, then at higher LET there should be energy wastage and RBE values less than unity; in contradiction to this, the observed RBE values for human fibroblasts are substantially greater than unity and are similar to those of established cell lines [40].

Goodhead [37] proposed that, in opposition to sublesion-interaction models, repair models were more consistent with the data—that is, that lesions arise predominantly by one-track actions in numbers proportional to dose, and are repaired by processes whose efficiency decreases with dose.

B. Dose-Rate Effect

Braby and Roesch [41] studied the predictions for the dose-rate effect of various models from the literature. The models were chosen because each represented a different concept of the nature of radiation damage and its repair. They tested the predictions with experiments using the eukaryotic unicellular green alga *Chlamydomonas reinhardi*, which in their opinion was an excellent subject for dose-rate and fractionation experiments because of its relatively unchanging radiosensitivity in the synchronization cycle.

The survival data for *C. reinhardi* were replotted as a $-\ln(S)/x^2$. For one of the models (what they called the accumulation model [42]) the data would fall on a single curve in this coordinate system, regardless of dose rate. The other models, on the other hand, predicted different curves for different dose rates. The results are shown in Fig. 12. Scatter in the data prevents complete confidence that they all lie on a single curve. Clearly, however, they do not lie on a family of curves with a consistent pattern of change with changing dose rate. For this reason the authors concluded that at least for for *C. reinhardi* the accumulation model best predicts the effect of dose rate on survival. Other models, such as the Swann-del Rosario [43] and Rajewsky-Danzer [44], include sublethal damage interaction, but they are based on the assumption that each cell is either undamaged, sublethally damaged, or lethally damaged. Therefore there is no provision for degrees of damage, so there can be no change in probability of transition from sublethal to lethal states with increase in dose. What does happen with increasing dose is that the fraction of the population in a damaged state increases. The Laurie-Orr-Foster [29] and Kappos-Pohlit [45] models do not include sublethal damage. Instead, a sigmoidal survival curve results from a decrease in ability to repair potentially lethal damage with increasing dose. Thus, these repair-saturation models do not lead to a correct prediction of the dose-rate effect.

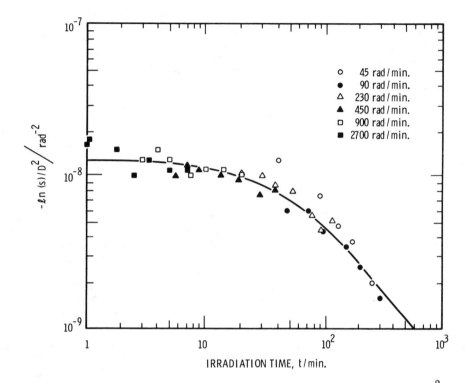

FIGURE 12   Survival data for *C. reinhardi* replotted as $-\ln(S)/D^2$.
Examination of (21), which is the accumulation model for the dose-
rate effect, shows that the ordinate depends only on the repair rate
(μ) not the dose rate, if $\alpha = 0$.   In fact, experimental results with
C. reinhardi indicate that lethality due to single events is very in-
frequent [41] and may be neglected.   Thus from (21) $\ln(S)/D^2 =$
$\beta g(\mu t)$ (From Ref. 41 with permission.)

V.   MODELS OF FRACTIONATION AND
DOSE-RATE EFFECTS

The preceding discussion has focused on cell-survival models for
the effect of single doses of radiation and has set out evidence that
would seem to favor the accumulation type of exponential-repair
model, e.g., the LPL model of Curtis [32].   Our present task is to
generalize a model of cell survival to the fractionated and low-dose-
rate settings.   We present first an empirical model, the incomplete-
repair model , on account of its mathematical simplicity, and then
show that it is equivalent to the generalized LPL model for small
doses per fraction and low dose rates [46].

A. The Incomplete-Repair (IR) Model

Lajtha and Oliver [17] observed that the increase in dose required
from a low-dose-rate exposure to achieve the same effect as a high-
dose-rate exposure could be satisfactorily explained by the concept
of an "effective dose" that decays exponentially in time or, equivalently, of a "dose-equivalent of incomplete repair" [47] in a split-
dose experiment. Oliver's [47] model is illustrated in Fig. 13,
where survival after two acute doses of size x is pictured. If repair is complete (long Δt), the initial shoulder is repeated (upper
curve in lower inset), and survival is described by a continuation
of the survival curve (lower curve) if no break occurs between
doses (Δt = 0). In intermediate cases it is envisioned that an initial

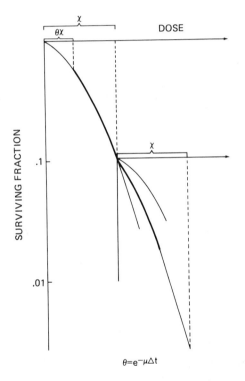

$$\theta = e^{-\mu\Delta t}$$

FIGURE 13 Dose-equivalent of incomplete repair [47]. The heavy
portion of the dose-survival curve is repeated after a second dose
of size x; the initial segment $\theta x = x \exp(-\mu\Delta t)$ is not repeated.
As Δt increases, an increasingly larger part of the initial segment
is repeated, until for large Δt the entire segment is recovered
(modified from Ref. 46).

segment of the survival curve, equivalent to the dose θx (where θ is a number between 0 and 1), is not repeated, and survival after the second dose is described by the heavy portion of the initial shoulder. The factor θ determines the rate at which repair proceeds, i.e., the repair kinetics. Oliver assumed an exponential form for θ:

$$\theta = \exp(-\mu \Delta t) \tag{14}$$

which is consistent with the behavior shown in Fig. 13.

Log survival after split doses (pictured in Fig. 13) is given by

$$\ln \text{s.f.}(2 \text{ doses of size } x, \text{ interval } \Delta t) = \ln f(x) + \ln \frac{f(x + \theta x)}{f(\theta x)}$$

$$\tag{15}$$

where $f(x)$ = surviving fraction after dose x.

If the doses x are small enough that survival is adequately described by the LQ model

$$f(x) = \exp(-\alpha x - \beta x^2) \tag{16}$$

then, after a little algebra, (15) becomes

$$\ln \text{s.f.}(2 \text{ doses of size } x, \text{ interval } \Delta t) = -2\alpha x - 2\beta x^2 - 2\beta x^2 \theta$$

$$\tag{17}$$

Thus, for long Δt, $\theta \sim 0$ and $\ln \text{s.f.} = -2\alpha x - 2\beta x^2 = 2 \ln f(x)$, i.e., there is an equal response from each dose because of complete repair and recovery of all the initial segment of survival curve (upper curve in lower inset, Fig. 13). If there is no break between doses ($\Delta t = 0$), then $\ln \text{s.f.} = -2\alpha x - 4\beta x^2 = \ln f(2x)$, i.e., the response to a single dose of size $2x$.

We now generalize (17) to n fractions, under the assumption that cell proliferation is negligible. After a third dose x, given at the same interval Δt after the second dose, the dose equivalent of incomplete repair is $\theta x + \theta^2 x$. The first term, $x \exp(-\mu \Delta t)$, represents unrepaired injury from the second dose. The second term, $\theta^2 x = x \exp -\mu(2\Delta t)$, represents unrepaired injury from the first dose, given $2\Delta t$ before the third dose.

These considerations suggest that the proper change in (15) to account for the third dose is

$$\text{ln s.f.(3 doses of size x, interval } \Delta t) = \text{ln } f(x) + \text{ln } \frac{f(x + \theta x)}{f(\theta x)}$$

$$+ \text{ln } \frac{f(x + \theta x + \theta^2 x)}{f(\theta x + \theta^2 x)}$$

Let

$$s_n(x, \theta) = \text{s.f.(n doses of size x, interval } \Delta t)$$

Then the generalization to n doses is

$$\text{ln } s_n(x, \theta) = \text{ln } f(x) + \text{ln } \left[\frac{f(x + \theta x)}{f(\theta x)}\right] + \left[\frac{f(x + \theta x + \theta^2 x)}{f(\theta x + \theta^2 x)}\right]$$

$$+ \cdots + \text{ln } \left[\frac{f(x + \theta x + \cdots + \theta^{n-1} x)}{f(\theta x + \theta^2 x + \cdots + \theta^{n-1} x)}\right] \tag{18}$$

In connection with (18), note that if Δt is large and thus $\theta = 0$, then $f(0) = 1$ and $s_n(x, 0) = f(x)n$; i.e., complete repair during interfraction intervals leads to equal decrements in survival. On the other hand, if $\Delta t = 0$, then $\theta = 1$, and

$$s_n(x, 1) = f(x) \left[\frac{f(x + x)}{f(x)}\right] + \left[\frac{f(x + x + x)}{f(x + x)}\right] \cdots = f(nx)$$

i.e., the response to a single dose of size nx.

To derive a mathematical expression for the IR model, we must choose a survival function. Because of its mathematical simplicity, and because of the presumably small doses per fraction x that occur in a multifractionated setting, the LQ model (16) is chosen. In fact, a model linear in its parameters is required in order to go further with the calculations. However, in addition to the assumptions of negligible cell regeneration and constant radiosensitivity during protracted exposure, there is the added assumption that doses per fraction are small enough that the LQ model is an adequate representation of the survival function $f(x)$. Moreover, the role of repair is unspecified, since the model is derived from assumptions concerning one- and two-track actions [24,48]. This role is made clear in the subsequent comparison with the LPL model.

Therefore, from [16] we have ln $(fx) = \alpha x - \beta x^2$, ln $f(x + \theta x) = -\alpha(x + \theta x) - \beta(x + \theta x)^2$, etc. Substituting into (18) we find

$$\ln s_n(x, \theta) = \sum_{k=0}^{n-1} \left\{ \ln f\left(x \sum_{i=0}^{k} \theta^i\right) - \ln f\left(x \sum_{i=1}^{k} \theta^i\right) \right\}$$

$$= \sum_{k=0}^{n-1} \left\{ -\alpha x \left(1 + \sum_{i=1}^{k} \theta^i\right) - \beta x^2 \left(1 + \sum_{i=1}^{k} \theta^i\right)^2 \right.$$

$$\left. + \alpha x \sum_{i=1}^{k} \theta^i + \beta x^2 \left(\sum_{i=1}^{k} \theta^i\right)^2 \right\}$$

$$= n(-\alpha x - \beta x^2) - 2\beta x^2 \sum_{k=0}^{n-1} \sum_{i=0}^{k} \theta^i \qquad (19)$$

When the summations of (19) are carried out, the result is

$$\ln s_n(x, \theta) = n \ln f(x) - n\beta x^2 h_n(\theta)$$

$$h_n(\theta) = \frac{2}{n} \left(\frac{\theta}{1 - \theta}\right) \left[n - \frac{1 - \theta^n}{1 - \theta}\right] \qquad (20)$$

Equations (19) and (20), mathematical representation of the IR model for fractionated doses, provide expressions for log survival after n doses of size x with intervals Δt between fractions. The following point may be made:

1. Incomplete repair affects only the β-component of killing, and not the α-component.
2. The limiting behavior of the function $h_n(\theta)$ in (20) is given by $h_n(0) = 0$ and $h_n(1) = 1$. Therefore $\ln s_n(x, 0) = \ln f(x)$ (complete repair), and $\ln s_n(x, 1) = \ln f(nx)$

A test of (20) is provided by the results of in vivo colony assays of the response of mouse jejunum to multifractionated irradiation, with variable Δt [49]. As illustrated in Fig. 14, the model provides reasonably accurate predictions of survival as dose fractionation is altered by changing either dose per fraction x or interfraction interval Δt [50].

An IR model for survival response after continuous exposures (with the assumptions of negligible cell proliferation and unchanging

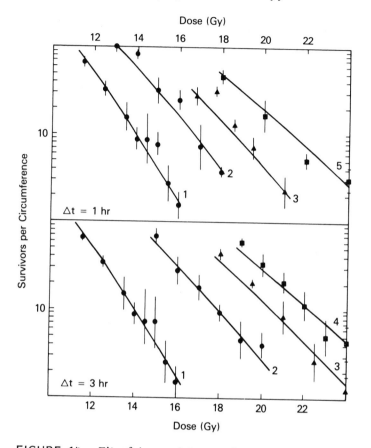

FIGURE 14   Fit of incomplete-repair model [(20) in text]. Goodness of fit to observed response of jejunal mucosa to fractionated regimens with intervals of 1 (upper) and 3 (lower) hr (modified from Ref. 50). Numbers beside lines indicate number of fractions.

radiosensitivity) may be derived from (20) in a limiting process whereby x and Δt are allowed to tend toward zero as n → ∞ but such that the total dose D = nx and overall time t = (n − 1)Δt remain constant. Put otherwise, (20) may be thought of as an approximation to the effect of continuous irradiation at dose rate v, so that total dose

$$D = vt = (\text{dose rate})(\text{exposure time})$$

is given in a sequence of n small doses of size x separated by intervals Δt. Therefore, after n doses of size x = vΔt = vt/n (we replace $n - 1$ by n, because the latter is assumed very large compared with 1), the log surviving fraction is given by (20).

We now seek the limit of $\ln s_n$ as $\Delta t \to 0$ ($n \to \infty$). For the first term we have

$$\lim_{n \to \infty} n \ln f(x) = \lim_{n \to \infty} n \left[-\alpha \left(\frac{vt}{n} \right) - \beta \left(\frac{vt}{n} \right)^2 \right] = -\alpha vt$$

This is the limiting response obtained when dose rate is so low that the initial slope is prolonged and survival is exponential. From the second term of (20) we have

$$\lim_{\Delta t \to 0} x^2 \frac{\theta}{1 - \theta} \left[n - \frac{1 - \theta^n}{1 - \theta} \right]$$

$$= \lim_{\Delta t \to 0} (v\Delta t)^2 \left[\frac{\exp(-\mu \Delta t)}{1 - \exp(-\mu \Delta t)} \right]$$

$$\times \left[\frac{t}{\Delta t} - \frac{[1 - \exp(-\mu \Delta t)^{t/\Delta t}]}{1 - \exp(-\mu \Delta t)} \right]$$

$$= (vt)^2 \left[\frac{\mu t - 1 + \exp(-\mu t)}{(\mu t)^2} \right]$$

Therefore, if we designate the limit of s_n by $S(vt, \mu)$, we have

$$S(vt, \mu) = \lim_{n \to \infty} s \left[\frac{vt}{n}, \exp(-\mu \Delta t) \right]$$

$$= \text{s.f.(continuous dose } vt \text{ delivered at (low) dose rate } v \text{ for time } t, \text{ with repair constant } \mu)$$

Then

$$\ln S(vt, \mu) = -\alpha(vt) - \beta(vt)^2 g(\mu t)$$

$$g(\mu t) = \frac{2[\mu t - 1 + e^{-\mu t}]}{(\mu t)^2}$$

(21)

The following points may be raised in connection with (21), which is equivalent to the "accumulation" model of Roesch [42]:

1. Dose rate affects only the β-component (through the function g). At ever smaller dose rates the survival curve tends toward the exponential with a slope identical to the initial slope of the acute-dose survival curve.

2. The function g has the value g(0) = 1 for very short exposure times and tends gradually toward zero (concave side up) as t increases
3. The previous emphasis on the adjective "low" to describe the dose rate v derives from averaging many (n) small, acute exposures over the time t. When the limit is taken, the dose rate is low during any finite time interval.

The IR model for continuous exposures (21) has been tested by Braby and Roesch [41], who studied the survival of *C. reinhardi* after exposures at different dose rates. A comparison of six dose-rate models found in the literature (c.f. Section IV) showed that only one of them, the accumulation model [identical to (21)], was consistent with the experimental results. The fit is illustrated in Fig. 15.

B. Comparison with Generalized LPL Model

1. Fractionation

Generalizing the LPL model to fractionated doses proceeds as follows. It is clear from the solution (14) of the initial value problem (13) that $N_B(t)$ and $N_C(t)$ are, in a sense, "propagated" from their initial values $\eta_{AB}x$ and $\eta_{AC}x$. In particular, we may define the propagators ψ and ϕ as follows:

$$N_B(t) = \psi_t[N_B(0)] \qquad N_C(t) = \eta_{AC}x + \phi_t[N_B(0)] \qquad (22)$$

where

$$\psi_t(N) = N \exp(-\varepsilon_{BA}t) \left[1 + \frac{N}{\varepsilon}(1 - \exp(-\varepsilon_{BA}t))\right] \qquad (23)$$

$$\phi_t(N) = N \left(1 + \frac{N}{\varepsilon}\right) \frac{1 - \exp(-\varepsilon_{BA}t)}{1 + (N/\varepsilon)[1 - \exp(-\varepsilon_{BA}t)]}$$

$$- \varepsilon\ln\left\{1 + \frac{N}{\varepsilon}[1 - \exp(-\varepsilon_{BA}t)]\right\} \qquad (24)$$

The function ψ propagates an initial number $N_B(0)$ of reparable lesions to the number present at time t; ϕ propagates $N_B(0)$ to the number that have been converted to irreparable lesions at time t.

The use of this notation, introduced to spare algebra, may be illustrated for the case n = 2 fractions. We are interested in survival after two doses x, separated by time interval Δt, at long times after the second dose (complete "PLD" repair), i.e., the traditional split-dose experiment. No distinction is drawn between lesions repaired between doses (sublethal) and those repaired after the

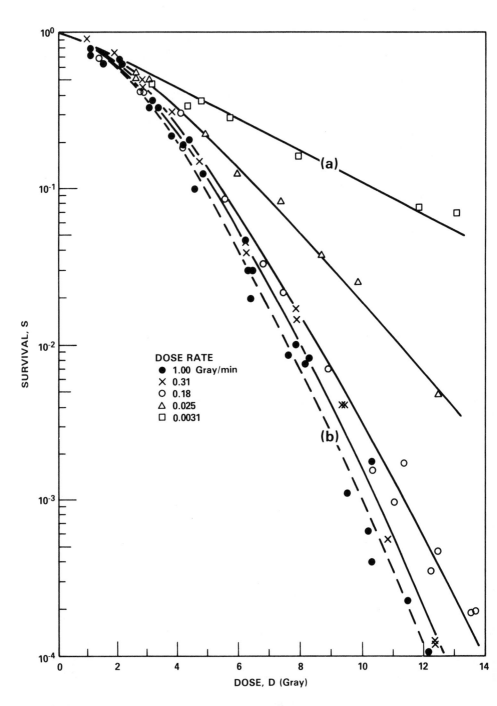

FIGURE 15   Experimental data for the survival of *C. reinhardi* at
six different dose rates.   (From Ref. 41 with permission.)

second dose (potentially lethal). From (22) we have, at time Δt after the first dose,

$$N_B(\Delta t) = \psi_{\Delta t}[N_B(0)] \qquad N_C(\Delta t) = \eta_{AC}x + \phi_{\Delta t}[N_B(0)] \quad (25)$$

When the second dose is given, the evolution of the system is again described by the differential equations (8), but with initial conditions

$$N_B(\Delta t) = \eta_{AB}x + \psi_{\Delta t}[N_B(0)]$$

$$N_C(\Delta t) = 2\eta_{AC}x + \phi_{\Delta t}[N_B(0)] \qquad (26)$$

Therefore, the solutions are given by (22) with $N_B(0)$ replaced by $N_B(\Delta t)$ and $\eta_{AC}x$ by $2\eta_{AC}x$.

It is clear that at long times all B-lesions are either fixed or repaired, i.e., $\lim_{t\to\infty}\psi_t = 0$, so split-dose survival with interval Δt is given by

$$\ln f(x, \infty) = -N_C(\infty) - \phi_{\Delta t}[N_B(0)]$$

$$= -2\eta_{AC}x - \phi_{\Delta t}[N_B(0)] - \phi_\infty(\eta_{AB}x + \phi_{\Delta t}[N_B(0)]) \qquad (27)$$

Before proceeding, we evaluate ψ and ϕ in the low-dose region, where

$$\frac{(\eta_{AB}x)^3}{\varepsilon^2} \ll 1 \qquad (28)$$

holds. In (24) we expand the quotient and logarithm:

$$\phi_t(N) = N\left(1 + \frac{N}{\varepsilon}\right)\frac{1 - \exp(-\varepsilon_{BA}t)}{1 + (N/\varepsilon)[1 - \exp(-\varepsilon_{BA}t)]}$$

$$- \varepsilon \ln\left\{1 + \left(\frac{N}{\varepsilon}\right)[1 - \exp(-\varepsilon_{BA}t)]\right\}$$

$$= N[1 - \exp(-\varepsilon_{BA}t)]\left\{1 - \left(\frac{N}{\varepsilon}\right)[1 - \exp(-\varepsilon_{BA}t)] + \cdots\right\}$$

$$+ \left(\frac{N^2}{\varepsilon}\right)[1 - \exp(-\varepsilon_{BA}t)]\left\{1 - \left(\frac{N}{\varepsilon}\right)[1 - \exp(-\varepsilon_{BA}t)] + \cdots\right\}$$

$$+ \frac{N^2}{2\varepsilon}[1 - \exp(-\varepsilon_{BA}t)]^2 + O\frac{(\eta_{AB}x)^3}{\varepsilon^2}$$

which simplifies to the approximation

$$\phi_t(N) \simeq \frac{N^2}{2\epsilon} [1 - \exp(-2\epsilon_{BA}t)] \tag{29}$$

Similarly, we obtain

$$\psi_t(N) \simeq N\exp(-\epsilon_{BA}t) - \frac{N^2}{\epsilon} \exp(-\epsilon_{BA}t)[1 - \exp(-\epsilon_{BA}t)] \tag{30}$$

We now employ (29) and (30) with (27), the expression for split dose survival:

$$\ln f(x, \infty) = -2\eta_{AC}x - \frac{(\eta_{AB}x)^2}{2\epsilon} [1 - \exp(-2\epsilon_{BA}\Delta t)]$$

$$- \left(\frac{1}{2\epsilon}\right) [\eta_{AB}x + \eta_{AB}x\exp(-\epsilon_{BA}\Delta t) + \cdots]^2 \tag{31}$$

$$\simeq -2\eta_{AC}x - 2\left(\frac{\eta_{AB}^2}{2\epsilon}\right)x^2 - 2\left(\frac{\eta_{AB}^2}{2\epsilon}\right)x^2\exp(-\epsilon_{BA}\Delta t)$$

This expression for split-dose survival is the same as that derived for the IR model (17), with the identifications of α and β given in (13) and

$$\theta = \exp(-\epsilon_{BA}\Delta t) \tag{32}$$

Having shown that this correspondence holds for $n = 2$, we now proceed to demonstrate by an induction argument that the IR model of response to n fractions, $n > 2$ [i.e., (7)] is equivalent to the n-fraction version of the LPL model (see later) at long times after the final dose, given the conditions (28).

For simplicity we use (32) in the sequel. Continuing the line of thinking that led to (25) and (26), we see that at long times after the third dose the number of remaining C-lesions is

$$N_C(\infty) = 3\eta_{AC}x + \underbrace{\phi_{\Delta t}(\eta_{AB}x)}_{\text{(from 1st dose)}} + \underbrace{\phi_{\Delta t}(\eta_{AB}x + \psi_{\Delta t}(\eta_{AB}x))}_{\text{(from 2nd dose)}}$$

$$+ \phi_\infty\{\eta_{AB}x + \psi_{\Delta t}[\eta_{AB}x + \psi_{\Delta t}(\eta_{AB}x)]\}$$

This last expression (which may be shown to be identical to (20) with n = 3) suggests that to arrive at the n-fraction version of the LPL model we simply continue to add terms in the brackets in an analogous way. Thus, for n fractions (with repair complete after the final dose)

$$
N_C(\infty) = n\eta_{AC}x + \left(\frac{\eta_{AB}^2}{2\epsilon}\right)x^2 \Bigg[(1 - \theta^2) + (1 - \theta^2)(1 + \theta)^2
$$

$$
+ (1 - \theta^2)(1 + \theta + \theta^2)^2 + \cdots + (1 - \theta^2)\left(\sum_{k=0}^{n-2} \theta^k\right)^2 + \left(\sum_{k=0}^{n-1} \theta^k\right)^2 \Bigg]
$$

$$
= \eta_{AC}(nx) + \left(\frac{\eta_{AB}^2}{2\epsilon}\right)x^2 \Bigg[(1 - \theta^2)\sum_{k=0}^{n-2}\left(\sum_{i=0}^{k} \theta^i\right)^2 + \left(\sum_{k=0}^{n-1} \theta^k\right)^2 \Bigg]
$$

Therefore, the n-fraction LPL analogue of (20) may be written

$$
\ln s_n^{LPL}(x, \theta) = -\eta_{AC}(nx) - \frac{\eta_{AB}^2}{2\epsilon}x^2 \Bigg[(1 - \theta^2)\sum_{k=0}^{n-1}\left(\sum_{i=0}^{k} \theta^i\right)^2
$$

$$
+ \theta^2\left(\sum_{i=0}^{n-1} \theta^i\right)^2 \Bigg] \tag{33}
$$

and the task is to show, from (18)-(20) and (33), that

$$
\ln s_n^{LPL}(x, \theta) = \ln s_n(x, \theta)
$$

given the low-dose condition (28) and the identifications (13) and (32).

Because of the forms of (19) and (33), it is sufficient to prove that

$$
n + 2\sum_{k=1}^{n-1}\sum_{i=1}^{k} \theta^i = (1 - \theta^2)\sum_{k=0}^{n-1}\left(\sum_{i=0}^{k} \theta^i\right)^2 + \theta^2\left(\sum_{i=0}^{n-1} \theta^i\right)^2 \tag{34}
$$

The proposition is established for n = 2 by the equivalence of (17) and (31) from the foregoing. Suppose for some value n = n* > 2, (34) holds. Then for n = n* + 1 we have

$$(1 - \theta^2) \sum_{k=0}^{n*} \left(\sum_{i=0}^{k} \theta^i \right)^2 + \theta^2 \left(\sum_{i=0}^{n*} \theta^i \right)^2$$

$$= (1 - \theta^2) \left[\left(\sum_{i=0}^{n*} \theta^i \right)^2 + \sum_{k=0}^{n*-1} \left(\sum_{i=0}^{k} \theta^i \right)^2 \right] + \theta^2 \left[\theta^{n*} + \sum_{i=0}^{n*-1} \theta^i \right]^2$$

$$= (1 - \theta^2) \sum_{k=0}^{n*-1} \left(\sum_{i=0}^{k} \theta^i \right)^2 + \theta^2 \left(\sum_{i=0}^{n*-1} \theta^i \right)^2 + (1 - \theta^2) \left(\sum_{i=0}^{n*} \theta^i \right)^2$$

$$+ \theta^2 \left[\theta^{2n*} + 2\theta^{n*} \sum_{i=0}^{n*-1} \theta^i \right]$$

By hypothesis, the first two terms equal

$$n* + 2 \sum_{k=1}^{n*-1} \sum_{i=1}^{k} \theta^i$$

so the proof reduces to showing that

$$1 + 2 \sum_{i=1}^{n*} \theta^i = (1 - \theta^2) \left(\sum_{i=0}^{n*} \theta^i \right)^2 + \theta^2 \left(\theta^{2n*} + 2\theta^{n*} \sum_{i=0}^{n*-1} \theta^i \right)$$

(35)

Equation (35) follows from manipulating the right-hand side (rhs) of (35):

$$\text{rhs}(35) = (1 - \theta^2)\left(\theta^{n^*} + \sum_{i=0}^{n^*-1} \theta^i\right)^2 + \theta^2\left(\theta^{2n^*} + 2\theta^{n^*} \sum_{i=0}^{n^*-1} \theta^i\right)$$

$$= (1 - \theta^2)\left[\theta^{2n^*} + 2\theta^{n^*} \sum_{i=0}^{n^*-1} \theta^i + \left(\sum_{i=0}^{n^*-1} \theta^i\right)^2\right]$$

$$+ \theta^2\left[\theta^{2n^*} + 2\theta^{n^*} \sum_{i=0}^{n^*-1} \theta^i\right]$$

$$= \left(\sum_{i=0}^{n^*} \theta^i\right)^2 - \theta^2\left(\sum_{i=0}^{n^*-1} \theta^i\right)^2$$

$$= \left[\sum_{i=0}^{n^*} \theta^i + \theta \sum_{i=0}^{n^*-1} \theta^i\right]\left[\sum_{i=0}^{n^*} \theta^i - \theta \sum_{i=0}^{n^*-1} \theta^i\right]$$

$$= \left[1 + \sum_{i=1}^{n^*} \theta^i + \sum_{i=1}^{n^*} \theta^i\right]\left[\sum_{i=1}^{n^*} \theta^i - \sum_{i=1}^{n^*} \theta^i\right]$$

$$= 1 + 2\sum_{i=1}^{n^*} \theta^i$$

2. The LPL Model for Continuous Exposures

The initial value problem given by (8) is modified to

$$\frac{dN_B}{dt} = \eta_{AB}v - \varepsilon_{BA}N_B - \varepsilon_{BC}N_B^2 \qquad N_B(0) = 0$$

$$\frac{dN_C}{dt} = \eta_{AC}v + \varepsilon_{BC}N_B^2 \qquad N_C(0) = 0 \tag{36}$$

In (36), v = dose rate (constant), assumed low enough that repair and fixation compete kinetically with the induction of new lesions by the radiation field.

The solution of the system (36) is

$$N_B = \frac{2\eta_{AB}v(1 - \theta')}{(1 - \theta')\varepsilon_{BA} + (1 + \theta')\sqrt{\varepsilon_{BA}^2 + 4\varepsilon_{BC}\eta_{AB}v}} \tag{37}$$

$$N_C = \eta_{AC}x + \varepsilon_{BC}\int_0^t N_B^2 \, dt'$$

in which

$$\theta' = \exp\left(-t\sqrt{\varepsilon_{BA}^2 + 4\varepsilon_{BC}\eta_{AB}v}\right) \tag{38}$$

Instead of proceeding with the rather complicated forms of (37) and (38), we invoke the condition that v is small and expand the radical:

$$\sqrt{\varepsilon_{BA}^2 + 4\varepsilon_{BC}\eta_{AB}v} = \varepsilon_{BA}\sqrt{1 + \frac{4\eta_{AB}v}{\varepsilon\varepsilon_{BA}}}$$

$$= \varepsilon_{BA}\left(1 + \frac{2\eta_{AB}v}{\varepsilon\varepsilon_{BA}} + \cdots\right) \underset{\sim}{\sim} \varepsilon_{BA}$$

if the condition

$$\frac{2\eta_{AB}v}{\varepsilon\varepsilon_{BA}} \ll 1 \tag{39}$$

is satisfied. When (39) is valid, solution (34) simplifies to

$$N_B = \frac{\eta_{AB}v}{\varepsilon_{BA}}(1 - \theta)$$

$$\tag{40}$$

$$N_C = \eta_{AC}x + \frac{\eta_{AB}^2}{\varepsilon}\left(\frac{v}{\varepsilon_{BA}}\right)^2\left[-\ln\theta - \frac{3}{2} + 2\theta - \frac{1}{2\theta^2}\right]$$

where

$$\theta = e^{-\varepsilon_{BA}t} \qquad (t = \text{exposure time at dose rate } v) \tag{41}$$

We now inquire about survival at long times after a continuous, low-dose-rate exposure for time t. This is equivalent to following survival for long repair times after an acute (high-dose-rate) exposure that resulted in the instantaneous induction of B- and C-lesions in numbers given by (40). That is, we require the solution of the system (8), but with initial conditions given by (40). Then if we let S(vt) denote the surviving fraction after dose vt, we have

$$\ln S(vt) = -N_C(t) - \phi_\infty[N_B(t)]$$

To exploit the simplified approximation for ϕ given by (29), we need a restriction different from that embodied by (28), since N_B is now defined by (40) with $N_B(0) = 0$. The additional restriction is

$$\frac{(\eta_{AB} v / \varepsilon_{BA})^3}{\varepsilon^2} \ll 1 \tag{42}$$

Therefore

$$\ln S(vt) \underset{\sim}{\sim} - N_C(t) - \frac{[N_B(t)]^2}{2\varepsilon}$$

$$= -\eta_{AC} vt - \frac{\eta_{AB}^2}{\varepsilon} \left(\frac{v}{\varepsilon_{BA}}\right)^2 \left[-\ln\theta - \frac{3}{2} + 2\theta - \frac{1}{2\theta^2}\right]$$

$$- \frac{1}{2\varepsilon}\left(\frac{\eta_{AB} v}{\varepsilon_{BA}}\right)^2 (1 - \theta)^2 \tag{43}$$

$$= -\eta_{AC}(vt) - 2\left(\frac{\eta_{AB}^2}{2\varepsilon}\right)(vt)^2 \frac{\varepsilon_{BA} t - 1 + e^{-\varepsilon_{BA} t}}{(\varepsilon_{BA} t)^2}$$

$$= -\eta_{AC}(vt) - \frac{\eta_{AB}^2}{2\varepsilon}(vt)^2 g(\varepsilon_{BA} t)$$

which agrees with (21), $\mu = \varepsilon_{BA}$, $\alpha = \eta_{AC}$, and $\beta = \eta_{AB}^2 / 2\varepsilon$.

VI.   CONCLUSIONS

A.   Effect of Repair in Fractionated Exposures

As a result of the equivalence of the generalized LPL model and the IR model, explicit radiobiological assumptions on which the former rests may be used to interpret the latter.

Nature of Repair: It is the repair of sublethal damage that is accounted for in the IR model, and its application requires the assumption that sufficient time has been allowed after fractionated or continuous radiation exposures that all post-treatment (potentially lethal) repair is complete.   The generalized LPL repair model accounts for both types of repair, although making no distinction between repair categories given differing operational definitions in experimental studies.

In the IR and generalized LPL models, repair kinetics is first order regardless of dose and cannot be saturated.   The shouldered survival curve results from hypothesis about one- and two-track actions in the IR model, since it assumes the LQ survival model while it results from the interaction of radiation-induced lesions in the LPL model.   Interestingly, it is not necessary to assume saturation of repair or depletion of critical factors to obtain the shouldered curve.   The shoulder arises rather from the damage-fixation [32] process, i.e., from the conversion of reparable lesions to irreparable lesions (cf. Fig. 7).   All of these lesions are potentially lethal, however, and may be fixed, e.g., by replating plateau-phase cells in fresh medium and causing their entry into the cell cycle, in which there are defined "fixation points" [51].

Dose Range Where Valid: Because of the simplicity of the IR model, it is important to have some estimates of the low-dose range where it is equivalent to the LPL model.   The restriction given in (28) defines the range in which the generalized LPL and IR models of response to fractionated radiation give the same results.   From experimental data on stationary phase Ehrlich ascites tumor cells [51], Curtis [32] calculated best-fit values of $\eta_{AB} = 1.10$ Gy^{-1} and $\varepsilon = 20.8$, so for these cells the restriction on the valid dose range is defined by the condition $0.003x^3 \ll 1$, where x = dose per fraction (Gy).   This restriction is nontrival (e.g., for $x = 4$, Gy, $0.003x^3 = 0.19$), suggesting that the LQ-approximation may not be strictly valid (without a cubic term) for doses well in excess of 4 Gy, if the LPL model correctly describes the survival response.

Conditions (39) and (42) both apply in defining the domain in which both continuous-exposure models, (21) and (43), are valid. Since we require that

$$\frac{(\eta_{AB}v/\epsilon_{BA})^3}{\epsilon^2} = \left(\frac{2\eta_{AB}v}{\epsilon\epsilon_{BA}}\right)\left(\frac{\eta_{AB}^2}{2\epsilon}\right)\left(\frac{v^2}{\epsilon_{BA}^2}\right) \ll 1$$

by the restriction (42), and the factor $2\eta_{AB}v/\epsilon\epsilon_{BA} \ll 1$ by (39), the remaining factors on the rhs cannot be large compared with 1, i.e.,

$$\frac{\eta_{AB}^2}{2\epsilon}\left(\frac{v^2}{\epsilon_{BA}^2}\right) \leqslant 1 \tag{44}$$

which is equivalent to a restriction on dose rates defining the domain where both continuous-exposure models are valid:

$$v(\text{dose rate}) \leqslant \frac{\mu}{\sqrt{\beta}} \tag{45}$$

In (45) $\mu = \epsilon_{BA}$ is the first-order repair constant, and $\beta = \eta_{AB}^2/2\epsilon$ is the LQ model parameter. This is also a nontrivial restriction, as shown by parameter estimates for jejunum [50]: $\mu = 1.4$ hr^{-1}, $\beta = 0.018$ Gy^{-2}, so the models apply when dose rates are not greatly in excess of 10.4 Gy hr^{-1}, i.e., 17 cGy min^{-1}.

B. Survival-Curve Interpretation or Smaller α/β Ratios in Late-Effects Tissues

It has been observed both clinically and experimentally that the slowly responding normal tissues are more sensitive to changes in size of dose per fraction than are those that respond rapidly to radiation injury. This finding may be simply interpreted in terms of a fundamental difference between the dose-survival curves of the target cells, with a smaller ratio α/β for late-effects target cells [52].

This view has been challenged by the proposition that differences in the post-irradiation kinetic behavior of target cells cause the dissociation of acute and late responses [53]. The difference in kinetic behavior was attributed to variable division probability of lethally injured cells, depending on size of dose per fraction. Thus it was envisioned that the higher division probability associated with smaller dose fractions would permit differentiation (and rescue from the division cycle and mitotic death) of relatively larger numbers of cells, thereby contributing to tissue function, and decreased value of α/β. This effect would be predominant in the late-responding

tissues, presumably by virtue of the slow rate of renewal of their
target cells and, furthermore, would cause a dissociation of functional and clonogenic measures of organ response.

When subjected to experimental test, however, this hypothesis
appeared to be questionable [54]. An alternative explanation of
the higher sensitivity of late-responding normal tissues to altered
dose fractionation is suggested by (11), an explanation based on
time available for repair before resuming or initiating movement in
the division cycle [46]. It is not unreasonable to expect that this
time is longer in the slowly proliferating target cells of the late-
responding tissues. Curtis et al. [55] observed a decline in chromosome
aberration frequencies in hepatocytes over a period of many months
after acute x-irradiation of mice, which they attributed to a slow
chromosomal repair process. These observations have been confirmed more recently by Tates et al. [56] and Scott et al. [57].

Therefore, even if it assumed that intrinsic sensitivity (η_{AB}
and η_{AC}) and repair constants (ε_{BA} and ε_{BC}) are the same in
each population of cells, the consequence of longer repair time
(before fixation of injury by movement in the division cycle) in
target cells of late-responding tissues is a smaller α/β, as may
readily be deduced from [cf. (11)]

$$\left(\frac{\alpha}{\beta}\right)_{acute} = \frac{\eta_{AC} + \eta_{AC}\exp(-\varepsilon_{BA}t)}{(\eta_{AB}^2/2\varepsilon)[1 - \exp(-\varepsilon_{BA}t)]^2} > \frac{\eta_{AC}}{\eta_{AB}^2/2\varepsilon}$$

$$= \left(\frac{\alpha}{\beta}\right)_{late} \tag{46}$$

The time t is not related to the interfraction interval; it is the time
between radiation injury and fixation of unrepaired lesions caused by
progression in the division cycle. This mechanism does not require
a dissociation of functional and clonogenic measures of tissue injury.

C. The Time Factor in Radiotherapy

At the outset of this chapter we saw that tissue recovery after low
dose rate and fractionated radiotherapy was approximated by power-
law relations involving the overall treatment time T [(1) and (2)].
On the assumption of negligible proliferation and constant radiosensitivity, as throughout our treatment, representations of the exponents p (dose-rate effect) and q (fractionation effect) in terms of
the parameters α, β, and μ can be derived. We begin by assuming
that "isoeffect equals isosurvival"; i.e., we fix ln $S(vt, \mu)$ [survival
after dose D = vt given at dose rate v, (21)] and ln $s_n(x)$ [survival
after n fractions of size x with complete repair, (20)] and differentiate.

Under the assumption that n is proportional to T, as with conventional fractionated radiotherapy, the results are

$$p = 1 + \frac{D(T\ dg/dT)}{\alpha/\beta + 2Dg(\mu T)} \tag{47}$$

$$q = \frac{x}{\alpha/\beta + 2x} \tag{48}$$

Here g and g' tend to zero for the long exposure times typical of radiotherapy; therefore, since dg/dT < 0, p would be a number slightly less than unity, as observed (cf. Section I). Since doses per fraction typical of radiotherapy are in the range 1.8–2 Gy, q would be a fraction less than 0.5, possibly in the range 0.2–0.3, as deduced by Strandqvist [6]. Finally, p + q would be near unity, as predicted from the empirical Schwarzschild law. We conclude that repair can account for a major portion of the recovery observed with dose fractionation and low dose rate, and that the predictions based on the target-cell hypothesis ("isosurvival equals isoeffect") are consistent with the clinical and experimental data.

ACKNOWLEDGMENTS

The author gratefully acknowledges the skillful assistance of Ms. Connie Seifert and Ms. Vickie Struwe in the preparation of this manuscript. This work was supported by Grants CA-11430 and CA-29026 from the National Cancer Institute, National Institutes of Health.

REFERENCES

1. Freund, L. Ein mit Rotgen-Strahlen behandelter Fall von Naevus pigmentosus piliferus. *Wien. med. Wsch.*, 47:428–434 (1897).

2. Perthes, G. Über die Behandlung des Karzinomas mit Rontgenstrahlen und über den Einfluss der Röntegenstrahlen auf die Zellteilung. *Münch. med. Wschr.*, 51:282–283 (1904).

3. Coutard, H. Roentgentherapy of epitheliomas of the tonsillar region, Hypopharynx, and larynx from 1920 to 1926. *Am. J. Roentgenol.*, 28:313–331 and 343–348 (1932).

4. Witte, E. Dosierung im biologischen Mass. *Strahlenther.*, 72: 177–194 (1941).

5. Wachsmann, F. Grundsätzliches zur Frage der Fraktionierung
    bei der Röntgenbehandlung bösartiger Geschwültse. *Strahlen-
    ther.*, *73*:636–648 (1943).

6. Strandqvist, M. Studien uber die kumulative Wirkung der
    Rötgenstrahlen bei Fraktionierung. *Acta Radiol. Suppl.*, *55*:
    1–300 (1944).

7. Cohen, L. Clinical radiation dosage. II. *Br. J. Radiol.*, *22*:
    706–713 (1949).

8. Cohen, L. Radiation response and recovery: Radiobiological
    principles and their relation to clinical practice, in *The Bio-
    logical Basis of Radiation Therapy* (E. E. Schwartz, ed.),
    Pitman, London, pp. 208–348 (1966).

9. Fletcher, G. H. and Barkley, H. T. Present status of the
    time factor in clinical radiotherapy. I. The historical background
    of the recovery experiments. *J. Radiol. Electrol.*, *557*:443–451
    (1974).

10. Thames, Howard D., Jr., Peters, Lester J., Withers, H.
    Rodney, and Fletcher, Gilbert H. Accelerated fractionation vs.
    hyperfractionation: Rationales for several treatments per day.
    Int. J. Radiat. Oncol. Biol. Phys., *9*:127–138 (1983).

11. Puck, T. T. and Marcus, P. I. Actions of x-rays on mammalian
    cells. *J. Exper. Med.*, *103*:653–666 (1956).

12. Elkind, M. M. and Sutton, H. X-ray damage and recovery in
    mammalian cells in culture. *Nature*, *184*:1293–1295 (1959).

13. Elkind, M. M. and Sutton, H. Radiation response of mam-
    malian cells grown in culture. I. Repair of x-ray damage in
    surviving Chinese hamster ovary cells. *Radiat. Res.*, *13*:
    556–593 (1960).

14. Fowler, J. F. and Stern, B. E. Dose-rate effects: some
    theoretical and practical considerations. *Br. J. Radiol.* *33*:
    389–395 (1960).

15. Fowler, J. F. and Stern, B. E. Dose-time relationships in
    radiotherapy and the validity of cell survival curve models.
    Br. J. Radiol., *36*:163–173 (1963).

16. Elkind, M. M. Cellular aspects of tumor therapy. *Radiol.*, *74*:
    529–541 (1960).

17. Lajtha, L. G. and Oliver, R. Some radiological considerations
    in radiotherapy. *Br. J. Radiol.*, *34*:252–257 (1961).

18. Munro, T. R., and Gilbert, C. W. The relation between tumor
    lethal doses and the radiosensitivity of tumor cells. *Br. J.
    Radiol.*, *34*:246–251 (1961).

19. Cohen, L. Radiotherapy in breast cancer. I. The dose-time relationship: theoretical considerations. *Br. J. Radiol.*, *25*: 636–642 (1952).

20. Fowler, J. F., Morgan, M. A., Silvester, J. A., Bewley, D. K., and Turner, B. A. Experiments with fractionated x-ray treatment of the skin of pigs. *Br. J. Radiol.*, *36*:188–196 (1963).

21. Withers, H. R. and Peters, L. J. Biological basis of radiotherapy, in *Textbook of Radiotherapy* (G. H. Fletcher, ed.), Lea & Febiger, Philadelphia, pp. 103–180 (1980).

22. Elkind, M. M. and Whitmore, G. F., *The Radiobiology of Cultured Mammalian Cells*, Gordon and Breach, New York, pp. 7–51 (1967).

23. Alper, T. Survival curve models, in *Radiation Biology in Cancer Research* (R. E. Meyn and H. R. Withers, eds.), Raven press, New York, pp. 3–18 (1980).

24. Kellerer, A. M. and Rossi, H. H. The theory of dual radiation action. *Curr. Topics Radiat. Res. Quaterly*, *8*:85–158 (1972).

25. Lea, D. E., *Actions of Radiation on Living Cells*, Cambridge University Press, Cambridge (1946).

26. Chadwick, K. H. and Leenhouts, H. P. A molecular theory of cell survival. *Phys. Med. Biol.*, *18*:78–87 (1973).

27. Leenhouts, H. P. and Chadwick, K. H., An analysis of radiation-induced malignancy based on somatic mutation. *Int. J. Radiat. Biol.*, *33*:357–370 (1978).

28. Alper, T., Implications of repair models for LET effects and other radiobiological phenomena. *Br. J. Cancer*, *49*, (Suppl. VI):137–143 (1984).

29. Laurie, J., Orr, J. S., and Foster, C. J. Repair processes and cell survival. *Br. J. Radiol.*, *45*:363–368 (1972).

30. Powers, E. L. Considerations of survival curves and target theory. *Phys. Med. Biol.*, *7*:3–28 (1962).

31. Tobias, C. A., Blakely, E. A., Ngo, F. Q. H., and Yang, T. C. H. The repair-misrepair model and cell survival, in *Radiation Biology and Cancer Research* (R. Meyn and H. R. Withers, eds.), Raven Press, New York, pp. 195–230 (1980).

32. Curtis, S. B. Ideas on the unification of radiobiological theories, Lawrence Berkeley Laboratory Report 13159 (1982).

33. Pohlit, W. and Heyder, I. R. The shape of dose-survival curves for mammalian cells and repair of potentially lethal damage analyzed by hypertonic treatment. *Radiat. Res.*, *87*:613–634 (1981).

34. Goodhead, D. T. Inactivation and mutation of cultured mammalian
     cells by aluminum-characteristic ultrasoft X-rays. III. Implica-
     tions for theory of dual radiation action. *Int. J. Radiat. Biol.,*
     32:43–70 (1977).

35. Goodhead, D. T., Thacker, J., and Cox, R. The conflict be-
     tween the biological effects of ultrasoft X-rays and microdosi-
     metric measurements and application, in *Proceedings of the*
     Sixth Symposium on Microdosimetry, Brussels (J. Booz, and
     H. G. Ebert, eds.), Commission of the European Communities,
     London, *EUR* 6046, pp. 829–843 (1978).

36. Goodhead, D. T., Thacker, J., and Cox, R. Effectiveness of 0.3
     keV carbon ultrasoft x-rays for the inactivation and mutation of cul-
     tured mammalian cells. *Int. J. Radiat. Biol., 36*:101–114 (1979).

37. Goodhead, D. T. Models of radiation inactivation and muta-
     genesis, in *Radiation Biology in Cancer Research* (R. E. Meyn
     and H. R. Withers, eds.), Raven Press, New York, pp. 231–
     247 (1980).

38. Kellerer, A. M. and Rossi, H. H., A generalized formulation
     of dual radiation action. *Radiat. Res., 75*:481–488 (1978).

39. Leenhouts, H. P. and Chadwick, K. H. Stopping power and
     the radiobiological effect of electrons, gamma rays, and pions,
     in, *Proceedings of the Fifth Symposium on Microdosimetry,*
     Verbania Pallanza, Italy (J. Booz, H. G. Ebert, and B. G. R.
     Smith, eds.) Commission of the European Communities, London,
     EUR 5452, pp. 289–308 (1975).

40. Cox, R., Thacker, J., Goodhead, D. T., and Munson, R. J.
     Mutations and inactivation of mammalian cells by various ionizing
     radiations. *Nature, 267*:425–427 (1977).

41. Braby, L. A. and Roesch, W. C. Testing of dose-rate models
     with *Chlamydomonas reinhardi. Radiat. Res., 76*:259–270
     (1978).

42. Roesch, W. C., in *Third Symposium on Neutron Dosimetry in*
     Biology and Medicine (G. Burger and H. G. Ebert, eds.)
     Commission of the European Communities, Luxembourg, p. 1
     (1978).

43. Swann, W. F. G. and del Rosario, C. The effect of radioactive
     emanations upon *Euglena. J. Franklin Inst., 211*:303–317 (1931).

44. Rajewsky, B. and Danzer, H. Über einige Wirkungen von
     Strahlen. VI. Eine Erweiterung der statistischen Theorie der
     biologischen Strahlenwirkung. *Z. Physik, 89*:412–420 (1934).

45. Kappos, A. and Pohlit, W. A cybernetic model for radiation reactions in living cells. I. Sparsely ionizing radiations; stationary cells. *Int. J. Radiat. Biol.*, 22:51–65 (1972).

46. Thames, Howard D. An "incomplete-repair" model for survival after fractionated and continuous irradiations. *Int. J. Radiat. Biol.*, 47:319–339 (1985).

47. Oliver, R. A comparison of the effects of acute and protracted gamma-radiation on the growth of seedlings of *Vicia faba*. II. Theoretical calculations. *Int. J. Radiat. Biol.*, 8: 475–488 (1964).

48. Gilbert, C. W., Hendry, J. H., and Major, D. The approximation in the formulation for survival $S = \exp(-\alpha D - \beta D^2)$. *Int. J. Radiat. Biol.*, 37:469–471 (1980).

49. Withers, H. R., in *Cell Survival after low doses of radiation: Theoretical and Clinical Implications* (T. Alper, ed.), John Wiley, Chichester, p. 369 (1975).

50. Thames, H. D., Jr., Withers, H. R., Peters, L. J. Tissue repair capacity and repair kinetics deduced from multifractionated or continuous irradiation regimens with incomplete repair. *Br. J. Cancer*, 49 (Suppl. VI):263–269 (1984).

51. Iliakis, G. Effects of β-arabinofuranosyladenine on the growth and repair of potentially lethal damage in Ehrlich ascites tumor cells. *Radiat. Res.*, 83:537–552 (1980).

52. Thames, H. D., Jr., Withers, H. R., Peters, L. J., and Fletcher, G. H. Changes in early and late radiation responses with altered dose fractionation: Implications for dose-survival relationships. *Int. J. Radiat. Oncol. Biol. Phys.*, 8: 219–226 (1982).

53. Wheldon, T., Michalowski, A., and Kirk, J. The effect of irradiation on function in self-renewing normal tissues with differing proliferative organization. *Br. J. Radiol.*, 55:759 (1982).

54. Thames, H. D., Brock, W. A., Bock, S. P., and Dixon, D. O. Effect of dose per fraction on the division potential of lethally irradiated plateau-phase CHO cells exposed to isoeffective fractionation regimes. *Br. J. Cancer*, 53 (Suppl. VII):376–381 (1986).

55. Curtis, H. J., Tilley, J., and Crowley, C. The elimination of chromsome aberrations in liver cells by cell division. *Radiat. Res.*, 22:730–734 (1964).

56. Tates, A. D., Broerse, J. J., Neuteboom, I., and de Vogel,
    N. Differential persistence of chromosomal damage induced in
    resting rat-liver cells by x-rays and 4.2-MeV neutrons. *Mutat.
    Res.*, *92*:275–290 (1982).

57. Scott, D., Gellard, P. A., and Hendry, J. H. Differential
    rates of loss of chromosome aberrations in rat thyroids after
    x-rays or neutrons. *Radiat. Res.*, *97*:64–70 (1984).

8

Modeling Resistance to Cancer Chemotherapeutic Agents

ANDREW J. COLDMAN   *Division of Epidemiology, Biometry and Occupational Oncology, Cancer Control Agency of British Columbia, Vancouver, British Columbia, Canada*

JAMES H. GOLDIE   *Division of Medical Oncology, Cancer Control Agency of British Columbia, Vancouver, British Columbia, Canada*

I. INTRODUCTION

During the past four decades a number of drugs have been identified and developed which have tumoricidal activity in both animals and man. Chemotherapy has been particularly effective in curing significant numbers of individuals with cancers of the hemopoietic and lymphatic systems. Progress in the solid tumor malignancies has been more limited with prolongation of survival times but limited increases in cure rates, except in early stage disease. The application of effective chemotherapy using currently available drugs is limited by two main factors: host toxicity and tumor resistance. Toxicity limits both the dose in which individual agents may be administered and the combinations of drugs which may be used in a single regimen. Observation on the tissue specific toxicity of drugs has permitted the combination of agents which do not have overlapping toxicity.

"Tumor resistance" is a rather vague clinical term which reflects the lack of response by a tumor to a chemotherapeutic agent. Many mechanisms have been identified, in experimental systems, which may lead to chemotherapeutic resistance. In this analysis we will be concerned with the acquisition of drug resistance, and, in particular, we will concentrate on a single mechanism for such resistance, that is, drug resistance acquired via somatic mutations.

Resistant tumor cells may be obtained in animals or tissue cultures by exposing the system to large and/or continuous doses of a chemotherapeutic agent. If the original tumor is large enough (where "large" is a function of the tumor and the drug), some cells will not be killed by the drug. If those cells are then regrown, the majority of the tumor cells will be resistant, and the tumor will not respond to the original drug. Many similar experiments have been carried out for different tumors and drugs. It appears that there exists an underlying process such that resistant cells spontaneously begin to appear at some critical size and that these cells transmit the property of resistance to the majority of their descendents. These observations suggest that this form of resistance is under genetic control, and, indeed, differences in the DNA of resistant cells compared to nonresistant (sensitive) cells has been observed [1]. For example, methotrexate-resistant cells have been isolated, which show amplified gene copies which code for the dihydrofolate reductase gene [2]. Since methotrexate competitively inhibits dihydrofolate reductase, the mechanism by which cells with an excess of the gene that codes for this enzyme exhibit resistance is readily apparent.

Similar phenomenon are also seen in bacteria, which can exhibit resistance to an antibiotic. In this case it was hypothesized that drug-resistant variant cells arose spontaneously via genetic mutations, and that such cells were then selected (for survival) from the total population of cells by the application of the drug. In a series of innovative experiments, Luria and Delbruck [3] estimated the rate at which cells spontaneously "mutated" to drug resistance (the mutation rate), and they showed that this model for the development of resistance was compatible with the data they collected.

These experiments have been repeated for in vitro tumor cell lines testing resistance to anticancer agents. Generally it appears that the experimental evidence supports the concept that drug-resistant tumor cells arise by the same process [1]. However, the evidence that tumors acquire resistance by the same mechanism in vivo is much more fragmentary [4]. We will develop a model for the spontaneous acquisition of drug resistance and discuss its implications for cancer chemotherapy. Before doing this, we must comment upon the growth of tumors, since we will require a model of tumor growth within which we can discuss the development of resistance.

II. A MODEL FOR TUMOR GROWTH

A large variety of kinetic and pathologic studies have shown that tumors are not composed of a homogenous collection of cells but may be partitioned into collections with greatly differing proliferative potential. In particular, Till et al. [5] have proposed a model whereby tumor cells may be classified into one of three mutually exclusive compartments [6]. These three compartments consist of stem cells, transitional cells, and end cells, defined as follows:

Stem cells (C_0): Stem cells are cells capable of unlimited proliferation. At each division a stem cell will give rise to two stem cells with probability p, two transitional cells with probability q, and one of each with probability $1 - p - q$.

Transitional Cells $(C_1, \ldots, C_n)$: Transitional cells are cells capable of limited proliferation. This class is made up of disjoint subclasses $C_1, \ldots, C_n$, where n is referred to as the clonal expansion number. Transitional cells which are the immediate result of a stem cell division are entered in subclass C_1. Upon dividing a single C_1 cell gives rise to two C_2 cells. These processes are repeated for $C_2, \ldots, C_{n+1}$.

End Cells (C_{n+1}): End cells are functionally dead cells incapable of further proliferation. Two end cells are formed by the division of a single C_{n+1} transitional cell.

The characteristics of this model which we will use are that the stem cell compartment controls the growth of the tumor, and that extinction of the stem cell compartment is equivalent to cure of the tumor. We will primarily be concerned with the behavior of the stem cell compartment and will consider the development of drug resistance only within this compartment. Further discussion of this model of tumor growth in the context of drug resistance and in a more general setting is available elsewhere [6].

III. THE DEVELOPMENT OF RESISTANCE TO A SINGLE DRUG

In this section we will assume that a stem cell may be in one of two mutually exclusive states: sensitive or resistant to a particular drug. Resistance is defined as a state in which a cell shows a reduced effect (compared to a sensitive cell) upon the application of a drug. In particular, we will assume that the probability that a resistant cell will survive administration of the drug is greater than the probability that a sensitive cell will. We will now describe the model to be developed.

We will assume that in a time interval of length Δt the probability that a single stem cell will divide to form two stem cells is $b\Delta t + o(\Delta t)$, that it will divide to form a stem cell and a transitional cell is $c\Delta t + o(\Delta t)$, and that it will migrate, die, or form two transitional cells is $d\Delta t + o(\Delta t)$. These events will be referred to as births, renewals, and deaths, respectively. The probability of two or more events occurring in a time interval of length Δt will be assumed to be $o(\Delta t)$. In what follows, b, c, and d will be assumed to be constants for a particular tumor. In common with the theoretical model of Luria and Delbruck [3], we will assume that there is a fixed probability α that a birth event in a sensitive cell will result in the addition of a single resistant cell and a probability $1 - \alpha$ that a sensitive cell will be added. Similarly, we assume that there is a probability β that a renewal event to a sensitive cell will result in the replacement of a sensitive stem cell by a resistant stem cell and a probability $1 - \beta$ that there will be no change in the number of sensitive cells. We will also assume that a sensitive stem cell may spontaneously mutate from sensitivity to resistance with probability $\gamma \Delta t + o(\Delta t)$ in an interval of length Δt. Resistant stem cells will be assumed to have the same parameters b, c, and d, and all progeny of resistant cells are assumed to remain resistant; i.e., transitions from the resistant to the sensitive state do not occur.

We will now go on to develop an expression for the joint probability generating function of the number of sensitive and resistant stem cells.

A. Calculating the Probability Generating Function

Let

$$R_0(t) = \text{number of sensitive stem cells at time t}$$

$$R_1(t) = \text{number of resistant stem cells at time t}$$

$$N(t) = R_0(t) + R_1(t)$$

$$P_{ij}(t) = P\{R_0(t) = i, R_1(t) = j\} \qquad \text{for } t \geqslant 0$$

From the previous discussion we may now use the Kolmogorov forward equations to obtain the following family of differential equations for $P_{ij}(t)$:

$$
\begin{aligned}
\frac{dP_{ij}(t)}{dt} = &-[(b + d)j + (b + d + c + \gamma)i]P_{ij}(t) \\
&+ b(1 - \alpha)(i - 1)P_{i-1j}(t) + c(1 - \beta)iP_{ij}(t) \\
&+ d(i + 1)P_{i+1j}(t) + \alpha biP_{ij-1}(t) \\
&+ (\beta c + \gamma)(i + 1)P_{i+1j-1}(t) + b(j - 1)P_{ij-1}(t) \\
&+ d(j + 1)P_{ij+1}(t)
\end{aligned}
\tag{1}
$$

for i, j $\geqslant$ 0, where $P_{ij}(t) \equiv 0$ for $i < 0$ or $j < 0$. Let $\phi(s_0, s_1; t)$ be the probability generating function of $\{R_0(t), R_1(t)\}$; that is,

$$\phi(s_0, s_1; t) = \sum_{i=0}^{\infty} \sum_{j=0}^{\infty} P_{ij}(t) s_0^{i} s_1^{j}$$

In what follows we will specify the initial distribution of cells by the probability generating function at time 0; that is

$$\phi(s_1, s_2; 0) = \psi(s_0, s_1)$$

and

$$\psi(s_0, s_1) = \sum_{i=0}^{\infty} \sum_{j=0}^{\infty} P_{ij}(0) s_0^{i} s_1^{j}$$

Then using equation (1), we may easily show (by multiplying by $s_0^{i} s_1^{j}$ and summing over i and j) that the probability generating function satisfies

$$\frac{\partial \phi}{\partial t} = [bs_0 - d][s_0 - 1]\frac{\partial \phi}{\partial s_0} + [\alpha b s_0 + \nu][s_1 - s_0]\frac{\partial \phi}{\partial s_0}$$

$$+ [bs_1 - d][s_1 - 1]\frac{\partial \phi}{\partial s_1} \tag{2}$$

where $\nu = \beta c + \gamma$. Using the method of characteristics [7], we get the general solution of (2):

$$\phi(s_0, s_1; t) = \psi(s_0^{0}, s_1^{0}) \tag{3}$$

where

$$s_1^{0} = \frac{d(1 - s_1) + (bs_1 - d)\exp(-\delta t)}{b(1 - s_1) + (bs_1 - d)\exp(-\delta t)} \tag{4}$$

$$s_0^{0} = s_1^{0} + \frac{f(t)}{[\delta^{2-\alpha}(s_0 - s_1)]^{-1} - b(1 - \alpha)\displaystyle\int_0^t f(v)\, dv} \tag{5}$$

and $f(v) = \exp\{-(\delta + \alpha d + \nu)v\}[b(1 - s_1) + (bs_1 - d)e^{-\delta v}]^{-2+\alpha}$.
Equation (4) is just the probability generating function for the
birth and death process with fixed parameters b and d.

As expected, substituting $s_0 = s_1 = s$ in (5) yields $s_0^0 = s_1^0$,
and thus the growth of the stem cell compartment as a whole is a
birth and death process with parameters b and d. Similarly, substituting $s_1 = 1$ in (5) shows that the sensitive stem cell compartment grows as a birth and death process with parameters $b(1 - \alpha)$
and $d + \nu$. For future use we will now calculate some elementary
properties of the process $\{R_0(t), R_1(t)\}$. By differentiating (2)
with respect to s_0 and s_1 and setting $s_0 = s_1 = s$, we obtain the
following ordinary differential equations for $m_0(t) = E[R_0(t)]$ and
$m_1(t) = [R_1(t)]$, respectively:

$$\frac{dm_0(t)}{dt} = (\delta - \alpha b - \nu)m_0(t)$$

$$\frac{dm_1(t)}{dt} = \delta m_1(t) + (\alpha b + \nu)m_0(t)$$

Solving gives

$$m_0(t) = m_0 \exp\{(\delta - \alpha b - \nu)t\}$$

$$m_1(t) = [m_1 + m_0(1 - \exp\{-(\alpha b + \nu)t\})]e^{\delta t} \tag{6}$$

where $m_0 = m_0(0)$, $m_1 = m_1(0)$, which are obtained directly from the
probability generating function at $t = 0$, $\psi(s_0, s_1)$. From (6) we
get

$$E[N(t)] = (m_1 + m_0)e^{\delta t}$$

Finally we note that the probability that a single stem cell, present
at some time $t = t'$, will not have any surviving progeny (either
sensitive or resistant) at $t = \infty$ is given by $\varepsilon = d/b$ [8]. Similarly,
since the stem cell compartment grows as a birth and death process
with parameters $b(1 - \alpha)$ and $d + \nu$, the probability that a single
sensitive stem cell will not have any surviving sensitive progeny at
time $t = \infty$ is $(d + \nu)/b(1 - \alpha)$. To consider the behavior of a
tumor subject to therapy, we must first examine the effects on the
tumor cells and on the normal tissue.

B. Effects of Drug Treatment

As mentioned previously, the development of resistance to a drug can arise as a mutational process. Evidence for some drugs from experimental tumors shows that this can be effectively absolute—for example, resistance to arabinosylcytosine (ara-C) in the L1210 mouse leukemia system. That is, treatment with any dosage of the drug on a cell resistant to it will have no effect. In other cases this is not true, and cells may be identified that show reduced sensitivity when compared to the parent sensitive line. To model the resistance phenomenon, we must first consider the response of a single cell to chemotherapy.

A large body of experimentation, notably by Skipper and his associates [9], has indicated that there exists a linear relationship between the delivered dose (in a single course of therapy) and the logarithm of the fraction of cells surviving for doses which do not result in death of the subject. Repeated courses of chemotherapy to the same population of cells are found to satisfy the same relationship with the same constant of proportionality as long as resistant cells do not emerge. This relationship holds for many different (non-phase-specific) drugs in several types of tumors and for a range of tumor sizes. From these observations it has been postulated that tumor cells subject to chemotherapy at dose D have an individual fixed probability, $\pi(D)$ say, of surviving chemotherapy, which may be expressed as $\pi(D) = \exp\{-kD\}$, where k is a constant of proportionality, and that the response of each cell is independent of that of the others. For drugs with phase-specific effect this relationship also applies, provided that cells are in the sensitive phase of the cell cycle. We will use this model of chemotherapeutic action in the development that follows.

Consider the random variable X, where X = 1 if the cell survives administration of a single course of the drug and X = 0 if it dies. If $\xi(s)$ is the probability generating function of X, then

$$\xi(s) = 1 - \pi(D) + \pi(D)s \tag{7a}$$

for a non-phase-specific agent, and

$$\xi(s) = 1 - p\pi(D) + p\pi(D)s \tag{7b}$$

for a phase-specific agent, where p is the probability that the cell is in the sensitive phase of the cell cycle.

We may use similar models to incorporate the effect of surgery or radiotherapy on the tumor cells. However, this must only be considered to be a crude first approximation. Models for response to radiation are presented elsewhere in this volume.

When a single drug is given alone via injection, we will assume that its effect is instantaneous and independent of other treatments. If t_j is the time of the jth application of chemotherapy ($j = 1, \ldots, J$), then we have

$$\phi(s_0, s_1; t_j) = \phi[\xi_0(s_0), \xi_1(s_1); t_j^-] \tag{8a}$$

where $\xi_0(s_0)$, $\xi_1(s_1)$ are the probability generating functions for cell survival for the sensitive and resistant cells, respectively, given by equations (7a) or (7b); i.e., $\xi_i(s) = 1 - \pi_i + \pi_i s$ (where the dependency on dose is suppressed) and t_j^- represents the time immediately before treatment. At some time t, where $t_j < t < t_{j+1}$, the probability generating function for the number of cells is

$$\phi(s_0, s_1; t) = \phi[s_0^0(t - t_j), s_1^0(t - t_j); t_j] \tag{8b}$$

where s_1^0 and s_2^0 are given by (5) and (4). In particular, the continuity of the functions ϕ, ξ_i and s_i^0 ($i = 0, 1$) in t implies that $\phi(s_0, s_1; t_{j+1}^-)$ is given by the right side of (8b), where $t = t_{j+1}$. Notice that these equations are also of the same form for phase-specific agents since the ξ are the same form. $\phi(s_1, s_2; t_1^-)$ is given by (3) with $t = t_1$.

These relationships may be used recursively to calculate the probability generating function for $\{R_0(t), R_1(t)\}$ after several courses of the same agent. The expected number of resistant and sensitive cells may be recursively calculated from

$$m_0(t_j) = \pi_0 m_0(t_j^-) \qquad \text{and} \qquad m_1(t_j) = \pi_1 m_1(t_j^-) \tag{9a}$$

From (9a) we also have

$$m_0(t_{j+1}^-) = m_0(t_j)\exp\{(\delta - \alpha b - \nu)(t_{j+1} - t_j)\}$$

$$m_1(t_{j+1}^-) = [m_1(t_j) + m_0(t_j)(1 - \exp\{-(\alpha b + \nu)(t_{j+1} - t_j)\})]\exp\{\delta(t_{j+1} - t_j)\} \tag{9b}$$

If the dosage is adjusted during therapy, then π_0 and π_1 would be adjusted accordingly in (8a) and (9a).

The complex form of (5) and the recursive nature of the operation needed to determine $\phi(s_0, s_1; t)$, when treatments have been applied, indicate the need for some simple measure which summarizes the effects of treatment. The expected values $m_i(t)$ provide one such summary; however, we will now develop a more useful summary measure.

C. Summarizing Treatment Effects

Using the previously described recursive relationships, we can calculate the probability generating function $\phi(s_1, s_2; t)$ for arbitrary t for any sequence of treatments. However, the relationships are difficult to invert, and thus it is not easy to calculate the $P_{ij}(t)$. We therefore require some quantities which will provide a useful summary of the behavior of the system. The expected values $m_i(t)$ provide some indication but do not tell the whole story. A quantity of some interest is $P\{N(t) \equiv R_0(t) + R_1(t) = 0\}$, since this is the probability that the treatment has been successful in eliminating the stem cells at time t. Since eliminating the stem cells implies that the tumor will eventually become extinct (or not grow sufficiently to kill the patient or animal), this may be thought of as the probability that the tumor has been cured at time t. The probability that there are no cells at time t is given by $\phi(0, 0; t)$, and this quantity may be easily calculated from (8a) and (8b). However, this quantity depends on t and thus does not represent the probability that the tumor has been cured by the treatment regimen, for if t_J is the time of the last treatment and $t_1' > t_2' > t_J$, then for the model under consideration

$$P\{R_0(t_1') = 0, R_1(t_1') = 0\} = \phi(0, 0; t_1') \geqslant \phi(0, 0; t_2')$$

$$= P\{R_0(t_2') = 0, R_1(t_2') = 0\}$$

with equality if d = 0.

Thus consider

$$P_{t_J} = \lim_{t \to \infty} E\{P[N(t) = 0 \mid N(t_J)]\}$$

We will refer to P_{t_J} as the probability of cure, which will depend on the regimen being used. Since each cell has a probability $\varepsilon = d/b$ of going spontaneously extinct (see discussion in Section III.A) and cells behave independently, the probability that N cells will go extinct is ε^N. Thus if N is a random variable with probability generating function $\phi_N(s)$ the probability that the cells will go spontaneously extinct is $\phi_N(\varepsilon)$. From this we may simply see that for a treatment regimen which gives the last cycle of therapy at time t_j,

$$P_{t_J} = \phi(\varepsilon, \varepsilon; t_J) \tag{10}$$

Note that P_{t_J} will not correspond exactly to the clinical likelihood of cure because it does not exclude sample paths, destined for extinction, which may nevertheless grow sufficiently to cause patient death. Such paths occur with vanishingly small probability in most practical situations, and P_{t_J} will be considered to be equal to the clinical probability of cure.

In some cases, as in the treatment of L1210 leukemia by the drug ara-C [10], resistance can be effectively absolute for any drug concentration which does not result in death; in this case there exists a possibility that a tumor cannot be cured by the drug no matter what dose is used. If we also assume that at the maximum therapeutic dosage $\pi_0(D) = 0$ (the probability of sensitive stem cell survival is zero), then it is only necessary to apply a single course of the drug (since subsequent courses will have no effect), and we have the probability of cure, P_{t_1}, is given by

$$P_{t_1} = \phi(\varepsilon,\ \varepsilon;\ t_1) = \phi(1,\ \varepsilon;\ t_1^{-}) \tag{11}$$

This equation may be viewed as an approximation to the probability of cure for cases in which $\pi_1(d) \sim 1$, $\pi_1(D) \sim 0$, and the treatments are applied frequently. Using equations (6)-(8b), we have

$$P_{t_1} = \psi[G(t_1),\ \varepsilon] \tag{12}$$

where

$$G(t_1) = \varepsilon + \frac{(1 - \varepsilon)(\delta + \alpha d + \nu)e^{-(\delta+\alpha d+\nu)t_1}}{(\delta + \alpha d + \nu) - \delta(1 - \alpha)[1 - e^{-(\delta+\alpha d+\nu)t_1}]}$$

and $\psi(s_0,\ s_1) = \phi(s_0,\ s_1;\ 0)$.

If $(\delta + \alpha d + \nu)t_1 \gg 1$, then

$$P_{t_1} \sim \psi(\varepsilon,\ \varepsilon) \tag{13}$$

Thus, for sufficiently large t_1, P_{t_1} is approximately equal to the probability that the tumor will go spontaneously extinct $\psi(\varepsilon,\ \varepsilon)$. Equation (12) may be used to assess the curability of an experimental tumor where the number of cells implanted has probability generating function $\psi(s_0,\ s_1)$, the drug parameters are $\pi_0(D) = 0$, $\pi_1(D) = 1$, and the tumor is treated at time t_1, where t_1 is large. However, it also illustrates that the theory developed to this point is of limited use in describing the treatment of large tumors (either clinical or experimental) since it includes spontaneous extinctions (which will largely have occurred in the early history of the neoplasm). The deficiency is especially marked for human disease, where it is generally believed that the tumor originates with a single stem cell, i.e., $\psi(s_0, s_1) = s_0$, and thus the probability of spontaneous extinction can be large (if ϵ is large).

When a clinical or experimental tumor is observed, the number of resistant stem cells is unknown. The total number of stem cells can be estimated either by direct experimentation or by using historical information for that tumor type. In both cases we will refer to the number of stem cells as being "observed" even though they may only have been estimated by historical experience. As previously mentioned, the theory developed in Section III.A describes the growth of the sensitive and resistant stem cells and includes cases where these cells go spontaneously extinct. By the time a tumor has reached a size where it is clinically detectable, the likelihood of spontaneous extinction is small. Thus to calculate the distribution of the number of resistant cells, it is appropriate for us to condition on the total number of stem cells—that is to determine $P\{R_1(t) \mid N(t)\}$. Unfortunately, this distribution is not easily obtained because the integral in (5) may not be expressed in terms of standard functions. Also, for human tumors there is the associated problem that t is unknown, and we wish to construct expressions independent of this parameter. Since this problem is of central importance in the construction of an appropriate distribution for $R_1(t)$, we will outline two approaches that provide approximate solutions to this problem under different circumstances.

D. Conditioning on N(t)—Approximation 1

In most cases of practical interest $\alpha \ll 1$ and $\nu \ll b$ (i.e., transitions to resistance proceed slower than growth), so for the majority of sample paths $R_1(t) \ll R_0(t)$ and thus $R_0(t) \underset{\sim}{\sim} N(t)$. This suggests that it may be reasonable to approximate the distribution $P\{R_1(t) \mid N(t)\}$ with the distribution $P\{R_1(t) \mid R_0(t)\}$. This approach has previously been considered by Birkhead [11]. This calculation is complex for general $\psi(s_0, s_1)$, and we will only consider the special case $\psi(s_0, s_1) = s_0$. Thus $\phi(s_0, s_1; t) = s_0^0$, as given in equation (5). Since $\phi(s_0, 1; t)$ is the probability generating function of the number of sensitive cells at time t, the coefficient of s_0^i in the expansion of s_0^0 (evaluated at $s_1 = 1$) in powers of s_0 gives the probability that there will be i sensitive cells at time t. Performing this expansion yields

$$P\{R_0(t) = i\} = \frac{\lambda^2 e^{-\lambda t}[b(1 - \alpha)(1 - e^{-\lambda t})]^{i-1}}{[b(1 - \alpha) - (d + \nu)e^{-\lambda t}]^{i+1}}$$

$$\text{for } i = 1, 2, \ldots \tag{14}$$

where $\lambda = \delta - \alpha b - \nu$. Similarly the coefficient of s_0^i in the expansion of s_0^0 (for general s_1 yields)

$$\sum_{j=0}^{\infty} P\{R_0(t) = i, R_1(t) = j\}s_1^j = \frac{\delta^{-2+\alpha} f(t)I(t)^{i-1}}{[\delta^{-2+\alpha} + s_1 I(t)]^{i+1}}$$

$$i = 1, 2, \ldots \qquad (15)$$

where $f(t)$ is given in (5) and $I(t) = b(1 - \alpha)\int_0^t f(v)\, dv$. Taking the ratio of (15) to (14) and setting $s_1 = s$ then yields the probability generating function $\zeta_i(s; t)$ of the distribution $P\{R_1(t) \mid R_0(t) = i\}$ as

$$\zeta_i(s; t) = \frac{\delta^{-2+\alpha} f(t)e^{\lambda t}[g(t)]^{i-1}}{\lambda^2[h(t)]^{i+1}} \qquad (16)$$

where

$$g(t) = \frac{I(t)}{b(1 - \alpha)(1 - e^{-\lambda t})}$$

and

$$h(t) = \frac{\delta^{-2+\alpha} + sI(t)}{b(1 - \alpha) - (d + \nu)e^{-\lambda t}}$$

We may use (16) to evaluate $E[R_1(t) \mid R_0(t) = i]$ by differentiating w.r.t. s and setting s = 1. However, the resulting expressions are complex and involve the difference of exponential functions. If $\delta \gg \alpha b + \nu$, then

$$E[R_1(t) \mid R_0(t) = i] = i\left[\frac{(2 - \alpha)(\delta - \alpha b - \nu)^2}{\delta(1 - \alpha)(2\delta - \alpha b - \nu)} e^{(\alpha b + \nu)t} - 1\right]$$

$$+ L_1 + L_2$$

$$\simeq i[e^{(\alpha b + \nu)t} - 1] + L_1 + L_2 \qquad (17)$$

where

$$L_1 = i\left[1 + \frac{d + \nu}{b(1 - \alpha)}\right]\left[\frac{(2 - \alpha)(\delta - \alpha b - \nu)^2}{(1 - \alpha)\delta(2\delta - \alpha b - \nu)}\right] e^{-(\delta - 2\alpha b - 2\nu)t}$$

$$+ O(ie^{-(\delta - \alpha b - \nu)t})$$

and

$$L_2 = \frac{b(2 - \alpha)(\alpha b + \nu)}{\delta(2\delta - \alpha b - \nu)} e^{\delta t} + O(e^{(\alpha b + \nu)t})$$

For large t ($\delta t \gg 1$) L_1 is dominated by the first term in (17). If $i \gtrsim E[R_0(t)]$, then $ie^{(\alpha b + \nu)t} \geq e^{\delta t}$, and L_2 is dominated by the first term of (17). However, if $i \ll E[R_0(t)]$, then L_2 may be comparable or larger than the first term in (17), and the approximation $R_0(t) \simeq N(t)$ may not be a good one. From (6), when $m_1(0) = 0$, as here, we have

$$E[E\{R_1(t)| R_0(t)\}] = E[R_0(t)](e^{(\alpha b + \nu)t} - 1)$$

which shows that the terms L_1 and L_2 in (17) have expectation O (approximately) with respect to R_0. The first term of (17) will in most cases (where $i = \geq E[R_0(t)]$) be a reasonable approximation to $E[R_1(t)| R_0(t)]$ for large t, except in situations where t is such that $E[R_0(t)] \gg i$.

For the special case $\pi_1(D) = 1$, $\pi_0(D) = 0$ we may calculate $P_{t_1}(i)$, the probability that the tumor (stem cells) will be cured by a single course of therapy at time t_1, when there are i sensitive cells present. Using the same argument as previously used in deriving equation (11), we have

$$P_{t_1}(i) = \zeta_i(\varepsilon; t_1)$$

Using (16) gives

$$\zeta_i(\varepsilon; t_1) = e^{-(\alpha b + \alpha d + 2\nu)t_1}$$

$$\left[\frac{(\delta + \alpha d + \nu)[b(1 - \alpha) - (d + \nu)e^{-(\delta - \alpha d - \nu)t_1}]}{(\delta - \alpha b - \nu)[b + \nu - d(1 - \alpha)e^{-(\delta + \alpha d + \nu)t_1}]}\right]^2$$

$$\cdot \left[\frac{(1 - e^{-(\delta + \alpha d + \nu)t_1})(b(1 - \alpha) - (d + \nu)e^{-(\delta + \alpha b - \nu)t_1})}{(1 - e^{-(\delta - \alpha b - \nu)t_1})(b + \nu - d(1 - \alpha)e^{-(\delta + \alpha d + \nu)t_1})}\right]^{i-1}$$

If $(\delta - \alpha b - \nu)t \gg 1$, we obtain the approximation

$$P_{t_1}(i) = \zeta_i(\epsilon; t_1)$$

$$\underset{\sim}{\ } e^{-(\alpha b + \alpha d + 2\nu)t} \left[\frac{(\delta + \alpha d + \nu)b(1 - \alpha)}{(\delta - \alpha b - \nu)(b + \nu)} \right]^2 \left[\frac{b(1 - \alpha)}{b + \nu} \right]^{i-1}$$

(18)

If, in addition, the individual mutation rates are small so that $(\alpha b + d + 2\nu)t \ll 1$ and $\delta \gg \alpha b + \nu$, then

$$e^{-(\alpha b + \alpha d + 2\nu)t} \underset{\sim}{\ } 1 \qquad \frac{(\delta + \alpha d + \nu)b(1 - \alpha)}{(\delta - \alpha b - \nu)(b + \nu)} \underset{\sim}{\ } 1$$

$$\frac{b(1 - \alpha)}{b + \nu} \underset{\sim}{\ } 1 - \frac{\nu}{\alpha b}$$

and thus

$$\zeta_i(\epsilon; t_1) = P_{t_1}(i) \underset{\sim}{\ } \left[1 - \alpha - \frac{\nu}{b} \right]^{i-1}$$

(19)

We see from (19) that $P_{t_1}(i)$ is independent of d. This may be contrasted with the expected proportion of resistant cells, which, by (17), is approximately given by $\exp\{(\alpha b + \nu)t\} - 1$. For higher death rates the mean age of the tumor increases; i.e., t increases. Thus the expected proportion of resistant cells is greater for higher values of d. The quantity (19) is plotted as a function of i, for particular α and ν/b in Fig. 1. It is apparent from the curves in Fig. 1 that the parameter $\alpha + \nu/b$ acts as a local parameter for $P_{t_1}(i)$.

If one point on the curve is known, then the remainder of the function may be plotted. However, clearly this can only be done realistically if the curability is known with some precision and it is not too close to either 0 or 1.

The preceding approximation is reasonable in cases where the age of the tumor at first treatment, t_1, is known. In clinical neoplasms this will seldom be the case, and an alternative approach is needed which removes the need to know t explicitly. Such an approach will be discussed in the next section.

E. Conditioning on N(t)—Approximation 2

The second approximation discussed here will consider not only the growth of tumors but also the rate at which they are produced.

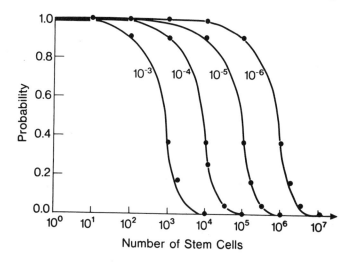

FIGURE 1   Plots of the probability of cure, P_N, (19) for four different values of $\alpha + \nu/b$. These curves are practically identical for all α and ν which sum to the same value. Notice that the parameter $\alpha + \nu/b$ behaves as a location parameter for the function, with each curve having a similar profile.

The basic approach will be to "integrate out" the time parameter present in the previous discussions and to develop formulas by summing across a distribution for $N(t)$. Again we will only consider the special case $\psi(s_0, s_1) = s_0$. Consider the following idealization of the detection of a tumor. An individual is selected at random at time t (the age measured in appropriate units), and a tumor is detected with the probability that depends on the number, n, of stem cells present. We wish to calculate $P_{r \mid n}(t)$, the probability that there are r resistant cells present at time t.

Let $f_t(r, n, u)$ be the joint distribution function of the number of resistant stem cells, total number of stem cells, and time at initiation u for a tumor detected at time t. Assuming the growth process of cells to be homogeneous in time, we have, using conditional probability,

$$f_t(r, n, u) = f(r, n \mid t - u)f_t(u)$$

where $f(r, n \mid t - u)$ is the distribution of the number of cells which have grown from a single cell in period $t - u$, and $f_t(u)$ is the marginal density for the time of initiation [$f_t(u) \equiv 0$ for $u < 0$ or $u > t$].

Then $f_t(r, n)$, the joint distribution function of the number of resistant stem cells r and the number of stem cells n in a tumor diagnosed at time t is

$$f_t(r, n) = \int_0^\infty f_t(r, n, u) \, du = \int_0^\infty f(r, n \mid t - u) f_t(u) \, du$$

Similarly, the distribution of stem cells in a tumor diagnosed at time t is

$$f_t(n) = \int_0^\infty f_t(n, u) \, du = \int_0^\infty f(n \mid t - u) f_t(u) \, du$$

and

$$P_{r \mid n}(t) = \frac{f_t(r, n)}{f_t(n)} = \frac{\int_0^\infty f(r, n \mid t - u) f_t(u) \, du}{\int_0^\infty f(n \mid t - u) f_t(u) \, du}$$

The form of $f_t(u)$ will naturally depend upon the animal and tumor under consideration. We will assume here that $f_t(u) = k = t^{-1}$. After a change of variable, $v = t - u$, we obtain

$$P_{r \mid n}(t) = \frac{\int_0^t f(r, n \mid v) \, dv}{\int_0^t f(n \mid v) \, dv}$$

For any finite nonzero n we have

$$\lim_{t \to \infty} \int_t^\infty f(n \mid v) \, dv = 0$$

Thus if the age of the animal is great, i.e., $t \gg 0$, we may put

$$\int_0^t f(n \mid v) \, dv = \int_0^\infty f(n \mid v) \, dv$$

A similar argument yields

$$\int_0^t f(r, n \mid v) \, dv \approx \int_0^\infty f(r, n \mid v) \, dv$$

Thus if the age of the animal is much greater than the likely time a tumor has taken to grow to size n, a reasonable approximation to $P_{r \mid n}(t)$ is

$$P_{r \mid n}(t) = \frac{\displaystyle\int_0^\infty f(r, n \mid v) \, dv}{\displaystyle\int_0^\infty f(n \mid v) \, dv} \tag{20}$$

In terms of notation developed earlier, this may be simply written as

$$P_{i \mid j} = \frac{\displaystyle\int_0^\infty P_{j-ii}(u) \, du}{\displaystyle\int_0^\infty P\{N(u) = j\} \, du} \qquad \text{for } i \leqslant j \tag{21}$$

$$P_{i \mid j} \equiv 0 \qquad \text{for } i > j$$

and as before $P_{ji}(u) = P\{R_0(u) = j, R_1(u) = i\}$.

When human disease is modeled, there is no unique size, j, at which a tumor is detected, but there is a distribution of such sizes. If we let g(j) be the probability that a tumor will be detected at size j (assuming no dependence on t the age of the patient), then the probability that a tumor will have i resistant cells at detection, P_i (where the dependence on g is suppressed), is

$$P_i = \sum_{j=1}^\infty g(j) P_{i \mid j}$$

where g(0) = 0; i.e., a tumor will not be diagnosed if it has no stem cells. We may pass g(j) through the integral sign in (21) to obtain

$$P_i = \int_0^\infty \sum_{j=1}^\infty g(j) \left\{ \frac{P_{j-ii}(t)}{\int_0^\infty P\{N(u) = j\} \, du} \right\} dt \qquad (22)$$

But $P\{N(u) = j\}$ is given by equation (14) with $\alpha = \nu = 0$ and $t = u$, since this is then the probability distribution for a birth and death process with parameters b and d. Integration gives

$$\int_0^\infty P\{N(u) = j\} = (bj)^{-1} \qquad \text{for } j > 0$$

and thus

$$P_i = \int_0^\infty \sum_{j=1}^\infty bjg(j)P_{j-ii}(t) \, dt$$

For general $g(j)$ P_i is difficult to evaluate because $P_{j-ii}(t)$ is not easily evaluated. However, consider the special case (which is similar to one considered by Day [12])

$$g(j) = \sum_{i=1}^r a_i q_i^{\,j} \qquad (23)$$

where $\Sigma_{i=1}^r a_i q_i^{\,j} \geqslant 0$ for all j, $q_i < 1$, $\Sigma_{i=1}^r a_i = 0$, and $\Sigma_{i=1}^r a_i q_i (1 - q_i)^{-1} = \Sigma_{j=1}^\infty g(j) = 1$.

Unfortunately functions $g(j)$ of the form (23) do not constitute a sufficiently rich set to accurately model an arbitrary distribution at diagnosis. However, for clinical neoplasms data is fairly coarse, and we may use $g(j)$ of this form to approximate the diagnostic distribution. The major limitation arises because these functions cannot give enough weight (99% or more probability) to a range of tumor stem cell sizes (Nmin, Nmax), where Nmax/Nmin $< 10^2$. This corresponds to a relative difference of fivefold in the linear dimensions of a spherical tumor, which definitely falls within the range commonly seen in a number of solid malignancies at diagnosis. Let $\theta(s)$ be the probability generating function for the distribution P_i, and let R_1 be the number of resistant cells, i.e., a random variable where $P\{R_1 = i\} = P_i$. It may be shown from the definition of the probability generating function that

$$\theta(s) = \sum_{j=0}^{\infty} P_j s^j = \sum_{i=1}^{r} a_i q_i b \int_0^{\infty} \left. \frac{\partial \phi \, (s_0, \ s_0 s; \ t)}{\partial s_0} \right|_{s_0 = q_i} dt \qquad (24)$$

where $\phi(s_0, \ s_0 s; \ t)$ is given by equation (3).

Now $\psi(s_0, \ s_1) = 0$, and we have, by integrating (5) with $s_1 = s_0 s$,

$$\int_0^{\infty} \left. \frac{\partial \phi \, (s_0, \ s_0 s; \ t)}{\partial s_0} \right|_{s_0 = q_i} dt = G(s) + H(s) \qquad (25)$$

where

$$G(s) = \frac{s}{b(1 - q_i s)} \qquad H(s) = \frac{\displaystyle\int_0^{\infty} h_1(s) h(s) \ dt}{1 - b(1 - \alpha) \displaystyle\int_0^{\infty} h(s) \ dt}$$

$$h_1(s) = \frac{1 - \varepsilon e^{-\delta t} + q_i s(1 - \alpha)(1 - e^{-\delta t})}{q_i[1 - \varepsilon e^{-\delta t} - q_i s(1 - e^{-\delta t})]}$$

and

$$h(s) = q_i(1 - s)(1 - \varepsilon)^{2-\alpha}[1 - \varepsilon e^{-\delta t} - q_i s(1 - e^{-\delta t})]^{-2+\alpha}$$
$$\cdot \ e^{-(\delta + \alpha d + \nu)t}$$

The term $G(s)$ in (25) is obtained by direct integration of the derivative (w.r.t. s) of the first term in (5). The second term, $H(s)$,
is most simply obtained by interchanging the order of differentiation
and integrating the second term in (5).

We may calculate the probability of cure for the special case
$\pi_0(D) = 0$, $\pi_1(D) = 1$ by evaluating (24) for $s = \varepsilon$. Then $E[R_1]$ and
$E[R_1^2]$ may be calculated by differentiating (24) w.r.t. s and
evaluating when $s = 1$. For general d and ν the resulting expressions must be evaluated numerically. When $q_i \sim 1$ (which is the
usual case), close attention must be paid to the accuracy with
which these integrals are evaluated. This is necessary because
most of the integrals have large absolute value; however, they do
not have the same sign, and the differences (in numeric value) are

comparatively small. Therefore it is of some practical interest to determine whether special cases exist which lead to simple forms for (24). Inspection of (24) shows that the special case $d = 0$ (no stem cell death) and $\nu = 0$ (mutations occur only at division) permits simplification

$$\phi(s) = \sum_{i=1}^{r} a_i q_i \left[\frac{s}{1 - q_i s} + \frac{s(1 - s)}{(1 - q_i s)^{2-\alpha} - (1 - s)(1 - q_i s)} \right]$$

Then the probability that the tumor is curable when $\pi_0(D) = 0$, $\pi_1(D) = 1$, $\theta(0)$, is

$$\theta(0) = \sum_{i=1}^{r} a_i q_i [1 - (1 - \alpha)q_i]^{-1} = \sum_{j=1}^{\infty} g(j)(1 - \alpha)^{j-1} \qquad (26)$$

and

$$E[R_1] = \theta'(1) = \sum_{i=1}^{r} \frac{a_i q_i}{(1 - q_i)^2} [1 - (1 - q_i)^{\alpha}]$$

$$E[R_1^2] = \theta''(1) + \theta'(1)$$

$$= \sum_{i=1}^{r} \frac{a_i q_i}{(1 - q_i)^3} \{[1 + q_i - 2(1 - q_i)^{\alpha}][1 - (1 - q_i)^{\alpha}]$$

$$+ 2\alpha q_i (1 - q_i)^{\alpha}\}$$

Table 1 gives results for $r = 2$, $q_1 = 0.99$, $q_2 = 0.9$ for general d and ν. The probability of cure (written Pg to emphasize its dependence on the distribution at diagnosis) and mean are calculated with the conditional model (Section III.D) for each tumor size j and are then averaged over $g(j)$ so that these quantities may be compared using the same underlying distribution of tumor size.

These quantities are not the same as the analogous quantities in the first approximation, since those depend on t. These two approaches may be contrasted in that the first assumes that the time of tumor induction has a degenerate distribution. The second approach assumes a uniform distribution of induction times. In

TABLE 1   Probability of Cure and Expected Number of
Resistant Cells for the Two Proposed Approximations to
$P\{R(t) \mid N(t)\}$[a]

d	α	ν	P_g		$E(R_1)$	
0.0	0.01	0.0	0.46	0.46	4.9	5.4
0.5	0.01	0.0	0.46	0.47	9.3	9.1
0.9	0.01	0.0	0.47	0.51	29.9	25.9
0.0	0.02	0.0	0.28	0.29	9.6	10.4
0.5	0.02	0.0	0.29	0.29	17.7	17.4
0.9	0.02	0.0	0.31	0.34	50.8	45.2
0.0	0.01	0.01	0.28	0.29	10.6	10.4
0.5	0.01	0.01	0.29	0.29	18.6	17.4
0.9	0.01	0.01	0.31	0.34	51.2	45.2

[a]The left-hand column represents calculations based on
the probability generating function given by (25), and
the right-hand column is that based on the model given
by (16) averaged over $g(j)$; see (23). P_g is the
probability of cure for the distribution at diagnosis $g(j)$,
where $r = 2$, $q_1 = 0.99$, and $q_2 = 0.9$.

modeling of a specific system the choice of functions depends on
which of these two cases is more realistic. Many human malignancies
show an increasing incidence with age, and thus neither of the
formulas developed would be appropriate. The method presented in
the approach is, in principle, generalizable to arbitrary distributions
of induction times; however, this will, in general, lead to rather
complex integrals, which make calculating the resulting probability
generating function for the number of resistant cells difficult. The
two approaches also assume different distributions for the total number of stem cells at diagnosis. The distribution (23) assumed in the
second approach is not as flexible as we like, but, given the relative
accuracy with which measurements may be made in human disease, it
is probably sufficient in many practical applications.

F.   Variation in the Resistance Parameters α, β, and γ

Up to this point we have assumed that α, β, and γ are fixed. In
passaged animal tumor systems this assumption appears reasonable

and has been assumed in all analyses of these systems. These tumor
systems also possess little variation in a number of other physical properties. This is not unexpected, since the process by which these tumors
are chosen for study tends to select those which maintain their characteristics after serial passaging. Spontaneous tumors, whether animal or
human, do not undergo such a selection process and may well exhibit a
greater variability in a number of physical characteristics than do passaged tumors. For example, experimental tumors display quite regular
growth rates specially when many cells are present. In constrast, human
tumors of almost every type display considerable variation in growth
rates. Possible variation in α, β, and γ can be thought of as occurring
in two distinct ways. First, these parameters may be considered to
"evolve" (either deterministically or stochastically) as a tumor grows.
One special case of this would be the possible effects of treatment on
these parameters. Radiation and many drugs used in cancer therapy
are known to be mutagenic, and the values α, β, and γ may be expected
to increase subsequent to treatment. Second, the parameters α, β, and
γ may vary between tumors within the same class with each class having
some distinct distribution of α, β, and γ.

Modeling the effect of mutagenicity of treatment is relatively
straightforward if we assume that the effect of treatment brings
about a deterministic change in the value of the mutation rates for
all the tumor cells. Since the probability generating function for
the appearance of new mutations to resistance is independent for
disjoint time intervals, we may use recursive relationships such as
(8) to determine the probability generating function after treatment.
If the effect of treatment is to induce a random change in the mutation rates of all the cells in a tumor (for a finite or an infinite time
period), then this is extremely complex to model. Here we will only
examine the effects of variations in the mutation rates between
tumors of a given class which are constant in time. Because we
know little regarding the relative magnitude of α, β, and γ (most
experiments measure the quantity $\alpha + \nu/b$), it does not seem appropriate to consider their joint distribution. If we let $\phi(s; t, a)$ be
the probability generating function of the distribution of the number
of resistant cells (computed using the approximation presented in
Section III.D), now viewed as conditional on $a = \alpha + \nu/b$, then the
unconditional probability generating function $\Psi(s; t)$ is

$$\Psi(s; t) = \int \phi(s; t, a) \, dF(a) \qquad\qquad (27)$$

where $F(a)$ is the cumulative distribution function for a.

Little is known about the distribution $F(a)$, since almost all
experiments have assumed a to be fixed. We will therefore choose
a convenient distribution which has support on a subset of $[0, 1]$.

An obvious choice for the distribution of a is the conjugate of
$P\{R(t) \mid N(t), a\}$; however, this probability distribution function
has not been determined. We propose to use the β-distribution,
which has support $[0, 1]$ and is conjugate to the Bernoulli distribution. We have already shown that the probability of cure at size
N for fixed a, where $\pi_0(D) = 0$, $\pi_1(D) = 1$, is $P_N(a) \sim (1 - a)^{N-1}$
[see (19)]. Then the cure probability, P_N, for the class of tumors
is

$$P_N \sim \int_0^1 (1 - a)^{N-1} \beta(a; u, v) \, da$$

where $\{u, v\}$ are parameters of the β-distribution, and we are
assuming that a and N are independent. It follows that

$$P_N = \frac{\Gamma(u + v)\Gamma(v + N - 1)}{\Gamma(v)\Gamma(u + v + N - 1)} = \prod_{x=0}^{N-2} \frac{v + x}{u + v + x} \qquad (28)$$

where Γ is the gamma function.
    It is a simple matter to evaluate this quantity. To estimate
the significance of variations in a on P_N, we must fix a frame of
reference. We choose here to assume that for some specified reference size there is a constant cure rate. Then we explore the effect
of different choices of u and v at sizes other than the reference
point. Examples are presented in Fig. 2; it may be seen that the
values of u and v can effect the shape of the curve considerably.
    Figure 2 shows that variation in a will affect the probability of
no resistant cells and thus affect the likelihood that the tumor will
be curable as a function of size. This observation seems important,
because not only does this formula relate to the probability of cure
in clinical disease, but it also related to current methods used to
estimate (assumed fixed) mutation rates in animal tumors. Experimental estimation of mutation rates are frequently based on destruc-
tive testing where it is assumed that $\pi_0(D) = 0$, $\pi_1(D) = 1$, and
the percentage of surviving animals is measured for various tumor
burdens; the mutation rate is estimated from an equation like (19).
Thus the fitting of this type of data to equation (28) allows one to
estimate the variability present in the mutation rates. However,
other factors which affect curability may also cause similar departures from (19); thus it is not possible to uniquely identify variability in mutation rates as the only cause. The curves in Fig. 2 are
strongly dependent upon the assumption of the β-distribution, the
curves of P_N may be quite different.

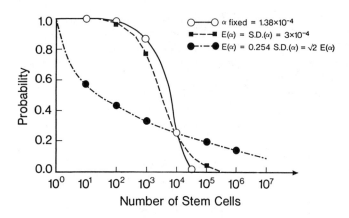

FIGURE 2   Plots of the probability of cure, P_N, as a function of the number of stem cells where the mutation rates are assumed to follow a β-distribution (28). The parameters were chosen so that the mean and standard deviation of a were as given. Each curve has been constructed to pass through the point $N = 10^4$, $P_N = 0.25$.

G. An Example

We will examine experimental data collected by Skipper, Schabel, and co-workers on the treatment of L1210 (mouse) leukemia by the drug cyclophosphamide (Cyc) [10]. The data to be used in the examination of response to Cyc alone is given in Table 2. All data is for single doses given up to the LD_{10}, which occurs at about 300 mg/kg. This information has been compiled from a number of clinical trials carried out by the investigators for intraperitoneally (IP) implanted L1210 leukemia. The data is collected from experiments in which a fixed number (usually between 100 and 1000) of cells are implanted in an animal. The growth of the tumor is known to be regular (for inoculums in this range), and the size at any time can be accurately estimated given the size of the original inoculum. Autopsies of animals indicate that 45-day survivors (after the completion of any treatment) are free of any measurable L1210 leukemia. The data presented in Table 2 give the number of 45-day survivors. The L1210 leukemia has been extensively studied, and many of its physical properties are well known. Observation of the tumor (using thymidine labeling) suggests that the median intermitotic time of the tumor is the same as the median doubling time. This implies that most cells must be actively dividing and, consequently, that the end cell compartment is small and cell loss is small. Limiting dilution assays suggest that a single cell is sufficient to cause animal death (from the leukemia). This implies that almost all the cells have stem cell capacity. We will assume that all cells are stem cells, and thus we have a model in which $c = d = 0$ (and there are no transitional cells). Data on cells from this tumor which have been selected for Cyc resistance suggests that such resistance is effectively absolute (resistant cells survive administration of the drug with probability 1); that is, $\pi_1(D) = 1.0$ for all achievable doses D. Data on the mode of therapeutic action of Cyc shows that it has general activity on all phases of the cell cycle. From this we see that the probability that a tumor of size S sensitive stem cells will be cured by administration of the drug at dose D is $[1 - \pi_0(D)]^S$, where $\pi_0(D)$ is the probability that a single sensitive cell will survive administration of the drug. The form of $\pi_0(D)$ may be estimated from observation on growth delay curves (time taken to reach some fixed size after treatments of varying dosages carried out at a common initial size). These observations indicate (assuming cells behave independently) that

$$\pi_0(D) = \exp\{-kD\} \tag{29}$$

for a range of doses up to the LD_{10}. There is some indication that (29) may not be accurate for doses approaching the LD_{10}, where the therapeutic effect may be less than predicted. This observation may be explained in at least two ways. First, it may be that the form of (29) should be modified at high doses because some mechanism (possibly drug transport into the cell) becomes saturated, so the effect of increasingly large doses is limited. Second, we note that estimates of $\pi_0(D)$ are based on observations of the whole tumor and not just on sensitive cells. Since large therapeutic effects can only be measured in large tumors, it is possible that resistant cells have emerged in these large tumors and contribute to the regrowth of the tumor. Thus a deviation from (29) would be expected in larger tumors where estimates of $\pi_0(D)$ are based on the response of the total tumor. Since it is known that resistant cells are present in large tumors, we will assume that the second explanation is the true one. Let t_1 be the time of treatment (only one cycle is given) and N the number of stem cells (all the tumor in this case). Then since $c = 0$, $d = 0$, we have

$$P_C \equiv P\{cure \mid N(t_1^-) = N\} = P\{R_0(t_1) = 0, R_1(t_1) = 0 \mid N(t_1^-) = N\}$$

Since $\pi_1(D) = 1.0$ and the cells are independent, we have

$$P_C = P\{R_0(t_1) = 0, R_1(t_1^-) = 0 \mid N(t_1^-) = N\}$$

$$= P\{R_0(t_1) = 0 \mid R_0(t_1^-) = N\}P\{R_1(t_1^-) = 0 \mid N(t_1^-) = N\}$$

$$\tag{30}$$

TABLE 2 Observed Survival of Animals with Intraperitoneally Innoculated L1210 Leukemia to Single Doses of Cyclophosphamide and Predicted Survival Rates for Fixed (Pred 1) and Variable (Pred 2) Mutation Rates

Dose (mg/kg)	Size at treatment	No. of animals treated	No. of survivors	Survival rates		
				Observed	Pred 1	Pred 2
300	8×10^7	94	7	0.074	0.000	0.109
	8×10^6	148	60	0.405	0.435	0.223
	8×10^5	39	30	0.769	0.920	0.446
230	8×10^6	50	7	0.140	0.393	0.218
	8×10^5	40	10	0.250	0.911	0.445
	8×10^4	50	41	0.820	0.992	0.778
200	8×10^7	109	3	0.028	0.000	0.008

8×10^6	160	11	0.069	0.145	0.173
8×10^5	60	11	0.183	0.824	0.435
8×10^4	10	8	0.800	0.981	0.776
8×10^3	10	10	1.000	0.998	0.964
150 8×10^7	30	0	0.000	0.000	0.000
8×10^6	19	0	0.000	0.000	0.000
8×10^5	20	1	0.050	0.003	0.066
100 8×10^7	10	0	0.000	0.000	0.000
8×10^6	20	0	0.000	0.000	0.000
8×10^5	144	0	0.000	0.000	0.000

Source: From Ref. 10.

Now the first term of (30) is

$$P\{R_0(t_1) = 0 \mid R_0(t_1^-) = N\} = [1 - \pi_0(D)]^N$$

since the probability of a single stem cell will survive therapy is $\pi_0(D)$. Using the approximation suggested in Section III.D—that is, replace $N(t_1^-)$ by $R_0(t_1^-)$ in the conditional probability [second term in (30)]—we have

$$P\{R_1(t_1^-) = 0 \mid N(t_1^-) = N\} \underset{\sim}{=} P\{R_1(t_1^-) = 0 \mid R_0(t_1^-) = N\}$$

$$= (1 - \alpha - \nu/b)^{N-1}$$

from (19). Since we cannot distinguish α and ν from one another (without further information), we set $a = \alpha + \nu/b$ and obtain

$$P_C \underset{\sim}{=} [1 - a]^{N-1}[1 - \pi_0(D)]^N$$

and from (29) we have

$$P_C \underset{\sim}{=} [1 - a]^{N-1}[1 - \exp(-kD)]^N \underset{\sim}{=} [1 - a]^N[1 - \exp\{-kD\}]^N$$

Then the approximate log-likelihood $L(a, k)$, for the data is

$$L(a, k) = \sum_{i=1}^{I} \sum_{j=1}^{J} n_{ij}[f_{ij} \ln P_{ij} + (1 - f_{ij})\ln(1 - P_{ij})] \qquad (31)$$

where

N_i = size of tumor at treatment, $i = 1, \ldots, I$

D_j = dosage of treatment applied, $j = i, \ldots, J$

n_{ij} = number of animals tested at size N_i and dosage D_j

s_{ij} = number of animals cured treated at size N_i with dosage D_j

f_{ij} = s_{ij}/n_{ij}, the observed proportion of cures

P_{ij} = probability of cure at size N_i and dose D_j

$\quad$ = $[1 - a]^{N_i}[1 - \exp\{-kD_j\}]^{N_i}$

The data for IP inoculation in Table 2 were first modeled by using the previous equations with a $\equiv 0$, which yielded a maximum likelihood estimate $k^* = 0.0678$ and a corresponding log-likelihood of $L(0, k^*) = -1262.94$. The full model was then fit, and the maximum likelihood estimates were $a^* = 1.04 \times 10^{-7}$, $k^* = 0.0780$ with $L(a^*, k^*) - -530.20$. Using the asymptotic χ^2 distribution for the difference in two log-likelihoods, we obtained that a test of $H_0{:}a = 0$ versus $H_1{:}a \neq 0$ has $\chi_1^2 = 1465.48$. The predicted values of P_{ij} using the maximum likelihood estimates a^* and k^* are given in Table 2 (Pred. 1). The data analysis provides evidence for the development of drug-resistant mutants. Coupled with observational evidence that drug (Cyc)-resistant cells may be selected from this tumor, we conclude that this analysis is compatible with the idea that these drug-resistant cells arise via spontaneous mutations.

In the analysis presented so far we have assumed that the mutation rates are fixed. In Section III.F we presented theory which modeled the mutation rates as varying according to a β-distribution. We may use this theory to determine whether this data provide evidence for variability in the mutation rates (of a type which may be approximated by the β-distribution) and estimate the parameters of the distribution. A technical problem arises because the probability of no resistant cells is given by (28), which requires computing the product of 8×10^7 terms (the largest size in the data); that is

$$P\{R_1(t_1^-) = 0 \mid R_0(t_1^-) = N\} \quad \prod_{x=0}^{N-2} \frac{v + x}{u + v + x}$$

where (u, v) are the parameters of the β-distribution. In the preceding analysis when rates were fixed, we found a $\sim 10^{-7}$. We would expect that the mean of this β-distribution, $u/(u + v)$, would be small and, thus, that $u \ll v$. If this is indeed the case, then we may approximate the product by

$$\prod_{x=0}^{N-2} \frac{v + x}{u + v + x} = \left(\frac{v + N - 2}{v} \right)^{-u}$$

and thus

$$P_C \simeq \left[\frac{v + N - 2}{v} \right]^{-u} [1 - \exp(-kD)]^N \tag{32}$$

Fitting this model to the IP data using the log-likelihood function (31), where

$$P_{ij} = \left[\frac{v + N_i - 2}{v}\right]^{-u} [1 - \exp(-kD_j)]^{N_i}$$

yielded the maximum likelihood estimates $u* = 0.301$, $v* = 0.578 \times 10^5$, and $k* = 0.0857$, with associated likelihood $L(u*, v*, k*) = -347.42$. The fixed-mutation-rate model is a special case ($u \to \infty$, $v \to \infty$ s.t. $u/u + v \to a$) of the variable-mutation-rate model, and we may construct a test assessing whether the fit of the model is improved by permitting variability. The evidence that variability exists must remain hypothetical, and we can only say that the analysis of the data presented here is compatible with this idea. This subject is worthy of future (experimental) study, although this will not be easy.

IV. THE DEVELOPMENT OF RESISTANCE TO TWO DRUGS

The previous section considered the development of resistance to a single drug among tumor stem cells. In the chemotherapy of many human malignancies several active drugs are available. Where possible these drugs may be combined to form regimens which are more effective than either of their individual constituents. The possible combinations (individual drugs and their dosages) are limited because of their effects on the host normal tissue systems. The construction of combined regimens depends on a variety of considerations. These include consideration of the activity of potential drugs on each component of the normal system of the host, pharmacokinetics of the drugs, and other factors relating to the "acceptability" of the resulting regimen. Naturally this will also include the use of modalities such as radiation and surgery. The construction of these regimens (especially in the light of the restricted and imperfect information available) requires consideration of factors which we do not propose to model here. Therefore, we will consider these combined regimens as fixed. It is of interest to examine the development of resistance to these combined regimens. We will consider a general framework for the development of resistance in stem cells and will provide a detailed examination of the case of two drugs.

Consider the case where there are n different antitumor agents available, $T_1, \ldots, T_n$. An individual tumor cell may then be characterized in one of 2^n mutually exclusive states with respect to these agents, according to which therapies it is resistant to. As before, a cell will be defined as resistant if it displays a log-kill less than its parent (sensitive) line upon administration of chemotherapy.

Let $R_{ij \cdots m}(t)$ be the number of stem cells at time t which are resistant to the set of drugs $\{T_i, T_j, \ldots, T_m\}$ and not resistant to any in the set $\{T_1, \ldots, T_n\}\backslash\{T_i, T_j, \ldots, T_m\}$. We refer to such cells as being in the state $R_{ij\cdots m}$. Those stem cells sensitive to all drugs will be identified as members of R_ϕ (ϕ is the empty set), which will be written R_0 to avoid confussion. The possible states for the individual tumor cells can be written as R_{A_i}, where A_i, $i = 0, 1, \ldots, 2^n - 1$ ($A_0 = \phi$) are the 2^n distinct subsets of $\{1, 2, \ldots, n\}$.

We will assume that when a stem cell in R_{A_i} divides to form two new stem cells, one of the will be in R_{A_i} and the other will be in R_{A_j} with probability α_{A_i, A_j}, where

$$\sum_{j=0}^{2^n-1} \alpha_{A_i, A_j} = 1$$

As in the single drug case, α_{A_i, A_j} ($i \geq 1$) will depend on the tumor type, the drug concentration, and the length of time the drug is administered. Similarly, we will define probabilities β_{A_i, A_j} as the probability that a stem cell transits from R_{A_i} to R_{A_j} when the cell divides to form a stem cell and a transitional cell. Also let $\gamma_{A_i, A_j}\Delta t + o(\Delta t)$ be the probability that a stem cell will mutate from R_{A_i} to R_{A_j} in the interval $(t, t + \Delta t)$. Transitions from the sensitive state R_0 to the resistant state R_{A_j} will have parameters α_{ϕ, A_j}, β_{ϕ, A_j}, and γ_{ϕ, A_j} for the three different types of transitions. We write these as α_{A_j}, β_{A_j}, and γ_{A_j}, respectively.

We now concentrate on the special case $n = 2$, i.e., two drugs. This case is both tractable and informative. As before, we will assume that the probability of two transitions between states occurring in a time interval of length h is about o(h). As in Section III, we will assume that the acquisition of resistance is permanent. This implies $\alpha_{1,2} = \beta_{1,2} = \gamma_{1,2} = \alpha_{2,1} = \beta_{2,1} = \gamma_{2,1} = 0$; $\alpha_{12,0} = \beta_{12,0} = \gamma_{12,0} = 0$; and $\alpha_{1,0} = \beta_{1,0} = \gamma_{1,0} = \alpha_{2,0} = \beta_{2,0} = \gamma_{2,0} = 0$. As before, we will only "keep track" of stem cells and the development of transitional and end cells (irrespective of their resistance status), and we will not be considered explicitly.

We will now discuss the calculation of the probability generating function for the process.

A. Calculating the Probability Generating Function

Define

$$P_{ijkl}(t) = P\{R_0(t) = i, R_1(t) = j, R_2(t) = k, R_{12}(t) = 1\}$$

and

$$N(t) = R_0(t) + R_1(t) + R_2(t) + R_{12}(t)$$

Let $\phi(s; t)$ be the probability generating function for the process; that is,

$$\phi(s; t) = \phi(s_0, s_1, s_2, s_3; t)$$

$$= \sum_{i=0}^{\infty} \sum_{j=0}^{\infty} \sum_{k=0}^{\infty} \sum_{l=0}^{\infty} P_{ijkl}(t) s_0^i s_1^j s_2^k s_3^l$$

Then proceeding as for the case of single resistance, we establish a partial differential equation which $\phi(s, t)$ must satisfy:

$$\frac{\partial \phi(s; t)}{\partial t} = \sum_{i=0}^{3} (bs_i - d)(s_i - 1) \frac{\partial \phi(s; T)}{\partial s_i}$$

$$+ \sum_{i=1}^{2} \left\{ (\alpha_{i,12} bs_i + \nu_{i,12})(s_3 - s_i) \frac{\partial \phi(s; t)}{\partial s_i} \right.$$

$$\left. + (\alpha_i bs_0 + \nu_i)(s_i - s_0) \frac{\partial \phi(s; t)}{\partial s_0} \right\}$$

$$+ (\alpha_{12} bs_0 + \nu_{12})(s_3 - s_0) \frac{\partial \phi(s; t)}{\partial s_0} \tag{33}$$

where

$$\nu_i = c\beta_i + \gamma_i, \quad \nu_{i,12} = c\beta_{i,12} + \gamma_{i,12} \text{ for } i = 1, 2, \text{ and}$$

$$\nu_{12} = c\beta_{12} + \gamma_{12}$$

The solution of (33) is not readily apparent, and therefore we choose to simplify the model. It has been previously shown (in the case of single resistance) that if t and $R_0(t)$ are known, then the distribution of the number of resistant cells can be reasonably well approximated by using a deterministic form for the growth of the sensitive cells [13]. From now on we assume that sensitive stem cells grow deterministically; to emphasize this, we set $R_0(t) = B(t)$; the compartments R_1, R_2, and R_{12} will grow as before. A less general form of this model has previously been considered elsewhere [13].

Let

$$P_{ijk}(t) = P\{R_1(t) = i, R_2(t) = j, R_{12}(t) = k\}$$

and let

$$\Phi(s; t) = \Phi(s_0, s_1, s_2, s_3; t) = \sum_{i=0}^{\infty} \sum_{j=0}^{\infty} \sum_{k=0}^{\infty} P_{ijk}(t) s_1^i s_2^j s_3^k$$

be the joint probability generating function for the number of resistant R_1, R_2, and R_{12} cells derived from sensitive stem cells (R_0) after time $t = 0$, excluding cells in R_1, R_2, or R_{12} present at time $t = 0$; that is, $P_{000}(0) = 1$, and thus $\phi(s; 0) = 1$. We retain s_0 in the vector s for future use. We may then derive a partial differential equation for $\Phi(s; t)$ in the same way as (33) was obtained, which yields

$$\frac{\partial \Phi}{\partial t}(s; t) = \sum_{i=1}^{3} [bs_i - d][s_i - 1]\frac{\partial \Phi(s; t)}{\partial s_i}$$

$$+ \sum_{i=1}^{2}\left\{ (\alpha_i b + \nu_i)(s_i - 1)B(t)\Phi(s; t) \right.$$

$$\left. + \frac{\partial \Phi(s; t)}{\partial s_i}(s_3 - s_i)(\alpha_{i,12}bs_i + \nu_{i,12})\right\}$$

$$+ (\alpha_{12}b + \nu_{12})(s_3 - 1)B(t)\Phi(s; t) \tag{34}$$

which can also be obtained by setting $s_0 = 1$, $\phi = \Phi$, and $\partial \phi/\partial s_0 = b(t)\Phi(s; t)$ in (33).

The solution of this equation is

$$\ln \Phi(s; t) = I_0 B_0 + \sum_{i=1}^{2} B_0(\alpha_i b + \nu_i) I_i(s_i) \tag{35}$$

where

$$I_0 = \left\{ \alpha_{12} b + \nu_{12} \sum_{i-1}^{2} \alpha_i b + \nu_i \right\} \delta(s_3 - 1) \int_0^t \frac{b'(t-v)\, dv}{b(1-s_3) + (bs_3 - d)e^{-\delta v}}$$

and

$$I_i(s) = \int_0^t \frac{B'(t-u) g_i(u)}{[\delta^{2-\alpha_{i,12}}(s-s_3)]^{-1} - b(1-\alpha_{i,12}) \int_0^u g_i(v)\, dv}\, du$$

with

$$g_i(v) = \exp[-\delta + \alpha_{i,12} d + \nu_{i,12})v][b(1-s_3)$$
$$+ (bs_3 - d)e^{-\delta v}]^{-2+\alpha_{i,12}}$$

$B'(u) = B(u)/B_0$, and $B_0 = B(0)$.

This function (35) is the probability generating function for the number of singly and doubly resistant cells derived from the growth of the sensitive cells over the interval $[0, t]$. To derive the overall probability generating function for an arbitrary distribution of sensitive and resistant cells at time $t = 0$, $\Psi(s; t)$, we note the following. Doubly resistant cells grow as a simple birth and death process and thus their probability generating function is given by (4). Singly resistant cells grow in a similar way to the sensitive cells when we are considering resistance to a single drug, and thus the probability generating function for the number of singly and doubly resistant cells derived from a single cell resistant to one drug is of the form of (5). Thus

$$\Psi(s; t) = \psi[1, \phi_1(s; t), \phi_2(s; t), \phi_3(s; t)]\Phi(s; t)\phi_0(s; t) \tag{36}$$

where $\psi(1, s_1, s_2, s_3) = \Psi(1, s_1, s_2, s_3; 0)$ is the probability generating function for the distribution of $\{R_1(t), R_2(t), R_{12}(t)\}$

at $t = 0$, $\phi_i(s; t)$ ($i = 1$, 2) is given by (5) with $\alpha = \alpha_{i,12}$, $\nu = \nu_{i,12}$, $s_0 = s_i$, $s_1 = s_3$, $\phi_3(s; t)$ is given by (4) and

$$\phi_0(s; t) = s_0^{[B(t)]} \tag{37}$$

where $[B(t)]$ is the integer part of $B(t)$.

For future reference we will now calculate the first moments of $R_1(t)$, $R_2(t)$, and R_{12}. Let $m_1(t) = E[R_1(t)]$, $m_2(t)] E[R_2(t)]$, and $m_{12} = E[R_{12}(t)]$. Now $m_1(t)$, $m_2(t)$, and $m_{12}(t)$ may be found explicitly when $B(u) = B_0\exp(ku)$ ($k \neq \delta - a_{i,12}$), which is the mean growth function for a birth and death process with fixed rates. Then

$$m_i(t) = \exp\{(\delta - a_{i,12})t\}\left(m_i(0) + \frac{a_i B_0[e^{(k-\delta+a_{i,12})t} - 1]}{k - \delta + a_{i,12}}\right) \tag{38a}$$

and

$$m_{12}(t) = e^{\delta t}\left\{ m_{12}(0) + \sum_{i=1}^{2} m_i(0)[1 - e^{-a_{i,12}t}]\right.$$

$$+ B_0 \sum_{i=1}^{2} \frac{a_i a_{i,12}}{k - \delta + a_{i,12}} \left[\frac{e^{(k-\delta)t} - 1}{k - \delta} - \frac{1 - e^{-a_{i,12}t}}{a_{i,12}}\right]$$

$$+ \frac{B_0 a_{12}}{k - \delta} [e^{(k-\delta)t} - 1]\right\} \tag{38b}$$

where $a_i = \alpha_i b + \nu_i$, $a_{i,12} = a_{i,12}b + \nu_{i,12}$ ($i = 1$, 2), and $a_{12} = \alpha_{12}b + \nu_{12}$

The choice $k = \delta - a_1 - a_2 - a_{12}$ yields expected numbers of singly resistant cells which are the same as those in the fully stochastic case, i.e., that with joint probability generating function satisfying (33).

B. Modeling Treatment Effects

To model the effects of chemotherapy upon stem cells, we will assume that the drugs obey the same laws of kill as outlined in Section II.B, and we will define the following quantities for A ε [$\{0\}$, $\{1\}$, $\{2\}$, $\{12\}$]:

$\pi_{i,A}(D) = P\{$a cell in R_A will survive administration of a single course of the drug T_i at dose D$\}$

for i = 1, 2

We will generally omit the dependence of $\pi_{i,A}(D)$ on D where it is understood to relate to some fixed but possibly unspecified dose. We define the variable $X_{i,A}$ as follows:

$$X_{i,A} = \begin{cases} 1 & \text{if a cell in } R_A \text{ survives administration of } T_i \\ 0 & \text{otherwise} \end{cases}$$

Then, $\xi_{i,A}(s)$, the probability generating function for $X_{i,A}$, is

$$\xi_{i,A}(s) = 1 - \pi_{i,A} + \pi_{i,A} \, s$$

Now if treatment T_i is given at time t_1, then

$$\Psi(s; t_1) = \Psi[\xi_i(s); t_1^-] \tag{39}$$

where $\xi_i(s) = [\xi_{i,0}(s_0), \xi_{i,1}(s_1), \xi_{i,2}(s_2), \xi_{i,12}(s_3)]$. This result is similar to (8a) for the single drug case. Equation (39) deserves some comment since $\Psi(s; t_1)$ contains one part in which the number of sensitive cells is deterministic and another in which it has a distribution. This arise because we had to assume $R_0(t) = B(t)$ in order to derive the probability generating function for the number of resistance cells derived from sensitive cells. We have also written a probability generating function for the number of sensitive cells at time t_1 (37) and used it to derive the probability generating function of the number of sensitive cells after treatment (37). We have done this because it more closely approximates the fully stochastic model. In intertreatment intervals we may consider stem cell growth to be stochastic, but to calculate the distribution of resistant cells which arise from sensitive cells (in that interval) we must use the deterministic growth function for $R_0(t)$. We know from Section III.A that for single resistance the stem cell compartment grows (stochastically) as a birth and death process with parameters $b(1 - \alpha)$ and $\nu + d$. Since the ultimate destination of cells is leaving the sensitive compartment irrelevant, we deduce that in the fully stochastic model for resistance to two agents, the sensitive cell compartment will grow as a birth and death process with parameters $b(1 - \alpha_1 - \alpha_2 - \alpha_{12})$ and $(d + \nu_1 + \nu_2 + \nu_{12})$.

We may use the stochastic model for sensitive cell growth to "update" the probability generating function for newly resistant stem cells as follows. In (35) we assumed that B_0 was constant, but it could have a distribution (but not be dependent on t), whereupon $\Phi(s; t)$ can be viewed as being conditional on B_0. If we emphasize this by writing $\Phi_{B_0}(s; t)$, then we see from (35) that

$$\Phi_{B_0}(s; t) = [\Phi_1(s; t)]^{B_0}$$

Furthermore if B_0 has a distribution with support on the nonnegative integers, then it has a probability generating function $\theta(s)$, say, and the unconditional generating function is $\theta[\Phi_1(s; t)]$.

In particular, this will be useful here, because after treatment the number of stem cells does have a distribution (defined on the nonnegative integers). We may write an expression for the probability generating function in an intertreatment interval as follows:

$$\Psi(s; t_j + v) = \Psi[\Phi_1(s; v)\phi_0(s; v), \phi_1(s; v), \phi_2(s; v),$$

$$\phi_3(s; v); t_j] \tag{40}$$

where $v < t_{j+1} - t_j$, t_j (j = 1, . . ., J) are treatment times, $\Phi_1(s; v)$ is given by (35) with $B_0 = 1$, $\phi_i(s; v)$ (i = 1, 2, 3) is as in (36), $\phi_0(s; v)$ is given by (4) with $s_1 = s_0$, birth parameter $b(1 - \alpha_1 - \alpha_2 - \alpha_{12})$, and death parameter $(d + \nu_1 + \nu_2 + \nu_{12})$.

We may therefore use equations (39) and (40) to calculate recursively the resulting probability generating function for the growth process for various treatment sequences by setting $v = t_{j+1} - t_j$ for the interval (t_j, t_{j+1}), where the initial probability generating function at time t_1^- is given by (36).

Notice that we may use (40) recursively at times where treatment is not given in order to improve the approximation to the fully stochastic model. In general, we would not do this prior to t_1 because it would then induce (a nondegenerate) distribution on $R_0(t_1)$ with all the attendant problems this produces.

The incorporation of a stochastic element to the growth of the sensitive stem cells is somewhat artificial; however, it does permit determination of $P\{N(t) = 0\}$, which would otherwise be undefined if $R_0(t)$ were left purely deterministic. The model can be expected to be a reasonable reflection of reality, because where there are large numbers of sensitive stem cells, growth can be expected to be quite regular and thus well approximated by the deterministic assumption. When the number of sensitive cells is small, the likelihood that new resistant cells will arise (from R_0) is small, and thus the assumption of deterministic growth should not cause a great distortion to the distribution of the number of resistant cells. As in Section III, we will now consider some special cases which illustrate the behavior of the model.

In many cases two drugs may not be given together because of their overlapping toxicity on normal tissue. Consider the special case where they may be given together, with $N(0) = R_0(0) = 1$ (origin from a single sensitive stem cell), $\pi_1 = \pi_2 = \pi_{1,2} = \pi_{2,1} = 0$, and $\pi_{1,12} = \pi_{2,12} = 1$ ($\pi_{1,1}$ and $\pi_{2,2}$ are arbitrary); i.e., when given together, all stem cells are killed except those in R_{12}. If both drugs are given at t_1, then the probability that the tumor will be cured, P_{t_1}, is $\Psi(1, 1, 1, \varepsilon; t_1^-)$ [see (11)], where $\Psi(s; t)$ is given by (36), which reduces to

$$P_{t_1} = \Phi(1, 1, 1, \varepsilon; t_1^-) \tag{41}$$

since $\psi(1, s_1, s_2, s_3) = 1$. If the tumor has N stem cells at time t_1, we may write $P_{t_1} = P_N$. Using (41), we find that when the rates a_i, $a_{i,12}$, and a_{12} are small, then

$$\ln P_N \simeq -(1 - \varepsilon)^{-1} N \left\{ a_{12}(1 - \varepsilon) + \sum_{i=1}^{2} a_i a_{i,12} \left[\ln\left(\frac{1 - \varepsilon}{a_{i,12}}\right) - 1 \right] \right\} \tag{42}$$

Note that (42) depends upon ε (i.e., d). If ε is large, say 0.9, the effect on P_N can be considerable. This would also be true for cases in which π_1, π_2, $\pi_{1,2}$, $\pi_{2,1}$ are not necessarily zero, although then the curability of the tumor will then depend on the treatment protocol under consideration.

This would seem to have wider implications for the general analysis of these processes. Resistance to some drugs appears to arise from a single discrete change in the genetic material. In such cases, resistance may be almost absolute. In other cases resistance may arise incrementally, such as in processes involving gene amplification. In these circumstances the acquisition of each gene copy may be viewed as a separate stage. Therefore the distribution of the numbers of cells prossessing a specified level of resistance (i.e., some minimum number of gene copies) will be that of a multistage process and not that of a single-stage process. This clearly represents a difficult problem when attempting to analyze experiments designed to estimate mutation rates to drug resistance. Indeed, in a multistage process there is no single parameter to estimate but rather a variable number depending on the number of stages involved. The number of stages would also need to be estimated (if not known) from such experiments, and, given the extremely variable nature of the basic process, it seems that estimating parameters will be quite difficult. Furthermore, even when the number of stages is known, it is not possible, in general, to write expressions for the distribution functions for the multistage process. This problem needs more detailed exploration.

C. Optimal Scheduling

When all the tumor and drug parameters are known, it is possible to examine the effect of various dosages and schedules of administration on the long-run curability of the tumor using equations (36), (39), and (40). This is useful for a number of experimental neoplasms; however, it is not so useful for clinical disease where these parameters are usually unknown and impossible to estimate with any accuracy from the very crude data collected in clinical studies. In this section we will only be concerned with examining treatment protocols whose object is to cure the patient. Protocols whose object is palliation will not be considered.

One special case which is of some practical interest is the situation where two drugs (or combinations) are available which are of approximately equal efficacy. This appears to arise in the treatment of Hodgkin's disease where there are two combinations, MOPP and ABVD, which produce similar cure rates and remission rates when delivered over the same time interval. These observations suggest that the development of resistance to each combination proceeds at the same rate and that cell kills of each regimen are similar. The evidence that is available also suggests that each regimen is equally successful in producing remissions and cures in tumors which have previously failed with the other therapy. This implies that each drug's effect is approximately the same in cells resistant to the other. As a first approximation, we may consider the two drug combinations as having equal values for the model parameters. In this situation we will refer to the two drugs as being equivalent, and by that we mean that each drug has identical values for all parameters. Explicitly two agents will be said to be equivalent if $\pi_{1,0} = \pi_{2,0}$, $\pi_{1,1} = \pi_{2,2}$, $\pi_{1,12} = \pi_{2,12}$, $\pi_{1,2} = \pi_{2,1}$, $\alpha_1 = \alpha_2$, $\nu_1 = \nu_2$, $\alpha_{1,12} = \alpha_{2,12}$, $\nu_{1,12} = \nu_{2,12}$, and $(t_{j+1} - t_j)$, $j = 1, \ldots, J - 1$, are constant. From the general definition of the resistant rates, we have $\pi_{i,0} < \pi_{i,i} \leqslant \pi_{i,12}$ for $i = 1, 2$. The tumor parameters b, c, and d are fixed and will not be explicitly specified.

As noted in Section III.B, in clinical disease chemotherapy is given in repeating cycles in which the doses and drugs used are fixed in advance. The intervening time between repeat applications is determined by the recovery time of the patients' normal tissues.

This recovery time is selected to be the minimum time for the necessary recovery. Protocols which administer the cycles at greater
than the minimum interval will be less effective than those giving
the same drugs at the same dose as frequently as permissible. To
see this, recall the objective of the protocol is to maximize the
probability of cure, and thus if the planned treatments are given
over the minimum time possible there is a minimum time for regrowth
between treatments. The term "probability of cure," P_N, will be
defined as the limit as $t \to \infty$ of $P\{N(t) = 0\}$ for a tumor first treated
at size N (stem cells) with a specified protocol with no further treatment (i.e., in the case of relapse, etc.). We will now consider the
construction of optimal rules for sequencing the administration of two
equivalent agents.

In attempting to find an optimal treatment plan, we must restrict
the rules considered in some way. One way is to consider only those
of some fixed length, i.e., some fixed number of times of treatments.
Notice that we can always "improve" any protocol—i.e., increase the
probability of cure—by adding further treatments to the end of the
regimen. The length of the regimen will therefore depend on the
value of any further increase in the probability of cure versus the
"costs" (both human and financial) associated with extra cycles of
treatment. By this reasoning any regime of length $J - 1$ (number
of cycles of therapy) will be no better than at least two of length J
(i.e., those which add a single cycle of either T_1 or T_2 to the previous protocol). We will therefore consider the problem of finding a
protocol of length J which maximizes the probability of cure P_N at
the completion of the planned therapy.

First we will fix J, the total treatment administrations in the
regimen. A therapeutic strategy will be represented by a vector
consisting of a sequence of J 1's or 2's, with each number referring
to the subscript of the treatment given (either T_1 or T_2) and the
sequence indicating the order in which they are given. There will
be 2^J such strategies, and we may index the strategies using the
natural ordering on the sequences; i.e., $\{1, \ldots, 1\} = 1$,
$\{1, \ldots, 1, 2\} = 2, \ldots, \{2, \ldots, 2\} = 2^J$. We will write $S(\kappa)$
for the strategy which occurs κth in the natural ordering, where
$1 \leqslant \kappa \leqslant 2^J$. Where more than one strategy is under consideration,
we will write the probability of cure as $P_N[S(\kappa)]$ to reflect the dependence on the strategy $S(\kappa)$. A solution to the fixed length
problem, which will depend on J, will be referred to as an optimal
strategy.

An optimal strategy exists because the number of fixed strategies
of length J is finite, and thus for at least one minimizes P_N. If

$$\Psi(s_0, s_1, s_2, s_3; 0) = \Psi(s_0, s_2, s_1, s_3; 0) \tag{43}$$

then for $t < t_1$ (the time of first treatment), we have

$$\Psi(s_0, s_1, s_2, s_3; t) = \Psi(s_0, s_2, s_1, s_3; t) \tag{44}$$

since the treatments are equivalent. Here will will assume (43) holds, which is reasonable, otherwise we would expect the response of the tumor to therapy by T_1 (alone) to be different from the response to T_2 (alone), and thus the treatments would not appear equivalent in any experiments carried out on the system.

From considering (43) we see that there must be at least two optimal strategies, since each stragety has a mirror image (i.e., 1's and 2's exchanged) with the same value of P_N because the drugs are equivalent.

We would like to show that there exists a unique (up to mirror image) strategy which is optimum for any pair of equivalent drugs; that is, there exist optimal strategies independent of the drug and tumor parameters. Unfortunately this is not true, which may be shown by producing an explicit counterexample. However, the object of therapy is to eradicate the tumor (stem) cells, and thus it seems reasonable to consider strategies which minimize $E[N(t_j)]$, where t_j is the time of the last treatment. Because the growth process is independent in disjoint time intervals, this is equivalent to considering strategies which minimize $E[N(t)]$ for a $t > t_j$. It is then possible to improve the following theorem.

Theorem. For two equivalent agents, $E[N(t)]$, $t > t_j$, is minimized by the two strategies which alternate therapy at each cycle among all strategies of fixed length. The proof is in [14].

The theorem illustrates that there is one "pattern" of strategies which is optimal (in terms of minimizing $E[N(t)]$) for any treatment parameters, providing the two drugs are equivalent. This property is extremely convenient, because in any situation where treatment must be stopped early (i.e., patient toxicity or perhaps refusal), the truncated regimen is then optimal for the number of treatments given. Similarly if it is decided to increase the treatment regimen, we may still construct the optimal plan of the required length by adding cycles of the drugs to the preexisting regimen.

As previously indicated, however, the probability of cure is not necessarily maximized by those strategies which minimize $E[N(t)]$ for $t > t_J$ when treatments are equivalent. This appears to occur in the particular set of circumstances when regrowth between treatments is large, so the treatment-regrowth process (for singly resistant cells) is not strongly subcritical. Such a situation is unlikely to be encountered in human disease, since growth over periods of one month (which is greater than most intertreatment intervals) is modest for most human tumors. However, such conditions may be encountered in several experimental cancers where doubling times of about 12 hr are not uncommon.

The theorem and preceding discussion indicate that in most cases of human cancer where two equivalent agents are available, which may not be used concurrently, the best way to use these two will be in alternating strategy. This result is of interest because of its generality (it does not depend on the particular parameter values) and because it is not current clinical practice.

In clinical medicine protocols are developed whereby active agents are combined, as much as possible, into regimens which are then repeated for a fixed number of cycles. Where two such regimens are available, the common practice is to use one continuously and then if there is evidence of relapse the other regimen is employed. Conversely, although we conclude that alternating strategies represent a departure from clinical practice it does not present a change in the clinical concept of combination chemotherapy. Combination chemotherapy uses drugs given at fixed times during a cycle and repeated a fixed number of times. In each regimen the drugs are frequently not given simultaneously but on different days. An alternating regimen can be viewed as combination chemotherapy with repeated cycles of the regimen $T_1 T_2$ or $(T_2 T_1)$ over a longer intertreatment interval.

The identification of optimal strategies (i.e., those which maximize P_N) for two drugs which are not equivalent represents a considerable problem in computation, if the parameters are all known. For example, when $J = 12$ there are 2^{12} possible strategies. Thus it is desirable to seek heuristics that reduce the set of strategies to be considered. For a strategy to be effective the treatments must be able to make the net growth of $R_0(t)$, $R_1(t)$, and $R_2(t)$ subcritical (over the treatment period); otherwise no cure is possible. In particular, the cells present at time t_1 in R_0, R_1, and R_2 must be eliminated with a "large" probability. Following this reasoning, we infer the expected number of these cells should be small at completion of the treatment regimen. That is, we would expect

$$E[R_i(t_1)][\pi_{1,i}^{n_1} \pi_{2,i}^{J-n_1}] < k \tag{45}$$

for $i = 0, 1, 2$, where n_1 is the number of times T_1 is given in the J cycles of therapy and k is chosen as a function of d [i.e., it will be larger if the death rate is larger; a possible choice is $k = 0.5(1 - \varepsilon)^{-1}$]. In certain cases the set of inequalities (45) may provide useful lower and upper bounds on n_1 (i.e., not 1 or J), thus restricting the number of strategies to be examined to determine an optimal one. These inequalities may also show that J is too small, so the search for an optimal rule of length J may not be of great use.

The search for optimal strategies has been examined in considerable detail by Day, where he considered 16 strategies for J = 12 and calculated their effect upon 256 different combinations of drug and tumor parameters [12]. He showed that it is possible to identify certain patterns in the best (of the 16) treatment strategies as the degree of asymmetry between the parameters of the two drugs increase. In a particular clinical problem strategies could be examined which were "close" to the best of the 16 determined by Day. The details of such a search remain to be worked out, the reader is referred to other chapters for further discussion of this problem.

D. An Example

A computer program was written which incorporates the relationships presented in (36), (38a), (38b), and (40). Numerical integration is performed using Simpson's approximation. The integrals are generally well behaved and may be evaluated to eight-figure accuracy by partitioning the interval of integration into no more than 100 subintervals.

The treatment parameters $\pi_{i,A}$, the probability of a cell in compartment A surviving administration of drug i, and T(i), the minimum recovery time after treatment i, must be entered for each drug. Five treatments are considered as follows:

i = 1,2 correspond to specific chemotherapeutic agents T_1 and T_2; i = 3 corresponds to the two agents (T_3) being given together; i = 4 represents a nonchemotherapeutic treatment (T_4) which affects all stem cells equally—that is, $\pi_{k,A}$ is the same for all A; and i = 5 represents a null treatment (T_5) where $\pi_{3,A} = 1.0$. It is assumed that no treatment may be administered within the (minimum) recovery time for the preceding treatment. T_5 is used so that other treatments may be applied at arbitrary times after the minimum recovery time. There is no implicit time scale used, but each parameter reflecting times [DT and T(i)] mujst be entered on the same scale (i.e., days, hours, etc.). The parameters input are given in Table 3 along with the values used in this example.

The output from the program includes $E[R_0(t)]$, $E[R_1(t)]$, $E[R_2(t)]$, $E[R_{12}(t)]$ evaluated at t_j^-, t_j, for j = 1, . . ., J. The following probabilities are also calculated: $P_0(t_j) = \phi(\epsilon, 1, 1, 1; t_j)$, $P_1(t_j) = \phi(1, \epsilon, 1, 1; t_j)$, $P_2(t) = \phi(1, 1, \epsilon, 1; t_j)$, $P_{12}(t_j) = \phi(1, 1, 1, \epsilon; t_j)$, and $P(t_j) = \phi(\epsilon, \epsilon, \epsilon, \epsilon; t_j)$ for j = 1, . . ., J. The first four quantities correspond to the marginal probabilities that cells in R_0, R_1, R_2, and R_{12}, respectively, at time t_j will go spontaneously extinct at some later time. $P(t_j)$ is the probability of cure. Notice that $P_0(t_j)$ is the probability that the sensitive cells at time t_j will go extinct (all cells derived from these cells go extinct) and not the probability that there will be no sensitive stem cells at

TABLE 3   Parameter Values for Simulations

Parameter	Value
N (number of stem cells at diagnosis)	10^7
DT (doubling time of tumor)	5 days
ε (=d/b)	0
c^* (=c/b)	0
α_1 (= α_2 = $\alpha_{1,12}$ = $\alpha_{2,12}$)	5×10^{-5}
ν_1 (ν_2 = $\nu_{1,12}$ = $\nu_{2,12}$)	0
α_{12}	0
ν_{12}	0
$\pi_{1,0}$ (= $\pi_{2,0}$ = $\pi_{1,2}$ = $\pi_{2,1}$)	10^{-2}
$\pi_{1,1}$ (= $\pi_{2,2}$ = $\pi_{1,12}$ = $\pi_{2,12}$)	1.0
T(1) [=T(2)] (minimum recovery times)	3 days
J (maximum number of cycles)	8

time $t = \infty$. This observation also applies (for the appropriate states) to $P_1(t_j)$, $P_2(t_j)$, and $P_{12}(t_j)$.

We will give an example with parameters chosen to be in the range of those seen in passaged experimental tumors. The parameters ε and c^* were chosen to be zero, implying that all cells are stem cells, which seems to be approximately true for some experimental tumors. The doubling times (DT) and intertreatment times [T(i)] were chosen to be five and three days, respectively. This doubling time represents the upper limit for most experimental tumors and the lower limit of these measured for human disease. However, as noted previously, the unit of measurement is irrelevant to these computations, and it is only the ratio (5/3) of the different quantities which is important. When the sum $\alpha_{A_i,A_j} + \nu_{A_i,A_j}$ is fixed, the various values of α_{A_i,A_j} and ν_{A_i,A_j} have little real effect on the probability of cure. Thus for simplicity we have chosen $\nu_{A_i,A_j} = 0$, and thus $\gamma^*_{A_i,A_j} = \beta_{A_i,A_j} = 0$. Similarly, for simplicity we have assumed that $\alpha_{12} = \nu_{12} = 0$; that is, single transitions from sensitivity to double resistance do not occur. The therapeutic parameters have been chosen so that resistant cells are absolutely resistant to the particular drug. For the purposes of illustration J = 8; that is, eight cycles of

TABLE 4 Probability of Extinction of Cells at Times of Treatment for Parameter Values given in Table 3 for Strategy S(1)

Time t	Treatment	$P_0(t)$	$P_1(t)$	$P_2(t)$	$P_{12}(t)$	$P(t)$
$\bar{t}_1$	—	0	0	0	0.641	0
t_1	T_1	0	0	0	0.641	0
t_2	T_1	0	0	0.500	0.573	0
t_3	T_1	0	0	0.984	0.487	0
t_4	T_1	0.707	0	1.000	0.386	0
t_5	T_1	0.995	0	1.000	0.277	0
t_6	T_1	1.000	0	1.000	0.172	0
t_7	T_1	1.000	0	1.000	0.087	0
t_8	T_1	1.000	0	1.000	0.033	0

TABLE 5 Probability of Extinction of Cells at Times of Treatment for Parameter Values Given in Table 3 for Strategy S(2)

Time t	Treatment	$P_0(t)$	$P_1(t)$	$P_2(t)$	$P_{12}(t)$	$P(t)$
t_1	—	0	0	0	0.641	0
t_1	T_1	0	0	0	0.641	0
t_2	T_1	0	0	0.500	0.573	0
t_3	T_1	0	0	0.984	0.487	0
t_4	T_1	0.707	0	1.000	0.386	0
t_5	T_2	0.995	0	1.000	0.277	0
t_6	T_2	1.000	0.059	1.000	0.275	0.022
t_7	T_2	1.000	0.934	1.000	0.275	0.263
t_8	T_2	1.000	0.999	1.000	0.275	0.275

TABLE 6 Probability of Extinction of Cells at Times of Treatment for Parameter Values Given in Table 3 for Strategy S(3)

Time t	Treatment	$P_0(t)$	$P_1(t)$	$P_2(t)$	$P_{12}(t)$	$P(t)$
t_1^-		0	0	0	0.641	0
t_1	T_1	0	0	0	0.641	0
t_2	T_2	0	0	0	0.573	0
t_3	T_1	0	0	0.369	0.571	0
t_4	T_2	0.707	0.254	0.368	0.569	0.044
t_5	T_1	0.995	0.254	0.968	0.569	0.155
t_6	T_2	1.000	0.955	0.968	0.569	0.537
t_7	T_1	1.000	0.955	0.999	0.569	0.550
t_8	T_2	1.000	0.999	0.999	0.569	0.568

therapy will be administered. Parameters were chosen so that the drugs satisfy the definition of equivalence given in Section IV.C.

Tables 4-6 show the effect of three treatment strategies on curability: $S(1) = (1, 1, 1, 1, 1, 1, 1, 1)$, $S(2) = (1, 1, 1, 1, 2, 2, 2, 2)$, and $S(3) = (1, 2, 1, 2, 1, 2, 1, 2)$. That is, $S(1)$ represents eight cycles of T_1 given at three-day intervals, with the first cycle being given when the tumor consists of 10^7 stem cells, etc. Since the treatments are equivalent, each strategy has its mirror image, which has the same probability of cure. Without loss of generality we will assume T_1 is given first.

Tables 4-6 show, for this example, that of the three strategies of length $J = 8$ which give a single drug per treatment, the probability of cure is maximized by the alternating strategy $S(3)$. As can be seen, all three strategies control (eliminate with high probability) the sensitive cells, but the strategies have differential effect in controlling the various resistant compartments. Strategies $S(2)$ and $S(3)$ successfully control both the singly resistant compartment but have a differential effect on the distribution of cells in R_{12}. Furthermore, since neither T_1 nor T_2 have any effect on cells in R_{12}, further treatment (after t_8) will not increase the curability to a value which exceeds $P_{12}(t_8)$. Tables similar to 4-6 are useful in constructing optimal strategies for arbitrary treatments for large J. Examining the response of each cell type to a variety of treatment strategies usually makes it a routine matter to identify the better ones and possibly the optimal ones.

V. CONCLUSION

Modeling the resistance process is useful in that it permits the identification and characterization of protocols designed to overcome the phenomenon. However, it must be stressed that many mechanisms lead to resistance and that here we have only concentrated on spontaneous mutations to resistance. A great deal of work remains to be done in integrating the modeling of various forms of resistance so that the clinical manifestation of resistance may be better understood. This will require the incorporation of some function which measures toxicity, because in practice there is an inverse relationship between these two phenomena; higher doses of drug lead to less resistance and greater toxicity, and vice versa. When this is done, it will then be possible to truly optimize treatment. We conclude that there is much fundamental work remaining to be done that is of practical and theoretical interest.

ACKNOWLEDGMENT

The authors gratefully acknowledge the patience and secretarial
assistance provided by Mrs. Shirley Morton.

REFERENCES

1. Ling, V. Genetic basis of drug resistance in mammalian cells,
    in *Drug and Hormone Resistance in Neoplasia*, Vol. 1 (N. Bruch-
    ovsky and J. H. Goldie, eds), CRC Press, Boca Raton (1982).

2. Schimke, R. T. Gene amplification, drug resistance and cancer.
    Cancer Research, *44*:1735–1742 (1984).

3. Luria, S. E. and Delbruck, M. Mutation of bacteria from virus
    sensitivity to virus resistance. *Gen.*, *28*:491–511 (1943).

4. Law, L. Origin of the resistance of leukemic cells to folic acid
    antagonists. *Nature (Lond.)*, *169*:628–629 (1952).

5. Till, J. E., McCulloch, E. A., and Siminovitch, L. A stochastic
    model of stem cell proliferation, based on the growth of spleen
    colony-forming cells. *Proc. Nat. Acad. Sci. USA*, *51*:29–36
    (1954).

6. Mackillop, W. J., Ciampi, A., Till, J. E., and Buick, R. N.
    A stem cell model of human tumor growth: implications for
    tumor cell clonogenic assays. *JNCI*, *70*:9–16 (1983).

7. John, F., *Partial Differential Equations*, 4th ed., Springer-
    Verlag, New York (1982).

8. Karlin, S. and Taylor, H. M. *A First Course in Stochastic
    Processes*, Academic Press, New York (1975).

9. Skipper, H. S., Schabel, F. M., and Wilcox, W. S. Experimen-
    tal evaluation of potential anti-cancer agents. XIV. Further
    study of certain basic concepts underlying chemotherapy of
    leukemia. *Cancer Chem. Rep.*, *45*:5–28 (1965).

10. Skipper, H. S., Schabel, F. M., and Lloyd, H. H. Dose re-
    sponse and tumor cell repopulation rate in chemotherapeutic
    trials, in *Advances in Cancer Chemotherapy*, Vol. 1 (A. Rozownki
    ed.), Marcel Dekker, New York, pp. 205–253 (1979).

11. Birkhead, B. G. Drug resistance and chemotherapy of residual
    tumours, draft report, Department of Statistical Science,
    University College, London (1985).

12. Day, R. A tumor growth model with applications to treatment policy and protocol choice, Ph.D. thesis, School of Public Health, Harvard University, Boston, Mass. (1984).

13. Coldman, A. J., Goldie, J. H., and Ng, V. The effect of cellular differentiation on the development of permanent drug resistance. *Math. Biosc.* 74:177–198 (1985).

14. Coldman, A. J. and Goldie, J. H. A model for the resistance of tumor cells to cancer chemotherapeutic agents. *Math. Biosci.*, 65:291–307 (1983).

9

Exploring Large Tumor Model Spaces
Drawing Sturdy Conclusions

ROGER S. DAY   *Department of Biostatistics, Harvard School of Public Health, Boston, Massachusetts*

I. INTRODUCTION

The goal in this chapter is to describe a few tools of sensitivity analysis that have proven their worth, or promise to do so, in some problems relating to treatment choice and timing in cancer therapy. The major focus is to present a modeling framework for exploring the consequences of one's favorite new piece of cancer biology, and to map out the computational and interpretational boundaries of usefulness for this framework. I will discuss why sensitivity analysis is important in tumor modeling and will review two examples of sensitivity analyses appearing in the literature, employed to generate fresh perspectives about cancer treatment and its limitations. The meat of the chapter presents sensitivity analysis in a broader sense; relaxing the basic assumptions about the fundamental types of cells and the ways that new kinds of cells arise. A capping discussion deals with the role of sensitivity analysis in the context of mathematical modeling in general.

A. Sensitivity Analysis in Tumor Modeling

Sensitivity analysis is used to gain confidence in the result when one is calculating something based on a mathematical model. There is always the suspicion that the chosen model is wrong enough to

produce misleading results. To cope with this, one can choose a
large set of mathematical models, typically by forswearing as many
simplifying assumptions as possible or by allowing some initial parameter choices to be varied across a range at least as broad as our
ignorance of their true values. Then if the result holds up across
the set of models, one feels much better about it. If not, the exceptions themselves can be illuminating.

Sensitivity analysis seems especially appropriate in cancer biology
and oncology. My orientation toward applying mathematical models to
cancer biology has been informed by an unpleasant recurrent pattern
in cancer research: bright ideas about the workings of this disease
and bright hopes for its cure have repeatedly been dimmed by
heterogeneity at every level. I have three levels in mind: the refusal of cancer to act like a single disease, the refusal of clinical
tumors with the same diagnosis and staging to respond uniformly to
treatment, and the refusal of tumor cells within a single tumor to be
identical. They all interfere with the discovery of general truths in
oncology.

Because of this multilevel variability, dependable conclusions are
accessible only if one asks modest questions, and asks them repeatedly in different settings. An oncology cooperative group will
test a promising new agent separately in groups of patients with
different disease sites and histologies. A cancer biologist gains confidence about the significance of a new observation only after it is
found in many different tumor cell systems or animal models. In
parallel with these cautious attitudes, a mathematical modeler, who
must respond to all three levels of heterogeneity, is impelled to
practice sensitivity analysis.

The simplest kind of sensitivity analysis to contemplate involves
simply varying parameters and observing the changes in outcome.
Two such applications are now briefly reviewed. Readers are en-
couraged to consult the original papers for full details.

B. Example 1: The Effect of Cell Death Rates

A simple example of a sensitivity analysis in tumor modeling is provided by Goldie and Coldman [1], who opened the door by investigat-
ing the effect of cell differentiation on the difficulties of treating a
tumor. Because tumor cells mimic normal differentiation to some extent, much of a tumor typically consists of cells incapable of dividing
indefinitely. Some time after these terminal cells or their progeny
die, they lyse and disappear. So it appears that for practical purposes, these terminal cells may be considered dead. The rest, the
"stem cells" (those which sustain the tumor through self-renewal),
are the true targets of treatment.

One reason that the distinction between terminal and stem cells is important is related to drug resistance. The resistance of tumors to drug treatment was originally ascribed to the idea that chemotherapeutic agents differ in their cycle specificity, some being effective mostly against actively dividing cells [2]. There was supporting evidence from the observation that slowly growing tumors are generally more resistant to treatment. However, another theory gained more credence. It was noted that in the clinic a common pattern was an encouraging regression of the tumor, followed by regrowth and unresponsiveness to the agents responsible for the regression. As new experimental techniques arrived, it was confirmed that the cells within a tumor differ in their responsiveness to treatment. In many cases the mechanisms of resistance have been elucidated and shown to be passed on to daughter cells when a cell divides. This provided an explanation for the observed pattern of treatment failure.

Goldie and Coldman wished to study the effect of cell death and differentiation on the rate of development of drug resistance. They considered a single drug and used a birth-death model [3] with two types of stem cells: sensitive and drug resistant. The "death rate" is the rate at which terminal or dead cells are generated. Because they took the birth rate to equal one, the cell death rate may be interpreted as the odds of a cell dying "naturally" (from nontreatment causes) before the cell divides. Thus a death rate equaling one would represent a so-called critical process.

If one assumes that the tumor stem cells have a zero death rate and assigns plausible values for other parameters in the model, one reaches a puzzling prediction: cancer should be much easier to cure [4,5] than it appears to be in reality. By relaxing an assumption, we reach an interesting insight into treatment failure.

Keeping fixed the growth rate (i.e., the net difference of birth and death rates), these authors were defining a class of tumor processes which would appear clinically nearly identical in rate of development. They then investigated the effect of varying death rates using four values for the death rate: 0, 0.50, 0.90, and 0.99.

They explored two distinct effects of cell death. A high cell death rate means that small residual tumor burdens remaining after treatment are susceptible to petering out, because the random nature of the process allows the possibility of an excess of deaths over births sufficient to eliminate all cells. This tends to increase the probability of cure. However, at the same time, the number of cell divisions from the first tumor cell to a given cell present at diagnosis must be higher, in compensation for the cell death. Consequently, there are proportionately more cell divisions in a given cell's history and a proportionately higher chance that one of the cell's ancestors had mutated to drug resistance. Thus a high cell death rate may bode ill for the prospects of cure.

The trade-off between these two effects was found to be rather balanced, in the sense that the probability of no resistant cells at the time of diagnosis depended little on the cell death rate. Curiously, though, in an extension considering resistance to two drugs rather than just one, it was found that the death rate is very important. The probability that a tumor at diagnosis has no doubly resistant cells (no cells resistant to both drugs) drops dramatically as the cell death rate increases. This discovery provides a new alternative explanation for the intractability of most adult tumors and the success against the quicker-growing childhood cancers: the more slowly growing tumors have higher cell death rates and therefore greater drug resistance. Here then, is another example where the answer changes when a broader model framework is considered. The importance of cell death and differentiation rates are negligible for single-agent therapy, but for combination chemotherapy or combined modality therapy its importance is great.

C. Example 2: Treatment Sequencing

The specific issue motivating my interest in sensitivity analysis [6] was originally raised in another seminal work by Goldie and Coldman [5], concerning the combination of more than one treatment in a cancer treatment regimen. This example is more complicated. To describe the setting will require some background.

The advent of combination chemotherapy is one of the successes of clinical cancer research [7]. The concept of resistance of tumors to chemotherapeutic treatment leads to a neat explanation for the synergism of cancer treatments, the idea being that cells resistant to one treatment could be killed by another treatment. In the last decade the idea of mutation to resistance as a central cause for treatment failure has profoundly affected clinical thinking.

Consequently, the strategy of combination chemotherapy has become almost universal in cancer drug protocols. Administering two active drugs concurrently when possible was intuitively appealing on theoretical grounds, whether phase specificity or drug resistance was responsible. Unfortunately, drug toxicity on normal tissues continues to limit chemotherapy.

Goldie and Coldman [4,5] extended the combination strategy by arguing that this picture of drug resistance as a major cause of treatment failure supports the use of different drugs in alternation when toxicity precludes the concurrent schedule. This would take the place of the more usual sequential schedule, which begins with one drug and switches to another just once, typically when there is a "recurrence," i.e., when it becomes clear that the first agent is no longer effective in restraining the cancer. An extensive citation list in the clinical literature reveals the extent to which the alternating strategy has been embraced by the clinical research community, though practice lags considerably behind theory.

1. Relaxing the Symmetry Assumptions

The arguments of Goldie and Coldman rest on a mathematical model for tumor growth and treatment incorporating mutation to drug resistance. Unavoidably, as with any mathematical model for a complex biological process, this model is built on simplifying assumptions which are known to be violated into reality. To do away with these assumptions and consider a very large class of plausible models seemed appealing on several grounds. First, if real clinical tumors violate the Goldie-Coldman assumptions sufficiently, one might be able to find strategies that perform substantially better than the strategy of administering two treatments in concurrent or alternating fashion. Second, one might instead find very little effect from relaxing assumptions; then one's confidence in the Goldie-Coldman strategy would increase, and a central place in new treatment protocols would be achieved more easily. Third, an astounding array of new laboratory equipment and techniques are promising that measurements of key parameters may soon be within reach; if sufficient accuracy and interpretability were gained, a mathematical model adequately reflecting the biology of the tumor might eventually be able to derive optimal strategies tailored to each individual patient, as some have suggested [8]. Finally, on the most pessimistic note, we might discover that the variability of tumor cells and cancer patients implies a fundamental limit on what can be accomplished in cancer treatment. This would be worth knowing, because it would bear on the debate between prevention advocates and treatment advocates over allocation of cancer research funds.

To extend the work of Goldie and Coldman, parameters determining the process of tumor growth and the effects of treatments were systematically varied, relaxing the "symmetry" assumptions of the original Goldie-Coldman model. Symmetry means, briefly, that the two drugs are equivalent in the sense that swapping one for the other throughout the treatment schedule would lead to identical results. Thus, all cell types have the same birth rates and death rates, all allowed mutations have the same rate, and, most importantly, each drug has equal potency on the cells sensitive to it. These assumptions seemed likely to fail in practice, and their failure seemed likely to result in major amendments to the conclusions.

2. Basic Setup

Here we summarize the design of the sensitivity analysis. The basic model is presented later in this chapter; for purposes of this investigation, the method of computation differs from the Goldie-Coldman

calculations only in that cell death is incorporated somewhat more
gracefully. The full details on the sensitivity analysis have been
published elsewhere [6].

I conformed to the basic setup and nomenclature of Goldie and
Coldman [5] with respect to drugs and cell types. There are two
drugs, called A and B, and four cell types: sensitive to both drugs
(S), resistant only to drug A (RA), resistant only to drug B (RB),
and resistant to both drugs (RAB). The tumor is assumed to begin
with a single sensitive (S) cell.

The doubling time of S-cells is taken to equal unity, which may
be thought of as one month. Treatment courses ("doses") are constrained to be one month apart, and are modeled as if the entire
course and all resultant cell death occurs at a single instant. Treatments are initiated at 30 doublings of the S-cell subpopulation, when
the tumor bulk is at roughly 10^9 cells. Justification for these choices
can be found in standard references [9,10].

The goal was to summarize the effectiveness of a large number of
two-drug treatment schedules on a large number of four-cell-type
tumor models. (Here "model" will refer to a particular assignment
of values to the parameters.) The problem was simplified by
circumscribing the models and schedules with a small number of carefully chosen representatives. A central symmetric model was defined
by choosing medium values for each parameter. High and low values
were chosen for varying these parameters in order to violate symmetry. A battery of 16 treatment schedules was chosen to represent
two important dimensions in the problem of combining two treatments:
the total number of courses of each drug (the dose mix), and the
timing of the first course for each drug (the time mix). For each
model and each treatment schedule, the probability that no tumor
cells remain at the end of treatment (the cure rate) was computed.
These probabilities were computed conditionally on the event that
the number of tumor cells at the time of treatment start is nonzero;
this is necessary because a positive death rate was allowed, creating
the possibility that the tumor dwindles away before it gets established.
From these cure rates, a "comparative cure index" was computed for
each schedule, comparing its cure rate to the cure rate of the other
schedules on the model under consideration on the logit scale; using
this scale and focusing on comparisons between schedules appear to
make the results insensitive to some of the vagaries and arbitrary
aspects of the model setup.

3.   Cube Vertices Versus Following Rays:
     Stages of the Investigation

Once a type of model is settled on and a range of plausible values
for parameters is chosen to define the universe of interesting models,
the most fundamental problem is to decide how to encompass and

explore this universe to be sure that one has a representative picture of it and that nothing important has been missed. In the tumor model example there are many parameters whose impact on the outcome of treatment needs to be assessed. Should we vary them one at a time, and plot the outcome for many values of the chosen parameter? This can be visualized as studying the behavior of the outcome along lines in the parameter space. Or should we consider only a very small set, perhaps as few as two values, for each parameter, but vary many parameters at a time in every combination? This can be visualized as the corners of a box in parameter space. Is there a compromise between these two extremes that most closely corresponds to exploring the potential assumption violations that worry us the most?

The solution chosen was to pick three values per parameter and relax assumptions in stages of progressively greater departures from symmetry. At each stage it was determined which types of tumor kinetics and resistance patterns favor the alternating strategies, which one favor interweaving but not strictly alternating strategies, which ones favor one-drug strategies, and which ones are indifferent. The performance of the optimal strategy was compared with the performance of alternating and one-drug strategies, and with the schedule choice indicated by a previous stage.

4. Results

The results were that under relevant violations of the symmetry assumptions, nonalternating treatment schedules frequently outperform alternation and combination substantially. The relative performance of schedules follows understandable patterns. A simple strategy was discovered (the "worst drug rule") which leads to profound improvements in outcome over a wide range of parameter values. This strategy involves choosing a treatment schedule in which the drug with the lower cell kill is actually given for more courses and/or earlier than the "better" drug. It initially appears counterintuitive and is contrary to current practice, but with some thought one finds the strategy consonant with common sense. There are two cell types consisting of singly resistant cells, and both compartments of cells must be eliminated to effect a cure; but each of these jobs can be accomplished by only one of the drugs, and, in particular, the worst drug will need more, or earlier, application to succeed.

Three potential protocol design strategies were derived from these results. When there is no knowledge of parameters, empirical trials in search of the best schedule can be contemplated, as long as patients with the same tumor type have similar parameters. Using minimal knowledge of cell kill parameters, application of the worst drug rule could have excellent results. Finally, an even larger improvement could result from predicting the best schedule based on detailed knowledge of the cell kinetics and drug kill parameters.

The issues surrounding these strategies have been explored in some depth [6].

The usefulness of these strategies is limited by two major sources of uncertainty about the target tumor, each with its own ramifications. The first is the difficulty of measuring the relevant parameters; as assay techniques improve, the last two strategies mentioned will become more attractive. The second type of uncertainty arises from the possibility of fundamental differences between the clinical tumors of patients who ostensibly have the same disease; if these differences turn out to be small, in a certain limited sense referred to as "pattern homogeneity," then the first two strategies become attractive. The role of pattern homogeneity appears to deserve careful consideration.

D. Sensitivity Analysis and Patient Heterogeneity

In our setting there is an additional boon to the use of sensitivity analysis. Facing the calculations for many models is a good reminder that each patient may need his or her own model. The observed differences among clinical tumors arise not just because the random aspect of the process (cell growth and mutation) leads to tumor variability but also because the process (e.g., the parameters) may differ across patients. The implication of the two sources of variability are quite distinct.

The first is accounted for by the stochastic model. But the second essentially cannot be modeled. The latter is precisely the second level of heterogeneity listed in the introduction to this chapter. It is the level of heterogeneity whose implications are most frequently overlooked. Fidler has suggested [11] that to the extent that the patterns and differences we see are a result of a random pattern, we have an opportunity to advance against cancer, because at least the degree of unpredictability is predictable. The proportion of patient variability explained by the randomness of the process, as opposed to haphazard differences in parameters, is thus a crucial question.

II. A COMPUTABLE FRAMEWORK FOR GENERAL
POPULATION STRUCTURES

A. Relaxing Assumptions: Varying Parameters
Versus Broadening the Model

The investigations described in the two examples relaxed assumptions about parameters already present or implicit in the simpler models which they were intended to extend. These assumptions are naturally described as conditions on parameters in a simple model already in use. One can make reasonable guesses about parameters, but then allow the parameters to depart from these guesses in some systematic way. The guesses may represent assumptions, such as setting one parameter equal to zero or requiring a pair of parameters to be equal.

A more challenging type of sensitivity analysis is demanded in response to the many discoveries in tumor biology concerning the different kinds of cells found in a tumor. One can make a conscious decision to ignore certain aspects of the biology whose incorporation would be inconvenient or too complicated. Alternatively, one can contemplate relaxing assumptions in the sense of extending or broadening the fundamental complexity of the model.

Some important phenomena to attend to include the presence of a single mutation leading to resistance to many drugs ("pleiotropic drug resistance"), the development of metastatic cells via mutational events, gene amplification as a multilevel mechanism of resistance, and autocrine and synocrine feedback relationships among and within tumor cell subpopulations. To help understand the implications of these biological discoveries, we would like a unifying framework for modeling them.

This section describes the framework in which the second example, the relaxation of symmetry assumptions, was performed. It allows much more complicated and general pictures of the structure of tumors, a capability that has yet to be fully exploited. The full solution for calculating the process is presented elsewhere [12]. It is most appropriate for cell colony subpopulation structures in which there are relatively rare events (such as mutation) with important biological consequences. A brief description is presented of the modeling framework and the algorithm used for the TREATS computer program developed at Dana-Farber Cancer Institute.

The suitability of this modeling framework is limited by several problems shared by other frameworks for tumor growth and mutation. As more complicated aspects of tumor biology are incorporated, one defines more types of cells in terms of their properties relative to cell kinetics and drug resistance and concretizes the definitions by setting appropriate ranges for the parameter values. (This will be illustrated later in examples). Two problems are raised by this procedure: (1) numerical stability and accuracy as the number of cell types increases, and (2) the choice of parameter values to represent the biological phenomena in the absence of direct measurement. Therefore we discuss numerical issues involving choice of iteration time intervals, the interpretation of the parameters, and two examples, namely the modeling of multiple levels of resistance and the modeling of differentiation for normal and neoplastic cells.

B. A Description of the Model

The basis for the model is a multitype branching process in continuous time, a general class of models described by Bellman and

Harris [13]. A cell colony is imagined to contain a small number of subpopulations, each one being homogeneous (of a single "cell type"). Each individual cell exists until one of the following events occur: renewal—replacement by two cells of the same type as the original cell; mutation—replacement by two cells, one of the same type and the other of a different type; conversion—replacement by one cell of a different type; diversion—replacement by two cells of different types; and death—the disappearance of the cell. Mutation, conversion, and diversion give rise to cells of new type; here we unify them under the term "origination," with apologies for the plethora of new terms required to simplify the presentation. The times of the events are independently distributed. This implies that any pair of cells at a point in time have statistically independent futures.

In this formulation the future of a cell at any instant depends only on the type of cell, not on the time since that cell's birth. Therefore the time until an event occurs to that cell is exponentially distributed and carries no information about which of the potential events may have occurred. This greatly simplifies the mathematics of the model, but introduces peculiarities in the interpretation of parameters. They are discussed later.

The model has certain other features. It allows "treatment" (binomial cell kill at distinct predetermined times). It allows conditioning on the sizes of subpopulations at arbitrary times (typically used to assure a diagnosable tumor at the start of treatment or to fit data). The rates at which the events occur are allowed to depend on the cell type and on chronologic time in a piecewise linear fashion. For simplicity the subsequent discussion will ignore these features.

C. Outline of Computation

The main computational goal is the probability generating function (p.g.f.) for the joint distribution of the number of cells of each cell type at a given time. In this section we give an overview of this computation.

Cell types will be denoted X and Y, and the number of cells will be denoted N_X, N_Y, etc. A vector containing the number of cells of each cell type will be denoted $N = (. . ., N_Y, . . .)$. The joint probability generating function for counts of all cell types at time t, evaluated at the dummy argument $s = (. . ., s_Y, . . .)$, is defined by

$$\Lambda_t(s) = E(\prod_Y s_Y^{N_Y(t)}) \tag{1}$$

where E signifies expectation over the distribution of N(t) and Y indexes of the cell types. We assume that Λ_0 is known (e.g., N is known at time 0).

The main use of the p.g.f. is to obtain the probability, $\Lambda_t(s)$, that there are no cells at the end of treatment. Other uses are described at length elsewhere [12].

The number of cells of type Y at the end of the interval [0, T] is

$$N_Y(T-) = \sum_x \sum_{j=1}^{N_X(0)} D_Y(T \mid X,j) \tag{2}$$

where the D's are random variables, each signifying the number of Y-type descendants of the jth X cell at time 0 after a time T has elapsed. Let Φ_T be the joint p.g.f. for all the progeny of a single X cell (e.g, the jth) present at the end of the interval, i.e., for [. . ., $D_Y(T \mid X,j)$, . . .] (the Y-coordinate is shown). Our assumption that cells at any given time have independent futures implies that any two D's representing progeny of two different cells will be independent. Therefore, the form of (2) allows the use of the composition rule for the p.g.f. of a random sum, which leads to

$$\Lambda_T(s) = \Lambda_0[. . ., \Phi_T(s), . . .] \tag{3}$$

Here the X-coordinate of the argument is shown.

Regrettably, the full solution for Φ_T is not tractable. However, it is possible to compute an approximation which omits all ancestral lines of cell descent for which two or more originating (mutation or conversion or diversion) events occur in [0, T]. In other words, we compute the solution which is exact for the process, augmented with the assumption that a second originating event in the same interval is fatal to the cell. Then this solution will be adequate for the original purpose if the probability of such a "double event" is very small. This is fulfilled if the interval is short enough. Therefore we make use of the iteration rule for p.g.f.s of random sums to rewrite (1); let $\Lambda(s) = (. . ., \Phi_T, . . .)$. Then the p.g.f. evaluated at time E = IT is obtained by applying Λ_0 to the I-fold iteration of Λ evaluated at s. This computational method is implemented in the TREATS program, which was developed by the author at Dana-Farber Cancer Institute and used in the study of treatment sequencing described in example 2 [6].

D. Assessing the Approximation: Uncounted Cells

This tactic will still disallow any ancestral line with two or more originating events within a single interval. Any such ancestral line in the true underlying process will be missing from the process as we have modeled it. The magnitude of the resulting error will depend on the population structure as well as kinetic parameters. The first two cell types of any temporal sequence of cell types will be properly counted; later cell types will be increasingly underrepresented. In practice we care about the bias if it is large enough to mask important differences or if it is shared unequally among the models we compare. To the extent that losing cells is roughly the same as having an increased cell death rate and decreased origination rates, the error will be unimportant. The most difficult situation to maintain accuracy is that in which there is a long sequence of originating events. This problem is ameliorated if T is chosen small enough. Such a solution increases the computation time, making it imperative to estimate the largest acceptable T.

We propose guidelines for maximum interval length, based on insights into a special case in which the answer and the error are easy to compute. Suppose a sequence of N + 1 cell types is labeled $S_0 \cdots S_N$. The initial condition is a single cell of type S_0. The N + 1 cell types are traversed in succession through conversion events at time intervals which are exponentially distributed with mean one. Other events are disallowed. This is a standard semi-Markov transition model. There should be exactly one cell at all times; the defect from this measures the probability of losing the cell due to the approximation. In genuine applications to tumor biology, originating events give rise to clones, not just single cells. As a consequence, two lines may share their early history, leading to correlation between the outcomes. The special case captures the essence of the problem and provides insight into the choice of interval. Adjusting for cell division will be discussed later.

A useful indicator of inaccuracy is the probability that a randomly chosen ancestral line ending in cell type S_N is lost through a double event. This is important because the last cell type of an evolving sequence often plays a special role; for example, it may represent the cells resistant to all therapeutic drugs, and one needs good accuracy in the probability that there are no cells of this type because it represents a cure rate. For a fixed time endpoint E and I intervals of equal length T = E/I, the probability of losing an S_N cell is the probability that more than one originating event occurs in a single interval, given that all N events occur by time E, the time of evaluation. If the transition to cell type S_N occurs exactly at E, this is

$$1 - \frac{I!}{(1 - N)!} \, I^{-N} = \frac{N(N - 1)}{2} \, I^{-1} + O(I^{-2})$$

(using Stirling's formula as I increases with N fixed). Note the lack of dependence on E. When E is relatively small (i.e., when the probability of an initial cell making it to S_N by time E is very small), this is a good estimate. It deteriorates as E increases; using the actual distribution of the time to S_N, we get

$$\text{prob(cell is lost)} \doteq \sum_{i=1}^{I} \frac{\int_0^E t^N e^{-t}[(N(N-1)/2)I^{-1} + O(I^{-2})]\, dt}{\int_0^E t^N e^{-t}\, dt}$$

$$= \frac{(N-1)(N+1)}{2} I^{-1} + O(I^{-2}) + O(E) \tag{4}$$

E will generally be small relative to the characteristic time for an originating event to occur, if the originating event is rare. Models of drug resistance and metastasis qualify in this regard; models for cell differentiation in which each mitosis leads to a new cell type, and models in which cells that are out of cycle are represented by a "quiescent" cell type, do not. The value of I must increase as the square of N to maintain fixed accuracy. In addition, computing time per iteration is proportional to N, so overall computing time varies with the cube of N. The length of sequences is limited in practice by these considerations when the destination cell type S_N is the focus.

Another index of inaccuracy is the probability that any cell, regardless of type at time E, is lost through a double event. If N were infinite, the probability of a double event within one of the intervals would be

$$\text{prob(the cell is lost)} = 1 - \prod_{i=1}^{I} \text{prob(0 or 1 event in the ith interval)} \tag{5}$$

$$= 1 - e^{-E}\left(1 + \frac{E}{I}\right)^I$$

This estimates the fractional underestimate of total burden. It forms a good upper bound even for small values of N. The probability of losing the cell converges to zero at the rate $(1/2)E^2 I^{-1} + O(I^{-2})$ as I increases.

Now suppose there is also cell division. One would like to know the fraction of lines lost when counted by the algorithm. The estimates of cell loss probability given earlier apply to each individual ancestral line. Any two cell lines intersect in their early history, and therefore if one is lost due to a double event in the intersection, the owther is well. We consider only type-N cells. Let G be the total number of generations from time 0 to E. For a pair of N-cells prob(the number of generations since the two lines separated is g) is equal to $2^{g-1}/2^G$. Also prob(both lines are lost | they separated at generation G − g) is roughly

$$\frac{1}{2}(N^2 - 1)I^{-1}\left(1 - \frac{g}{G}\right) + \left[\frac{1}{2}(N^2 - 1)I^{-1}\frac{g}{G}\right]^2$$

Using the facts

$$\sum_{g=1}^{G} 2^{g-1} = 2^G - 1$$

$$\sum_{g=1}^{G} g2^{g-1} = (G - 1)2^G + 1$$

$$\sum_{g=1}^{G} g^2 2^{g-1} = (G^2 - 2G + 3)2^G - 3$$

we can show that the probability that both cells are lost is

$$\frac{1}{2}(N^2 - 1)I^{-1}\frac{1}{G} + \left[\frac{1}{2}(N^2 - 1)I^{-1}\right]^2\left(1 - \frac{2}{G} + \frac{3}{G^2}\right) + O(2^{-G})$$

$$(6)$$

The first term indicates the degree of correlation in the outcome for the two cells. For quickly growing cells it is proportional to the cycle time.

To refine initial choices for interval length based on the given approximations, above, one can alter each equation in the algorithm by adding or subtracting the maximum bit noise of each arithmetic operation in the algorithm. This gives an upper and lower bound for each answer. Interval length is adjusted to meet accuracy needs. The bounds are conservative and involve substantial programming and computational overhead. This technique is most appropriate when one needs great accuracy, as in fitting a model to data.

The answer can be sharpened considerably by repeating the computation twice with different time intervals and fitting linear convergence in T [14]. This method, ad hoc as it is, works surprisingly well in many situations. It fails if higher-order terms in the convergence are not negligible for the computation using the largest interval. For example, if an ancestral line can traverse nine cell types, but only eight time intervals are used, the computation will ascribe zero probability to the initial cell's traversing to the ninth cell type, regardless of the rates of origination. Therefore it is generally wise to use more than two choices for T to check for linearity.

E. The Meaning of Kinetics Parameters

In setting kinetics parameters for a model, one must be aware that the relationships between these parameters and commonly used kinetics terms are not straightforward. The quantities which are natural in the model are the instantaneous rates to the events of cell division, to cell death, to mutation, to conversion, to diversion. One would like to make a direct connection between "simple" concepts (familiar ones such as cycling time, doubling time, growth fraction, or quantities which are at least, in principle, measurable experimentally).

First, let us understand the instantaneous rates. Each type of event has a characteristic rate dependent on the cell types involved. For notation let $\lambda_{X;S}$ equal

$$\frac{1}{dt} \Pr[\text{cell type X is replaced by the collection S of cells in } (t, t + dt)]$$

(independent of time t). The rate for ordinary mitosis is $\xi_X = \lambda_{X;X,X}$. The rate for mutation to cell type Y is $\mu_{X \to Y} = \lambda_{X;X,Y}$. The rate for conversion to cell type Y is $\beta_{X \to Y} = \lambda_{X;Y}$. The rate for cell death is $\delta_X = \lambda_{X;\text{dead cell}}$.

There are two ways of thinking about these rates. One is the "competing risks" formulation borrowed from epidemiology. It is helpful in understanding the mathematics but of little use in helping us to choose parameters. A fiction is maintained that for each event that can happen to a cell Nature chooses (randomly) a time at which it will occur if something else does not happen first. The occurrence actually takes place if that time is the first of all the potential event times chosen for the cell; otherwise the time is moot. The second involves summing the rates for all potential events that could occur to the cell. This sum is the rate at which any event occurs (regardless which event), once it is known that it occurs; only the probability of each particular event is dictated by the relative contribution of the associated rate to the sum. This raises the important point that the time of occurrence of the event is completely independent of which type of event occurs. The reasonableness of this characteristic depends on the application; generally, unless there is a tumorwide

synchronization phenomenon, it is perfectly adequate, because it is
the overall behavior of the tumor, not the behavior of individual cells,
that is important.

As a consequence, we have the first rule for choosing parameters;
the rates for events occurring to a cell must be proportional to the
fraction of cells of that type undergoing that event.

Generally there will be one event which is more common than any
other, usually ordinary mitosis. Its rate makes the largest contribution to the overall sum of rates. Choosing it establishes the time
scale at which the tumor evolves. Our suggestion is to identify
these rates with the behavior that one would observe if population
sizes equaled population means. In this way we draw connections between the rates, which are mathematical artifices, and cell-kinetic
quantities usually discussed. Thus

1. Cycling time of cell type X is the time to the doubling of the
   X population if there were no cell loss from death and conversion events and no contribution from other cell types via
   conversion or mutation $= \ln(2)/\xi_X$.
2. Doubling time of cell type X is the time to the doubling of X,
   taking into account cell loss, if contributions to X were
   ignored $= \ln(2)/\lambda_X$ where $\lambda_X = \xi_X - \delta_X - \sum_Z \beta_{X \to Z}$ is the
   growth rate of X.
3. Mutation rate from type X to type Y is the probability that in a
   given division of an X-cell, one of the daughters is a mutant
   of type Y $= \mu_{X \to Y}/\xi_X$. (Note that this is not truly a rate
   but a probability.)

One last aspect remains to be described: conversion rates (e.g.,
into and out of quiescence). Finding an intuitively appealing description, or even an operationally clear one, is difficult. The reasons
are

1. It must be applicable when the source X for the conversion
   is itself quiescent to allow for recruitment into cycle. Since
   there may be no competing events, a concept of conversion
   rate based on the fraction of events which are conversions is
   not applicable. Only the time scale remains.
2. In the exponential formulation, conditioning on a particular
   type of event, say conversion, makes the time to that event
   exponential, with a rate equal to the rate at which any event
   occurs. Therefore a description based on the event time
   conditional on the occurrence of the event is useless.
3. One might want to consider the ratio of source cell counts
   to recipient cell counts in an attempt to generalize the
   "growth fraction" concept. There is an asymptotic ratio

$X(\infty)/Y(\infty)$, but this is nontrivial only if the growth rate of X is greater than the rate of Y.

It is more straightforward to specify the

$$\text{conversion time from X to Y} = \frac{\ln(2)}{\beta_{X \to Y}}$$

In general, identifying something which can plausibly be called a "conversion time" is difficult. The first problem listed above arises as well with mutation, when X → XX mitoses do not occur. These matters will be considered further when examples are discussed.

Parameters may also vary with time for a variety of reasons. Birth rates may decrease, and/or death rates may increase as the tumor gets large. Or exposure to a treatment may affect the time a cell spends in each phase of the cell cycle. Or since many drugs used in the clinic are effective only on cells in a specific phase of the cell cycle, there is the potential for selecting cells with different cycling characteristics (e.g., a shorter S phase or a longer G_1) from the overall population as well as for synchronizing cells. Or treatment may stimulate remaining cells to rapid growth through decreased competition for nutrients or through immunosuppression. Finally, treatment with a mutagenic drug may hasten the development of resistance. These effects can all be accommodated in the model.

F. Example: Multiple-Level Drug Resistance

A major use of the class of models discussed here is the study of drug resistance, especially for malignant tumors. Suppose a sequence of cell types $\tau_1 \cdots \tau_N$ represents increasing levels of drug resistance. Let them first represent successive additions of resistance to active agents, as an extension of the Goldie-Coldman two-drug model [5]. (This sequence may be regarded as embedded in 2^N cell types representing all possible combinations of resistance to N drugs, assuming resistance takes on only two values for each drug.) Then E might typically be around 30 times the doubling time for the tumor (supposing a death rate of zero), and the characteristic time for an origination event from τ_i to τ_{i+1} would be, say, 10^4. Total cell loss will be negligible. It works out to $(30/10^4)2/2 = 0.005$ even for I = 1. For probability of loss less than 10% for the τ_N cells, one needs I = 75 for N = 4, which is quite manageable, but I = 315 for N = 8, which is large enough to dampen the interactive quality of the algorithm. Regardless of N, since G = 30, the probability of losing two cells is 1.33% instead of 1%, not a great enough departure from independence to cause concern about estimated cure rates.

The cell types can be given a different interpretation. Another occasion for considering such a sequence of resistance levels is the gene amplification mechanism. In that case it is surmised that there are several stages of intermediate resistance. The rate for each step is presumably greater than 10^{-4}. Therefore the overall cell loss will be greater but still negligible. Unless the "mutation" rate is very high, the effective value of E (G times mutation rate) will still be small enough to make the above estimates for τ_N cell loss valid. The role of τ_N, the cell type most subject to undercounting, is less important in this case.

G. Example: Differentiation

As another example we discuss differentiation. A differentiation model is regarded here as a classification of cell types into stem cells, transitional cells, and end cells. The distinction is especially useful when the stem cells are not the overwhelming majority of cells. Any explanation must account for the relative paucity of stem cells, the mortality of transitional cells, and the eventual overgrowth by stem cells in the case of neoplasm. Each of these manifestations has multiple explanations. Some putative models for stem cell kinetics are

1. Mutation model: ordinary divisions of stem cells, resulting in two stem cells, are relatively rare; most divisions result in one stem cell and one differentiating cell. Ordinary mitosis will balance stem cell death in normal cells but over-compensate in neoplasia.
2. Conversion model: all divisions are ordinary, but conversions to differentiating cells are very frequent, competing with ordinary mitosis, and replacing the role of cell death in No 1 in balancing the stem cell population.
3. Quiescence model: all divisions are ordinary, but stem cells (S) spend a great deal of time in a resting state (Q), and conversion to a differentiating cell (D) can occur from this resting state.

The expression of these models in terms of kinetic parameters is not completely intuitive. For No. 1, one sets ξ for the stem cell to be much smaller than μ from stem cells to differentiating cells, in proportion to the relative frequency of the two events. Here the usual concept of "mutation rate" as a proportion is a bit unusual; it will be close to 1. This does not imply that one thinks of the stem-cell-renewing cycle as very long; it is simply a trick which is adequate for most applications. The time characteristic of overall stem cell mitosis is $(\ln 1)/(\xi + \mu) \approx (\ln 2)/\mu$. For No. 2 the "cycle time" for stem cells may be a sensible value for a cycle time, and the conversion time should be chosen in proportion to the relative frequency but which a stem converts before mitosis; this will be 0.5 for normal differentiation but larger for a tumor. For No. 3 there are no immediately apparent intuitive choices for the rates into and out of the resting state. In reality, it may depend on the stage of the tumor; late stages of solid tumors are expected to have more cells in a resting state, but they may be end cells or distressed differentiating cells.

In computation, the cost of using model 3 will be substantial, because even though there are only two cell types involved in the transaction, there are long potential pathways; unless the stay in the quiescent state is very long ($\beta_{Q,S}$ is tiny) the computational need for very short intervals is great.

Some explanations for the mortality of differentiating cells include:

1. Ladder model: there is a sequence of distinct cells in differentiation $S_1 \cdots S_N$, which divide by "diversion" only; each mitosis is of the form $D_i \rightarrow D_{i+1}D_{i+1}$.
2. Kinetics model: differentiating cells have high mitotic rates but even higher rates of conversion to end cells.

The first will require short intervals. Since the period of time covered by the model is many times the usual time taken to traverse the differentiation ladder, the computational need for short intervals may be excessive.

These models also need to account for the eventual overgrowth in a tumor by stem cells. Explanations for this include crowding effects resulting in time-dependent or feedback models for changing kinetic parameters, or else a shift in the mix of stem cells, towards cells which favor renewal of stem cells over differentiated cells, due to competition among stem cells in a compressed natural selection. Introducing time dependence of kinetic parameters can be done with no penalty on computing time. Taking feedback into account is available, though one may pay a premium of a factor of 10 in computing time even for a rudimentary solution [12]. The latter explanation requires definition of cell types to describe the heterogeneity of heritable renewal. If the rate of origination of more "selfish" stem cells is slow, then the considerations laid out for resistance levels apply, and computing the competition model is straightforward.

III. THE GENERAL ROLE OF SENSITIVITY ANALYSIS

A suitable way to cap my plea for sensitivity analysis is to consider the general nature of mathematical modeling and the part played by

sensitivity analysis. The usefulness of a model is governed by the
relationship between parameter values and predictions. There are
two extremes in this relationship, each with its own peril and promise.
Sometimes widely disparate parameter choices lead to similar conclusions. This interferes with model fitting (parameter estimation and
hypothesis testing) because even a small error in the data is enough
to compromise the data's ability to discriminate between models that
are distinctly different in important ways. But it can be a good
situation for prediction, because quite fuzzy information about the
true value of the parameters may be enough to come to sturdy and
dependable conclusions. This is subject to the provision that the
model is similar enough to the reality it is intended to reflect.

On the other hand, sometimes small changes in parameters lead
to huge changes in the predicted behavior. In this case, parameters
would have to be known very precisely to make particular predictions
possible, but model fitting could potentially provide precise, useful,
interpretable estimates of parameters governing the biological process,
provided again that the model is adequate.

It makes sense, then, to plan a general exploration of an important part of the parameter space before attempting to fit data or
to make predictions as an early step in the application of a new
mathematical model. As one attempts to demarcate the ranges in
which either of the two somewhat contradictory goals of prediction
and estimation can realistically be met, it is crucial to keep in mind
what degree of uncertainty about the parameters there is, and what
degree of uncertainty about a prediction would still be sharp enough
to be useful.

What can be gained from this exercise? Why not just assign reasonable or widely accepted values of parameters and leave it at that?
One may imagine a hierarchy of models ranging from the absurdly
simple to the uncomputably complex. One passes to greater degrees
of complexity by relaxing assumptions. At the same time the diversity, both in behavior and in structure of the processes at one's
disposal, grows tremendously. As this happens, various thresholds
are passed:

It becomes difficult to estimate parameters from data or to judge
goodness of fit.
It becomes difficult or costly even to compute the model predictions.
A good match between reality and the model is achieved, if one
chooses the right parameter values and/or structure.
A good match between reality and the model is achieved for some
incorrect sets of parameter values and/or structure.

The first threshold precedes the second, but otherwise no ordering is compelled. For the most complex biological phenomena these
thresholds will be passed in an unfortunate order; either the model

becomes impossibly difficult to handle before it becomes a good imager of reality, or multiple explanations (parameter choices) for observed data appear which are equally suitable, or both. Judicious choice of the order in which assumptions are made, balancing increased mathematical difficulty with increased realism at each step, may lead to a satisfactory model choice somewhere on the hierarchy.

Another way to increase the likelihood of a happy choice is to weaken the goal of prediction, foregoing the hope of predicting the behavior of a particular system (e.g., choosing a priori the optimum treatment for a particular tumor) in favor of finding broad patterns in the model system's behavior. This is done when, for example, we require our tumor model to tell us correctly which of two treatment plans will work better, but not to predict the degree of improvement accurately. These resulting models, obtained by relaxing some assumptions but not others, is somewhat closer to biological reality than simpler models. This does not guarantee that the resulting predictions are closer to the behavior of real tumors. But it does offer more confidence, and provides some notion of what can realistically be expected from further applications of these models.

ACKNOWLEDGMENT

Supported by NIEHS grant #T 32-ES 07142-03 and NCI grant #CA-39640.

REFERENCES

1. Goldie, J. H. and Coldman, A. J., Quantitative model for multiple levels of drug resistance in clinical tumors. *Cancer Treat. Rep.,* 67:923-931 (1983).

2. Norton, L. and Simon, R. Tumor size, sensitivity to therapy, and design of treatment schedules. *Cancer Treat. Rep., 61*: 1307-1317 (1977).

3. Parzen, E., *Stochastic Processes,* Holden Day, San Francisco (1962).

4. Goldie, J. H. and Coldman, A. J., A mathematical model for relating the drug sensitivity of tumors to their spontaneous mutation rate. *Cancer Treat. Rep., 63*:1727-1733 (1979).

5. Goldie, J. H. Coldman, A. J., and Gudauskas, G. A., Rationale for the use of alternating non-cross resistant chemotherapy. *Cancer Treat. Rep. 66*:439-449 (1982).

6. Day, R. Treatment sequencing, uncertainty, and asymmetry: protocol strategies for combination chemotherapy. Cancer Research 46:3876-3885 (1986).

7. Frei, E. III. Combination cancer therapy: presidential address. *Cancer Research* 32:2593-2607 (1972).

8. Salmon, S. E., Hamburger, A. W., Soehnlen, B., Durie, B. G. M., Alberts, D. S., and Moon, T. E. Quantitation of differential sensitivity of human-tumor stem cells to anticancer drugs. *N. Eng. J. Med.*, 298:1321-1327 (1978).

9. Steel, G. G., *Growth Kinetics of Tumors*, Clarendon Press, Oxford (1977).

10. Schackney, S. E., McCormack, G. W., and Cuchural, G. J. Growth rate patterns of solid tumors and their relation to responsiveness to therapy. *Ann. Intern. Med.*, 89:107-121 (1978).

11. Fidler, I. J. and Hart, I. R. Biological diversity in metastatic neoplasms: origins and implications. *Science*, 217:998-1003 (1982).

12. Day, R. A branching process model for heterogeneous cell populations. *Math. Biosci.*, 78:73-90 (1986).

13. Harris, T. E., *The Theory of Branching Processes*, Springer-Verlag, Berlin (1963).

14. Noye, J. Finite difference methods for partial differential equations, in *Numerical Solutions of Partial Differential Equations* (J. Noye, ed.), pp. 124-126, Elsevier North-Holland, New York (1982).

10

SIMEST
An Algorithm for Simulation-Based Estimation of Parameters Characterizing a Stochastic Process

JAMES R. THOMPSON   *Department of Statistics, Rice University, Houston, Texas*

E. NEELY ATKINSON and BARRY W. BROWN   *Department of Biomathematics, University of Texas System Cancer Center, M.D. Anderson Hospital and Tumor Institute, Houston, Texas*

I. INTRODUCTION

The axioms defining stochastic processes are generally simple. However, estimating the parameters of a process from data is extremely difficult if customary techniques are used. This is due to the complexities involved in obtaining closed forms of likelihoods and evaluating them. We develop an estimation technique which selects those parameters that produce simulations that best mimic the data. SIMEST makes stochastic process modeling in oncology (and other fields) an attractive alternative to such currently popular alternatives as ad hoc regression models.

   The first published work dealing with the estimation of a cumulative distribution function was John Graunt's tabulation of the probability of survival until given ages [1]. Thus the first analysis of probabilities based on the real number system used time data. This initial use may be connected with the empirical ordering of time. Unlike the three spatial variables, which are unordered in direction, the time dimension is not only ordered but irreversible. It is likely that this psychologically strong ordering property of time drew Graunt to use failure analysis as the world's first example of the representation of continuous data.

   Graunt's approach was empirical, representational, and without axiomatic underpinings. It was over 150 years later that Poisson [2]

began the study of the underlying mechanisms which generated stochastic processes. For the simplest cases, the parameters characterizing these mechanisms lend themselves readily to estimation from
data; but the more difficult models that can be used to model, for
example, an economy or a tumor system, have proved generally in-
tractable to such estimation. Hence, workers in these areas tend to
use empirical models, which are frequently linear, to describe
phenomena. This empirical approach has been generally fustrating,
frequently unstable, and all too often misleading. The inability to
perform satisfactory parameter estimation using the axiomatic approach
of Poisson has been taken for granted for so long that stochastic
process modeling is little used in fields where it is *the* natural
approach.

The position we take here is that it is the emphasis on obtaining
closed-form solutions of differential-difference-integral equations
resulting from the axiomatic approach that has caused its lack of
utilization. The usual axioms of stochastic processes describe
changes in the order in which they occur in time. In contrast, the
derivation of a likelihood function requires a backwards approach;
for each end state of the process, all paths which might have led to
it must be traced backwards in time. We propose as an alternative to
closed-form solutions the simulation of stochastic processes directly
from the assumptions used in their definition. Parameter estimation
is accomplished by systematically varying the values of the parameters of the process under investigation until the simulated values
are maximally concordant with the data.

Two sets of questions arise from this brief statement of the
method. First, how are the simulations to be performed and how is
the degree of agreement between simulated values and data to be
assessed? Second, what methods for systematically varying parameter values lead to an optimal accord with the data? Most of this
investigation is concerned with the numerous ramifications of the first
question. The second question, which can be restated as the problem of minimizing a function whose values can only be estimated with
error, is under intensive investigation. Some preliminary suggestions
are offered.

The primary advantage of the simulation method over closed-form
solutions is that it can be used even in cases in which closed-form
solutions are unknown. In addition, the intellectual effort necessary
to perform simulation from assumptions is much less than that required to derive exact likelihood equations. This is of great importance for cases in which a series of related models is examined.
The similarity of models generally assures that the simulation algorithims
implementing them are also similar; in contrast, the exact likelihood equation may change greatly with minor changes in the model.

Simulation methods are computationally intensive and require a
digital computer. As a practical matter, however, a computer is also
required for maximizing exactly obtained nonlinear likelihoods.

The methods described here were first presented in Atkinson et al. [3,4]. A statement of the overall problem very similar to that presented here appears in Diggle and Gratton [5]. Their simulation solution involved density estimation at each set of parameter values. A likelihood is then calculated from the estimated density. We feel that the density estimation is unnecessary (and it is computationally expensive); in addition, a bad choice of the smoothing parameter in the density estimation can cause instability in the estimation, leading to real time defaults to the user. There are simpler, cheaper, and more easily automated alternatives.

II. DISCUSSION

A. Poisson Modeling

Let us consider Poisson's simplest model. We shall be interested here in the number of failures as a function of time. Following Poisson, we use the following axioms:

(A1) The probability that one failure takes place in a time interval $[t, (t + \Delta t)]$ is given by $\theta \Delta t$.

(A2) The probability that two or more failures take place in $[t, (t + \Delta t)]$ is given by $o(\Delta t)$
(where $\lim_{\Delta t \to 0} o(\Delta t)/\Delta t = 0$.

(A3) (First-order stationarity)
$\Pr[k \text{ failures in } [t, (t + s)] = \Pr[k \text{ failures in } [u, u + s)]$
for all k, t, u, and s.

(A4) $\Pr[k \text{ failures in } [t, t + s] \text{ and } \ell \text{ failures in } [u, u + v)] = \Pr[k \text{ failures in } [t, t + s)] \Pr[\ell \text{ failures in } (u, u + v)]$
when the two intervals have no points in common.

We denote by $x(t)$ the number of failures in $[0, t)$. Then

$$\Pr[x(t + \Delta t) = k] \tag{1}$$

$$= \Pr[x(t) = k]\Pr[x(\Delta t) = 0] + \Pr[x(t) = k - 1]\Pr[x(\Delta t) = 1]$$
$$+ o(\Delta t)$$

$$= \Pr[x(t) = k][1 - \theta \Delta t] + \Pr[x(t) = k - 1]\theta \Delta t + o(\Delta t)$$

This yields

$$\frac{\Pr[x(t + \Delta t) = k] - \Pr[x(t) = k]}{\Delta t} = \theta[\Pr[x(t) = k - 1]$$
$$-\Pr[x(t) = k]] + \frac{o(\Delta t)}{\Delta t} \tag{2}$$

Letting $\Delta t \to 0$, we obtain the differential-difference equation

$$\frac{dPr[x(t) = k]}{dt} = \theta\{Pr[x(t) = k - 1] - Pr[x(t) = k]\} \tag{3}$$

By using integrating factors for $k = 0, 1, 2$, and 3, we can guess the solution

$$Pr[x(t) = k] = \frac{e^{-\theta t}(\theta t)^k}{k!} \tag{4}$$

which can be checked as correct by noting that (4) satisfies (3). We can use (4) to obtain the probability of at least one failure on or before t via the cumulative distribution function

$$F(t \mid \theta) = 1 - Pr[x(t) = 0] = 1 - e^{\theta t} \tag{5}$$

The density function for the first failure is readily obtained by differentiation to give

$$f(t \mid \theta) = F'(t \mid \theta) = \theta e^{-\theta t} \tag{6}$$

We note that the expectation (average) of t is given by

$$\mu = E(t) = \int_0^\infty tf(t \mid \theta)dt = \int_0^\infty t\theta e^{-\theta t}dt = \frac{1}{\theta} \tag{7}$$

In many situations we will have n independent observations $\{t_1 \leqslant t_2 \leqslant \cdots \leqslant t_n\}$ from which we wish to estimate the characterizing parameter(s) (in the example given, θ). There are a number of procedures available for this purpose

B. Method of Moments Estimation

Perhaps the oldest estimation technique, extensively investigated by Pearson [6], but in actuality used hundreds of years earlier, is the "method of moments." To explicate this view, we consider the empirical finite distribution which has probability function

$$p(t) = \frac{1}{n} \text{ if } t = t_j \text{ for } j = \{1, 2, \ldots, n\} \tag{8}$$

$$= 0, \text{ otherwise}$$

The expected value of t for this distribution is give simply by the sample mean

$$\bar{t} = \sum_{j=1}^{n} t_j p(t_j) = \frac{1}{n} \sum_{j=1}^{n} t_j \tag{9}$$

If we make the oversimplifying assumption that the empirical finite distribution represents not only what has occurred but what could occur, then we could use as the estimate for μ in (7) simply $\bar{t}$. This gives immediately

$$\hat{\theta} = \frac{1}{\bar{t}} \tag{10}$$

Although the method of moments is frequently satisfactory when the parameter θ being estimated is of low dimensionality, there are problems with its usage as the dimensionality increases. This is due, in part, to the fact that $1/n \sum_{j=1}^{n} t_j^m$ becomes less and less satisfactory as an approximation to $\int_0^\infty t^m f(t \mid \theta) \, dt$ as m increases.

C. Bayesian Estimation

Another estimation in frequent use is that based on Bayes theorem [7]. Here, we assume that, prior to any observation of failure times, our feelings as to the true value of $\theta = (\theta_1, \theta_2, \ldots, \theta_m)$ can be characterized by a *prior* probability density function $g(\theta)$. The joint density of θ and $(t_1, \ldots, t_n)$ is then given by

$$g(\theta) \prod_{j=1}^{n} f(t_j \mid \theta) = g(\theta) L(\theta \mid t_1, \ldots, t_n) \tag{11}$$

The term $L(\theta \mid t_1, \ldots, t_n)$ is called the *likelihood*.

Subsequent to the recording of the failure times, the *posterior* density of θ is

$$g(\theta \mid t_1, \ldots, t_n) = \frac{g(\theta) \prod_{j=1}^{n} f(t_j \mid \theta)}{\int \cdots \int g(\theta_1, \ldots, \theta_m) \prod_{j=1}^{n} f(t_j \mid \theta) \, d\theta_1 \cdots d\theta_m} \tag{12}$$

For reasons of "closure" as well as computational convenience, it is frequently decided to pick $g(\theta)$ so that $g(\theta \mid t_1, \ldots, t_n)$ will

be of the same functional form as $g(\theta)$. In such a case, g is called
a *natural conjugate* prior.

In the example considered in (6), the natural conjugate prior is
the gamma density

$$g(\theta) = \frac{\beta^{\alpha}}{\Gamma(\alpha)} e^{\theta\beta}\theta^{\alpha-1} \qquad 0 < \theta \qquad (13)$$

The posterior density given the n failure times is simply

$$g(\theta \mid t_1, \ldots, t_n) = \frac{g(\theta)\Pi_{j=1}^{n} f(t_j \mid \theta)}{\int_0^{\infty} g(\theta)\Pi_{j=1}^{n} f(t_j \mid \theta) \, d\theta}$$

$$= \frac{(n\bar{t} + \beta)^{n+\alpha}}{\Gamma(n+\alpha)} e^{-\theta(n\bar{t}+\beta)}\theta^{n+\alpha-1} \qquad (14)$$

Using the posterior distribution in (14), we have several candidates
for estimating θ. For example, the posterior mean is

$$E(\theta \mid t_1, \ldots, t_n) = \int_0^{\infty} \theta g(\theta \mid t_1, \ldots, t_n) \, d\theta = \frac{n+\alpha}{n\bar{t}+\beta} \qquad (15)$$

The value of θ which maximizes $g(\theta \mid t_1, \ldots, t_n)$ is the posterior
mode.

$$PM(\theta \mid t_1, \ldots, t_n) = \frac{n+\alpha-1}{n\bar{t}+\beta} \qquad (16)$$

We note that as n becomes very large, both these estimators become
approximately equal to $1/\bar{t}$.

One problem with Bayesian estimators is that it is frequently
difficult to incorporate "prior information" into a prior density $g(\theta)$.
Another difficulty is that if we do not have a ready conjugate prior
for θ, then Bayesian estimation frequently becomes cumbersome,
both computationally and perceptually.

D. Maximum Likelihood Estimation

If our information about θ is very vague, we may use (12) to derive
an estimator based purely on the likelihood. We assume that the
prior density $g(\theta)$ is

$$g(\theta_1, \ldots, \theta_m) = \prod_{i=1}^{m} \frac{1}{b_i - a_i} \qquad \text{when } a_i < \theta_i < b_i \text{ for all } i$$

$$= 0 \qquad \text{otherwise} \qquad (17)$$

We take a_i to be so small and b_i to be so large that we are practically certain that θ_i is contained in the interval (a_i, b_i). Then (12) becomes

$$g(\theta \mid t_1, \ldots, t_n) = \frac{\prod_{i=1}^{m}(b_i - a_i)^{-1}\prod_{j=1}^{n}f(t_j \mid \theta)}{\prod_{i=1}^{m}(b_i - a_i)^{-1}\int \cdots \int \prod_{j=1}^{n}f(t_j \mid \theta)\, d\theta}$$

$$\qquad (18)$$

$$= C(t_1, \ldots, t_n) \prod_{j=1}^{n} f(t_j \mid \theta)$$

$$= C(t_1, \ldots, t_n)L(\theta \mid t_1, \ldots, t_n)$$

Clearly, then, to maximize $g(\theta \mid t_1, \ldots, t_n)$ (i.e., to obtain the posterior mode of θ), we find the value of θ which maximizes the likelihood of $L(\theta \mid t_1, \ldots, t_n)$. Such an estimatior $\hat{\theta}$ is called a *maximum likelihood* estimator for θ. This type of derivation of the method of maximum likelihood is attributed by Fisher [8] to Gauss. For the example given in (6), then, the likelihood is

$$L(\theta \mid t_1, \ldots, t_n) = \theta^n \exp[(-n\bar{t}\,\theta)] \qquad (19)$$

The maximum likelihood estimator for θ is simply equal to $1/\bar{t}$.

A major difficulty with all the estimation procedures considered so far is their dependence on the assumption that the density $f(t \mid \theta)$ is known. As we shall demonstrate shortly, such an assumption is frequently unjustified. In his famous attacks on Bayesian estimation, R. A. Fisher [8] rejected the reasonableness of the Bayesian assumption of knowledge of a prior density $g(\theta)$. However, he was quite willing to presuppose that $f(t \mid \theta)$ would be available.

E. Simulation-Based Estimation

We return to the case in which $f(t \mid \theta)$ is not readily available, but there is a means of simulating failure times according to axioms presumed to govern the data. Using the sample $0 < t_1 < t_2 < \cdots < t_n$, we divide the time axis into k bins, the ℓth of which contain n_ℓ

observations. Assuming a value for Θ, we use the simulation mechanism SM(Θ) to generate a large number N of simulated failures $0 < s_1 < s_2 < \cdots < s_N$. The number of these observations which fall into the ℓth bin will be denoted by $\nu_{k\ell}$. If our selection of Θ was close to the truth, then the simulated bin probabilities

$$\hat{p}_{k\ell} = \frac{n_\ell}{n} \tag{20}$$

should approximate the corresponding proportion of data in the same bin,

$$\hat{p}_\ell = \frac{n_\ell}{n} \tag{21}$$

We shall call the asymptotic value of $\hat{p}_{k\ell}(\Theta)$ as N goes to infinity, $P_{k\ell}(\Theta)$.
Criteria are needed for assessing the deviation of the $\hat{p}_{k\ell}(\ell)$ from the $\hat{p}_\ell$. One criterion is the multinomial log-likelihood:

$$S_1^1(\Theta) = \ln n! - \sum_{j=1}^{k} \ln n_j! + \sum_{j=1}^{k} n_j \ln \hat{p}_{kj} \tag{22}$$

The simulated observations are used to estimate the probability, $\hat{p}_{kj}$, that an observation will fall in the jth bin. The expression shown is then the logarithm of the probability that for each j the jth bin will contain n_j observations. The first two terms in the expression for S_1 do not depend not on Θ but on the binned observations n_j. Consequently, we can drop them and use as the criterion the equivalent expression

$$S_1(\Theta) = \sum_{j=1}^{k} n_j \ln \hat{p}_{kj} \tag{23}$$

This log of the multinomial likelihood is maximized when

$$\hat{p}_{kj} = \frac{n_j}{n} = \hat{p}_j \tag{24}$$

i.e., when the simulated cell probabilities match those from the original sample.

The determination of the relative sizes of the k bins used to discretize the data has not be specified. There are reasons for using a binning scheme with equal numbers of observations in each bin. For example, this minimizes the chance of empty cells in the simulation. Moreover, setting $p_j = 1/k$ gives the Min Max $\text{Var}\{\hat{p}_k\}$. And equal binning (setting $p_j = 1/k$) guarantees that the expectation of $S_1(\Theta)$ does not increase for small perturbations of Θ from truth (i.e., the Gateaux variation is not positive). However, there are circumstances in which equal-sized binning is not practical. For example, the values of the dependent variable may be clustered because of inaccuracies in measurement or rounding. In this case the estimation procedure is enhanced if the division points for discretizing the data are chosen between clusters.

Now, expanding $\ln(\hat{p}_{ki})$ in a Taylor's series about p_{ki}, we have, discarding terms of $O(1/N^2)$, the following formula for the asymptotic variance of S_1:

$$\text{Var}[S_1(\Theta)] = \sum_{i=1}^{k} \sum_{j=1}^{k} \left. \frac{\partial S_1}{\partial \hat{p}_{ki}} \right|_{p_{ki}} \left. \frac{\partial S_1}{\partial \hat{p}_{kj}} \right|_{p_{kj}} \text{Cov}(\hat{p}_{ki}, \hat{p}_{kj}) \Big|_{p_{kij}p_{kj}}$$

$$= \sum_{i=1}^{k} \frac{1 - p_{ki}}{N p_{ki}} n_i^2 - 2 \sum_{i=1}^{k-1} \sum_{j=i+1}^{k} \frac{p_{ki}p_{kj}}{N p_{ki}p_{kj}} n_i n_j$$

$$= \frac{1}{N} \left[\sum_{i=1}^{k} \frac{1 - p_{ki}}{p_{ki}} n_i^2 - (n^2 - n_1^2 - n_2^2 - \cdots - n_k^2) \right]$$

(25)

which is minimized for $p_{ki} = n_i/n$ for all i.

Suppose for the remainder of this discussion that the bins are chosen so that $\hat{p}_i = 1/k$ for all i; then if Θ is close to the truth, the simulated bin probabilities should each approximate $1/k$. If for a given k, there is only one value of Θ such that for each ℓ

$$\lim_{\substack{n \to \infty \\ N \to \infty}} \hat{p}_{k\ell} = \frac{1}{k}$$

(26)

then we shall say that Θ is *k-identifiable*.

For the simple Poisson case in (5), the bin boundaries b_{n0}, $b_{n1}, \ldots, b_{nk}$ converge almost surely to

$$b_\ell \doteq \frac{-\ln(1 - \ell/k)}{\theta_0} \tag{27}$$

where θ_0 is the true value of θ. Suppose there is only one bin ($b_0 = 0$ and $b_1 = \infty$). Now for any value of θ all the simulated failures will fall into the bin. Consequently, in this case, θ is not 1-identifiable. For two bins, $b_0 = 0$, $b_2 = \infty$, and

$$b_1 = \frac{-\ln(1/2)}{\theta_0} \tag{28}$$

There is no value of θ other than θ_0 for which

$$\lim_{N \to \infty} \hat{p}_{k1}(\theta) = \frac{1}{2} \tag{29}$$

Consequently, for the simple Poisson distribution, θ is 2-identifiable. Moreover, for values of $k \geqslant 2$, θ is k-identifiable. If SM(θ) is k-identifiable, then a natural procedure for estimating θ is to pick the value that maximizes

$$S_2(\theta) = \sum_{1=1}^{k} \ln \hat{p}_{k\ell}(\theta) \tag{30}$$

Note that maximizing S_2 is equivalent to maximizing S_1 when all of the n_j are equal.

Typically, n, the size of the sample will be relatively small compared to N, the size of the simulation. It is clear that the number of bins, k, is a natural smoothing parameter. For example, for $k = 1$, $\text{Var}(\hat{p}_{11}) = 0$ for all n and N. The variability of $S_2(\theta)$ can be approximated by the asymptotic formula

$$\text{Var}[S_2(\theta)] = \sum_{i=1}^{k} \sum_{j=1}^{k} \left.\frac{\partial S_2}{\partial \hat{p}_{ki}}\right|_{p_{ki}} \left.\frac{\partial S_2}{\partial \hat{p}_{kj}}\right|_{p_{kj}} \text{Cov}(\hat{p}_{ki}, \hat{p}_{kj})\Big|_{p_{ki}, p_{kj}}$$

$$= \sum_{i=1}^{k} \frac{1}{p_{ki}^2(\theta)} \frac{p_{ki}(\theta)[1 - p_{ki}(\theta)]}{N}$$

$$- 2 \sum_{i=1}^{k-1} \sum_{j=k+1}^{k} \frac{p_{ki}(\theta)p_{kj}(\theta)}{N p_{ki}(\theta)p_{kj}(\theta)}$$

$$\sim \frac{1}{N} \left[\sum_{i=1}^{k} \frac{1 - \hat{p}_{ki}}{\hat{p}_{ki}} - k(k - 1) \right] \tag{31}$$

Now

$$E[S_2(\Theta)] \sim \sum_{i=1}^{k} \ln \hat{p}_{ki} \tag{32}$$

Thus we have a ready measure of a signal-to-noise ratio by

$$SN_2(k) = \frac{\left| E[S_2(\Theta)] \right|}{\sqrt{Var[S_2(\Theta)]}} \tag{33}$$

$$\sim \frac{\left| \sqrt{N} \, \Sigma_{i=1}^{k} \ln \hat{p}_{ki} \right|}{\sqrt{\Sigma_{i=1}^{k}(1 - \hat{p}_{ki})/\hat{p}_{ki} - k(k - 1)}}$$

Let us suppose that

$$\frac{\text{Max} \{p_{k\ell}\}}{\text{Min} \{p_{k\ell}\}} = M \tag{34}$$

Suppose ℓ of the bins have probability η and k-ℓ have probability $M\eta$. Then

$$Var[S_2(\Theta)] = \frac{1}{N} \left[\frac{(M - 1)\ell + k}{M\eta} - k^2 \right] \tag{35}$$

This variance is maximized for $\ell = k/2$. So for the "worst case,"

$$Var[S_2(\Theta)] = \frac{k^2}{N} \left[\frac{(M + 1)^2}{4M} - 1 \right] \tag{36}$$

and

$$E[S_2(\Theta)] = \frac{R}{2} mM - k \ln \left[\frac{(M + 1)k}{2} \right] \tag{37}$$

Thus

$$SN_2(k, M) = \frac{\sqrt{N} \, \left| \ln \{2\sqrt{M}/[k(M + 1)]\} \right|}{\sqrt{(M + 1)^2/(4M) - 1}} \tag{38}$$

Table 1   Values of $SN_2(k, M)/\sqrt{N}$

		M		
k	5	10	50	100
5	2.13	1.52	0.83	0.65
10	2.90	2.00	1.03	0.79
20	3.68	3.14	1.23	0.93
100	5.48	3.63	1.70	1.26

In Table 1 we show values of $SN_2(k, M)/\sqrt{N}$ for various k and M. Equation (38) gives us an indication of instabilities introduced by the simulation process for values of Θ away from the truth. For example, for M = 100 and 20 bins, a simulation size of 11,562 will be required to achieve a signal-to-noise ratio of 100. For M = 10, a simulation size of 1014 will achieve a SN_2 of 100. At any stage of the optimization algorithm we can use $Max\{\hat{p}_{kj}\}/Min\{\hat{p}_{kj}\}$ as a pessimistic estimate of M to achieve conservative estimates of the signal-to-noise ratio.

In practice there will be occasions where we have two values of Θ, say Θ_1 and Θ_2, and wish to know whether

$$\lim_{N_1 \to \infty} S_2(\Theta_1) > \lim_{N_2 \to \infty} S_2(\Theta_2) \tag{39}$$

Now, suppose for a particular pair of simulated sample sizes we do have

$$S_2(\Theta_1) > S_2(\Theta_2) \tag{40}$$

How do we know that this difference is significant? From (31) we can obtain $Var[S_2(\Theta_1)]$ and $Var[S_2(\Theta_2)]$. The variance of the difference is given approximately by

$$Var[S_2(\Theta_1) - S_2(\Theta_2)] = Var[S_2(\Theta_1)] + Var[S_2(\Theta_2)] \tag{41}$$

Thus, if

$$S_2(\Theta_1) - S_2(\Theta_2) > 2\sqrt{Var[S_2(\Theta_1) - S_2(\Theta_2)]} \tag{42}$$

we are reasonably confident that the difference is real and not due to simulation noise.

Example

Suppose we have two Θ's: Θ_1 and Θ_2. We have divided the sample of n failures into 10 bins and carried out simulations with sizes $N_1 = 900$ and $N_2 = 2500$. Suppose, moreover, the estimated cell probabilities are as shown in Table 2.

From (31) and (41) we have

$$\text{Var}[S_2(\Theta_1) - S_2(\Theta_2)] = \frac{3.5786}{900} + \frac{14.304}{2500} = 0.009678 \qquad [43]$$

giving

$$2\sqrt{\text{Var(Diff)}} = 0.196955$$

Moreover, from (30), $S_2(\Theta_1) = -23.1966$ and $S_2(\Theta_2) = -26.6579$. Since $S_2(\Theta_1) > S_2(\Theta_2) + 2\sqrt{\text{Var(Diff)}}$, we can be reasonably confident that the apparently preferred performance of Θ_1 is not simply due to simulation noise. If, however, the difference between $S_2(\Theta_1)$ and $S_2(\Theta_2)$ is not significant, we may increase the two simulation sizes to increase the signal-to-noise ratio. We note that if any cell is empty, $S_2(\Theta) = -\infty$ and is essentially not informative. Accordingly, we need a procedure to avoid using a mesh structure which is not

Table 2   Estimated Bin Probabilities

	Θ_1	Θ_2
$\hat{p}_{10,1}$	0.12	0.09
$\hat{p}_{10,2}$	0.08	0.11
$\hat{p}_{10,3}$	0.10	0.05
$\hat{p}_{10,4}$	0.12	0.08
$\hat{p}_{10,5}$	0.08	0.09
$\hat{p}_{10,6}$	0.09	0.05
$\hat{p}_{10,7}$	0.11	0.15
$\hat{p}_{10,8}$	0.07	0.11
$\hat{p}_{10,9}$	0.12	0.12
$\hat{p}_{10,10}$	0.11	0.15

too fine, particularly at the beginning of the iteration procedure, when we may be far from the optimum. One such procedure is to examine the $\{\hat{p}_{kj}\}$ for a choice of k (say 100). We then find the largest $\hat{p}_{kj}$, say M. Then starting at the leftmost bin if $\hat{p}_{kj} < M/100$, then combine bin j with bins to the right until the combined bins have total $\hat{p}_{k,j} + \hat{p}_{k,j+\ell} + \cdots + \hat{p}_{k,j+\ell} \geq M/100$. When this has been achieved, we replace each of $\hat{p}_{k,j}, \hat{p}_{k,j+1}, \cdots, \hat{p}_{k,j+\ell}$ with $(\hat{p}_{k,j} + \cdots + \hat{p}_{k,j+\ell})/(\ell + 1)$.

Another convenient criterion function is Pearson's goodness of fit

$$S_3(\theta) = \sum_{j=1}^{k} \frac{(\hat{p}_{kj} - \hat{p}_j)^2}{\hat{p}_j}$$

(44)

Obviously, this function is minimized when $\hat{p}_{kj} = \hat{p}_j$, for all j.

The function S_3 has an advantage over both S_1 and S_2. Suppose both $\hat{p}_2 = c\hat{p}_1$ and $\hat{p}_{k2} = c\hat{p}_{k2}$. Then S_3 is unchanged when the two cells are combined into a single cell.

Now we observe that the variability of each of the three criterion functions considered is nondecreasing in the number of cells, k (in the completely noninformative case when k = 1, each of the three criterion functions has zero variability). On the other hand, increasing k increases our ability to discriminate between the effectiveness of various θ's to produce simulations which mimic the behavior of the actual sample of failure times.

To demonstrate this fact, let us suppose that we consider the effect of combining the first two cells when S_3 is used. Let us suppose the "miss" of $\hat{p}_{k1} + \hat{p}_{k2}$ from $\hat{p}_1 + \hat{p}_2$ is an amount η. Then for the pooled sample, the contribution to S_3 is

$$\frac{\eta^2}{\hat{p}_1 + \hat{p}_2}$$

(45)

Now, for these cells uncombined, let

$$\hat{p}_{k1} = \hat{p}_1 + \frac{\hat{p}_1}{\hat{p}_1 + \hat{p}_2}\eta + \varepsilon\eta \qquad \hat{p}_{k2} = \hat{p}_2 + \frac{\hat{p}_2}{\hat{p}_1 + \hat{p}_2}\eta - \varepsilon\eta$$

(46)

In the uncombined case, the contribution to S_3 is

$$\frac{[\hat{p}_1/(\hat{p}_1 + \hat{p}_2) + \varepsilon]^2 \eta^2}{\hat{p}_1} + \frac{[\hat{p}_2/(\hat{p}_1 + \hat{p}_2) - \varepsilon]^2 \eta^2}{\hat{p}_2}$$

$$= \frac{1 + \varepsilon^2(\hat{p}_1 + \hat{p}_2)^2/\hat{p}_1\hat{p}_2}{\hat{p}_1 + \hat{p}_2} \eta^2 \geqslant \frac{\eta^2}{\hat{p}_1 + \hat{p}_2} \tag{47}$$

We note that only in the case where η is split between the two cells in proportion to $\hat{p}_1$ and $\hat{p}_2$ does a decrease in the number of cells fail to decrease S_3. Hence a decrease in the number of cells decreases our ability to tell us how well a simulation is mimicking the actual data. A similar argument holds for S_1 and S_2.

Naturally, a number of cells greater than the size of the actual sample would be a bad idea. As a practical matter, using the sufficient statistic $(t_1, t_2, \ldots, t_n)$ to give the cell boundaries $(0, t_1)$, $(t_1, t_2), \ldots, (t_n, \infty)$ would generally be extreme. We recall that our strategy is to select a value of Θ which gives a simulation mimicking the sample. But, in a broader sense, we seek to mimic samples which *could have happened*. For n large, $F(t \leqslant t_j)$ will be very near j/n *except for j nearly 0 or for j close to n.* For these values of j, the t_j are poor estimators for the j/n'tiles of $F(\cdot)$. Thus for the leftmost and rightmost bins, we might be well advised to see to it that at least 1% of the sample observations are included in each.

We now address the issue of a practical means of obtaining a 95% confidence set for the true value of Θ. Once the algorithm has converged to a value, say $\hat{\Theta}$, we then use this value to generate M simulated data sets of size n. We then determine

$$\bar{S}_j = \frac{1}{M} \sum_{i-1}^{M} S_j(\hat{\Theta}, T_i) \tag{48}$$

$$s_{S_j}^2 = \frac{1}{M} \sum_{T=1}^{M} [S_j(\hat{\Theta}, T_i) - \bar{S}_j]^2 \tag{49}$$

where T_i denotes the ith simulated data set of size n and T_0 is the actual sample. Then with roughly 95% certainty

$$S_j(\Theta) = \bar{S}_j \pm \frac{2}{\sqrt{M}} s_{S_j} \tag{50}$$

Next, using $\hat{\Theta}$ as the center of a rotatable design, we fit the quadratic curve

$$S_j(\Theta) = A + B\Theta + C\Theta'\Theta \tag{51}$$

The 95% confidence set for Θ can now be approximated by

$$S_j(\hat{\Theta}, T_0) - \frac{2}{\sqrt{M}} s_{S_j} \leqslant A + B\Theta + C\Theta'\Theta \leqslant S_j(\hat{\Theta}, T_0) + \frac{2}{\sqrt{M}} s_{S_j} \tag{52}$$

III. AN APPLICATION

A. Metastatic Versus Systemic Secondary Tumor Generation

Let us now consider a stochastic process model for the description of the occurrence and growth of secondary tumors. The model was motivated by Ref. 10, in which there was an indication that the hazard of discovery of secondary tumors after removal of the primary appeared to be nearly constant in time. This led to the postulating of a model [11] in which secondary tumors were sometimes produced by a systemic mechanism with constant intensity in addition to, rather than solely by, an accepted metastatic process whose intensity is proportional to primary tumor size. We had data sets in which we had records of the time from the removal of the primary tumor to the first discovery of a secondary tumor. The model was based on four axioms:

H1. For each patient each tumor originates from a single cell and grows exponentially at rate α.

H2. The probability that a tumor of size $Y_j(t)$, not previously detected and removed to time t, is detectable in $[t, t + \Delta]$ is $bY_j(t)\Delta + o(\Delta)$.

H3. Until the removal of the primary the probability of metastasis in $[t, t + \Delta]$ is a $Y_0(t)\Delta$.

H4. The probability of systemic occurrence of a tumor in $[t, t + \Delta]$ is $\lambda\Delta + o(\Delta)$, independent of the prior history of the patient.

We note that these axioms are simple, rather like the axioms of the simplest Poisson process given in A1–A4. Clearly, the item of major interest is the estimation of the four parameters: α, b, a, and λ. Now if we seek to use maximum likelihood as the estimation technique, we find ourselves confronted by a complex multiterm expression. One of these terms is

$$P(T_1 = S', T_2 > S) = \int\int e^{w(S-S')} p(t; 1)p(S'; e^{\alpha u})[\lambda + ae^{\alpha(t-u)}]$$

$$\times \exp\left[-\lambda(t - u) - \frac{a}{\alpha}(e^{\alpha(t-u)} - 1)\right]$$

$$\times H[v(S - S'); S'; e^{\alpha u}]H[v(S - S')e^{\alpha S'};u,e^{\alpha(t-u)}]$$

$$\times du\ dt + \int\int e^{w(S-S')}p(t; 1)\exp\left[-\lambda t - \frac{a}{\alpha}(e^{\alpha t} - 1)\right]$$

$$\times \lambda e^{-\lambda u}p(S' - u; 1)H[v(S - S'); S' - u; 1]\ du\ dt$$

$$(53)$$

where

$$H(s;t,z) = \exp\left\{\frac{az}{\alpha}e^{\alpha t}(e^s - 1)\log[1 + e^{-s}(e^{-\alpha t} - 1)] \right. \quad (54)$$

$$\left. + \frac{\lambda s}{\alpha} - \frac{\lambda}{\alpha}\log[1 + e^{\alpha t}(e^s - 1)]\right\} \quad (55)$$

$$p(t; z) = bze^{\alpha t}\exp\left[-\left[\frac{bz}{\alpha}(e^{\alpha t} - 1)\right]\right]$$

$$w(y) = \lambda\left[\int_0^y e^{-v(u)}du - y\right] \quad (56)$$

and v(u) is determined from

$$u = \int_0^v (a + b + \alpha s - ae^{-s})^{-1}\ ds \quad (57)$$

The order of computational complexity here is roughly that of four-dimensional quadrature. This is near the practical limit of contemporary mainframe computers. The CPU time required (using STEPIT [11]) in the estimation algorithm was approximately 2 hours on the CYBER 173.

The other classical estimation procedures mentioned in this paper also present enormous complexities. We see at a glance the reason that stochastic process modeling has proved so marginal as a practical device in oncology, economics, etc. Typically, the simple axioms associated with these models lead to incredible tangles in the likelihood, moment generating functions, etc. The very problem of getting to the quadrature representation of the likelihood requires enormous human labor. And if another parameter is added in the axioms, we can expect yet another quadrature dimension.

Hypotheses H1–H4 lend themselves very well to a simulation of the times of occurrence of secondary tumors. This is hardly surprising, since they were formulated to describe the probabilities that events will or will not occur at a specified time.

To give a flowchart of the simulation process, let us first define some relevant random variables.

$$W_D = \text{time of detection of primary} \tag{58}$$

$$W_M = \text{time of origin of first metastasis}$$

$$W_S = \text{time of origin of first systemic tumor}$$

$$W_R = \text{time of origin of first recurrent tumor}$$

$$W_d^* = \text{time from } W_R \text{ to detection of first recurrent tumor}$$

$$W_D^* = \text{time from } W_D \text{ to detection of first recurrent tumor}$$

We generate all random variables by first generating u from a uniform distribution on the interval [0, 1]. Then we set $t = F^{-1}(u)$, where F is the appropriate cumulative distribution function. The tumor volume at time t is

$$v(t) = ce^{\alpha t} \tag{59}$$

Here, c is the volume of one cell. It follows from the hypotheses that

$$F_D(t) = 1 - \exp\left[-\int_0^t bce^{\alpha t}\, dt\right] = 1 - \exp\left[-\frac{bc}{a} e^{\alpha t}\right] \tag{60}$$

$$F_M(t) = 1 - \left[\exp\ -\frac{ac}{\alpha} e^{at}\right] \tag{61}$$

$$F_S(t) = 1 - \exp[-\lambda t] \tag{62}$$

$$F_d^*(t) = 1 - \exp\left[-\frac{bc}{\alpha} e^{\alpha t}\right] \tag{63}$$

We can now write our simulation algorithm straightaway:

SM   Input α, λ, a, b

   Repeat until $s > 0$

   Generate W_D

   Generate W_M

   If $W_M > W_D$, then $W_M \leftarrow \infty$

   Generate W_S

   $W_R \leftarrow \min(W_M, W_S)$

   Generate W_d^*

   $W_D^* \leftarrow W_R + W_d^* - W_D$

   $s = W_D^*$

   If $s < 0$, discard

   End repeat

   Return s (64)

Using the actual sample $t_1 < t_2 \leq \cdots < t_n$, we can generate k bins, each with apparent probabilities $\hat{p}_1, \hat{p}_2, \ldots, \hat{p}_k$. Now letting $\Theta = (\alpha, a, b, \lambda)$, we can use $SM(\Theta)$ N times to generate a simulation of N recurrences $s_1 < s_2 < \cdots < s_N$.

The numbers of simulated detections in each of these bins will be denoted by $\nu_{k1}, \nu_{k2}, \ldots, \nu_{kk}$. The simulated bin probabilities $\hat{p}_{k1}, \hat{p}_{k2}, \ldots, \hat{p}_{kk}$ are then computed by

$$\hat{p}_{kj} = \frac{\nu_{kj}}{N} \tag{65}$$

Now, using $S_1(\Theta)$, $S_2(\Theta)$, $S_3(\Theta)$, or some other reasonable criterion, we are in a position to ascertain how well our guessed value of Θ mimics the behavior of the sample.

The simulation SM embodies a simplifying assumption utilized by Bartoszyński, Brown, and Thompson [10], which employed a "closed-form" likelihood approach. This assumption is that the first secondary tumor generated is the first secondary tumor observed. Even with this assumption, the terms in the likelihood are almost too complicated for practical computational purposes [see (53)].

Note that with simulation this assumption can be easily be eliminated by the flowchart

SM2   Generate W_D (66)

        $j = 0$

        $i = 0$

        Repeat until $W_M(j) > W_D$

        $j = j + 1$

        Generate $W_M(j)$

        Generate $W_{dM}^*(j)$

        $W_{dM}^*(i) \leftarrow W_{dM}^*(i) + W_M(i)$

        If $W_{dM}^*(j) < W_D$, then $W_{dM}^*(j) \leftarrow \infty$

        Repeat until $W_S(i) > 10W_D$

        $i = i + 1$

        Generate $W_{dS}^*(i)$

        $W_{dS}^*(i) \leftarrow W_{dS}^*(i) + W_S(i)$

        If $W_{dS}^*(i) < W_D$, then $W_{dS}^*(i) \leftarrow \infty$

        $s \leftarrow \min[W_{dm}^*(j), W_{dS}^*(i)]$

        Return s

        End Repeat   (67)

In (67) we generate an array of metastasis detection times $\{W_{dM}^*(j)\}$ and systemic detection times $\{W_{dS}^*(i)\}$ and pick the smallest of these as the first detection time of a secondary. The SIMEST approach enables us to increase the complexity of the underlying model at modest cost to the simulation algorithm. For example, suppose we wished to add a fifth axiom:

H5   A fraction, γ, of the patients ceases to be at systemic risk at the time of removal of the primary tumor if no secondary tumors exist at that time. A fraction, $1 - \gamma$, of the patients remains at systemic risk throughout their lives.

The revised set of axioms H1–H5 can then be simulated via

SM3   Generate u from $U(0,1)$

        If $u > \gamma$, then proceed as in SM2

        If $u < \gamma$, then proceed as in SM2 except replace the step

"Repeat until $W_S(i) > 10W_D$"

with the step

"Repeat until $W_S(i) > W_D$"

An endless array of other modifications to the axiomatic system can be made at little cost to simulation complexity. Most of these modifications would cause an investigator essentially to start from the beginning to come up with a new closed-form likelihood function. This is a simple manifestation of the fact that simulation follows the forward and modular nature of the axioms, whereas the determination of the likelihood does not.

Moreover, SIMEST allows for easy collection of additional useful information. For example, by simple bookkeeping, we can observe what fraction of the discovered secondary tumors are metastatic in origin. We can also record the sizes of simulated tumors at their times of detection.

B. Optimization Methods

The problem of minimizing functions whose value can only be observed subject to noise is under intense investigation at M. D. Anderson Hospital. In the present application, parameter estimation in stochastic processes, the noise is simulation induced. Consequently we have the option of noise reduction by increasing the simulation size. When we are using equal-sized bins from the original sample, the signal-to-noise ratio is high near the true value of Θ. When we are so far from Θ that the simulation bin probabilities are vastly different, simulation noise is a serious problem.

In this study we have used robust, although slow, direct search optimization methods in our investigation of the methods presented. The two algorithms which have been most used are the simplex method of Nelder and Mead [12] and the more sophisticated method STEPIT [11] of John Chandler. We are examining modifications of these methods to handle noise, but we have not progressed to the point of reporting these modifications.

More recently developed algorithms such as the optimal locally constrained methods of Gay [13] are, in general, considerably faster than direct search methods. However, these algorithms rely upon derivative information calculated either explicitly from formal differentiation or implicitly by function evaluation. The effect of noise on derivative information can be catastrophic unless regression is used instead of finite differences. Such modifications are being pursued but are in an early stage of development. Because methods relying on derivatives are not expected to work at all well without extensive modification, they are not further pursued here.

In the examples presented in the next section, STEPIT was used, unmodified for the presence of noise. Noise can cause this method (and any other method not designed to handle noise) to veer off in incorrect directions and to converge prematurely. However, STEPIT's behavior in the presence of noise appears reasonably robust.

A brief outline of the algorithm employed by STEPIT (taken from its documentation) is as follows. At each base point, STEPIT varies each parameter value individually up and down. If either variation yields an improvement, the step size is doubled and another step is taken. The number of such steps allowed is limited. When a local minimum has been bracketed by this process, quadratic interpolation is used to attempt to refine the position of the minimum. Should this process yield a better value, the base point is moved to this value. If varying the individual parameter values leads to no improvement in the objective function, the step size is decreased. The algorithm terminates when the step size becomes smaller than a user-specified minimum.

If the examination of one parameter at a time yields a change in at least two different values, the resultant direction of the changes is calculated, and steps in this direction are attempted. Again, success causes the step size to be doubled, and quadratic interpolation is attempted when a minimum has been bracketed. The steps taken in this fashion sometimes oscillate, and STEPIT attempts to detect and shortcut these zigzags.

1. Numeric Examples

Since the intent of this work is to explicate a class of methods rather than to demonstrate results from cancer data, simulated data from the metastatic-systemic model is used. A real cancer data base is analyzed in [3]. The parameter values chosen for this simulation are taken from a data set which was fit using the cumbersome exact likelihood equations, namely $\alpha = 0.31$, $b = .23 \times 10^{-8}$, $\beta = 0.17 \times 10^{-9}$ and $\lambda = 0.003$. These values are appropriate for time in units of months and tumor volumes in units of number of cells.

With these values, about 91% of the secondary tumors are due to the systemic process, and only the remaining 9% are due to the volume-dependent metastatic process. This poses a somewhat difficult problem for fitting, because the first three model parameters produce only a minor effect on the vast majority of the data.

In the fit, one-half was added to all bins after each simulation with a specified set of parameters in order to avoid attempts to take a logarithm of zero in calculating the criterion function value. Initial step sizes were set at half of the initial value of the parameters; convergence is achieved when these step sizes decrease to 1% of the initial parameter values. Starting values were produced by varying a subset of the parameters upward or downward by a factor of 3 from the values used to simulate the data. In the explorations conducted it required 50 to 100 function evaluations to obtain convergence.

Censoring was not considered when simulating data sets to be fit; i.e., there is an unlimited follow-up time, and all cases eventually fail. Of course, with actual clinical data, censoring is very much a problem, and there are two ways that it can be handled. One, suitable for the quasi-likelihood criterion, S_1, is to add terms to the criterion representing the probability that the time is at least that observed. This corresponds precisely to the modification of the usual likelihood for censoring.

The second method, suitable for all of the criteria discussed, is to spread the failure time of each censored observation equally among the failure times that are larger than the censoring time. Should a censoring time exceed all failure times, it can be given an arbitrarily large value; since the last bin includes all large values, the particular choice of this value is not important. Whether or not the data contains censored observations, the simulations performed in fitting the data should not, because such censoring would amount to throwing away information available from the axioms and choise of parameter values.

Five hundred cases were generated with the parameters stated; these were used as the data in exploring the fitting methods. The data were placed into 20 bins, the boundaries of which were chosen so that each contained 25 data points. Five thousand cases were simulated at each parameter value to evaluate the criterion used, which was the quasi-likelihood S_1. Replication of the criterion evaluation at the values used to generate the data gave a standard deviation of the criterion of 1.1.

The behavior of the fitting algorithm is quite evidently strongly determined by the starting values used for the fit. For example, initial estimates of $(0.103, .8 \times 10^{-9}, .57 \times 10^{-10}, .003)$ converged to parameter values of $(.309, .22 \times 10^{-8}, .81 \times 10^{-10}, .003)$. (The vector notation used lists parameter values in the order α, b, β, and λ.) These values are quite near those used to generate the data, the quasi-likelihood at these values was less than one greater than the mean value obtained at the values used to generate the data, and a chi-square goodness of fit test yields an acceptable value. Hence, the fit is quite good. However, starting from $(.93, .69 \times 10^{-8}, .51 \times 10^{-9}, .003)$, the fitting algorithm converged to $(2.84, .42 \times 10^{-7}, .26 \times 10^{-9}, .0029)$. The quasi-likelihood was 26 units less than that obtained from the values used to generate the data, and the goodness of fit statistic did not show an acceptable fit. (Note that this criterion can be used with actual data for which the true parameter values are not known.) This perplexing behavior

caused an attempt to reduce the dimensionality of the problem in
order to obtain some understanding of the behavior of the fitting
algorithm.

The parameter λ is easily estimated from the data. It is the
slope of the logarithm of the survival curve for large times. Experimentation with the stated data set and others indicated that fitting
from a variety of starting points produced good estimates of this
parameter even when the others were bad. Having this estimate reduces the dimension of the fitting problem from four parameters to
three.

Additional information is available, both from clinical observation
and the simulation; this is the size of the primary tumor at detection,
and it can be used to connect parameters α and b by the following
argument:

By hypothesis H1, the volume of the primary tumor at time t
after its origination, $Y_0(t)$, is

$$Y_0(t) = \exp(c\alpha t) \tag{69}$$

where c is the volume of a single cell (which is 1 in the units being
used). By hypothesis H2 the detection of the primary tumor is a
nonhomogeneous Poisson process with intensity $bY_0(t)$. Thus the
probability of no detection of the primary tumor to time t

$$\exp\left(-\int_0^t bY_0(u) \, du\right) = \exp\left(-\int_0^t bc \exp(\alpha u) \, du\right)$$

$$= \exp\left(-\frac{b}{\alpha} [Y_0(t) - Y_0(0)]\right) \tag{70}$$

The term $Y_0(0)$, which equals c, the volume of a single cell, is
negligible compared to $Y_0(t)$, the volume of the tumor at detection.
Dropping this term, using the fact that in the units used c is 1.0,
and taking the negative derivative with respect to Y_0 show that the
density of the volume of the primary tumor at detection at any size
y to be

$$\frac{b}{\alpha} \exp\left[-\frac{b}{\alpha} y\right] \tag{71}$$

This is recognized as an exponential distribution with mean α/b.
Consequently, the mean observed volume of the primary tumor at
detection is a maximum likelihood estimate of α/b. For the simulated
data, this mean is 1.36×10^8 cells. (When using clinical data, we assume

that there are 10^9 cells/cm^3.) For comparison, the ratio obtained from the values used to simulate the data is 1.348×10^8.

The reduction in dimension for starting estimates of the param-eter does not solve the problem of the bad fits that were obtained before, because the starting values for the fits met the constraints of the reduction. Enforcement of these constraints is also not a solution, because the behavior of the fitting method is much the same with and without such constraints. The problem appears to be fundamentally difficult.

The separate estimation of λ and α/b allows contours of the quasi-likelihood surface to be produced. Figures 1 and 2 show these con-tours as a function of α and β (β is multiplied by 10^9 in the fig-ures). Figure 1 uses the same seed for the random number generator for each parameter value. Figure 2 allows this seed to vary from value to value and thus shows the fluctuation of quasi-likelihood value due to the simulation process.

It is evident from these figures that the likelihood is well be-haved in a reasonably sized neighborhood of the true values, par-ticularly for small values of α. In this region it steeply climbs to its optimal value. Outside of this region, however, the behavior is erratic, and the criteiron changes very slowly. This maps well to the findings from the fits.

In an attempt to discover whether this behavior is due to random behavior in generating the data set, another data set of 20,000 ob-servations was generated with the same parameters. This data was categorized into 99 bins. The behavior on this data set was close to that of the original. Using the same starting values that led to bad estimates in the original, the estimates obtained are (7.91, .59 $\times 10^{-7}$, .51 $\times 10^{-9}$, .003), and the fit was not acceptable.

2. Two-Dimensional Binning

Another attempt to improve the situation was to use the volume of the primary tumor at detection as well as the time to the secondary tumor in estimating the parameter values from 500 simulated observa-tions; handling a two-dimensional outcome is a straightforward exten-sion of the methods presented. The observed volumes were divided into 4 equally sized categories, the times to secondary tumors into 10 categories; the data was binned into the 40 divisions formed by the cartesian product of these categories, and the binned data was then fit by simulation using the quasi-likelihood criterion. This re-sulted in a modest improvement in performance over the time data alone, in that the estimates obtained were not as far from those used to generate the data as when time alone was used. These estimates were (3.75, 0.28 $\times 10^{-7}$, .54 $\times 10^{-9}$, .003); however, these estimates were not acceptable.

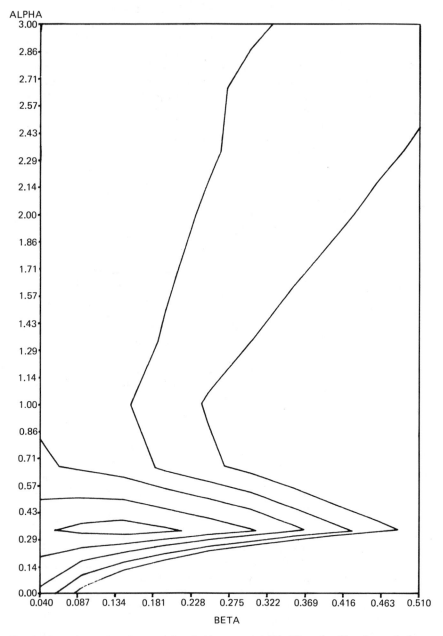

FIGURE 10.1   Contours of relative quasi-likelihood, fixed seed for random number generation.

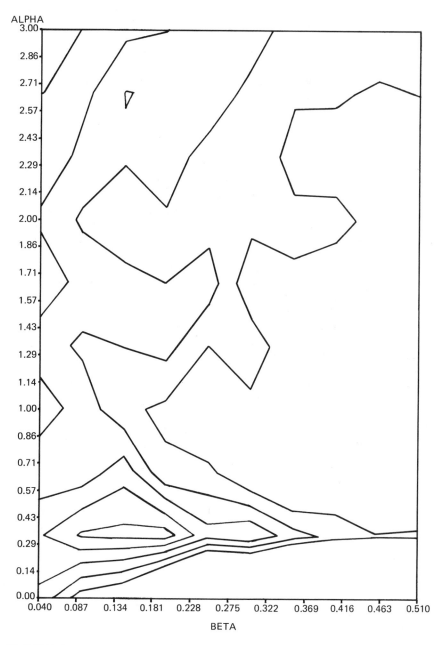

FIGURE 10.2   Contours of relative quasi-likelihood, varying seed
for random number generation.

This finding would tend to indicate that most of the information in the volume data has been extracted in estimating α/b, so the use of this data does not add appreciably to time alone. However, in many cases it will not be possibly to simply extract the relevant information for auxiliary variables, and using such variables as additional outcome information will greatly enhance the ability to estimate the process parameters.

IV. CONCLUSIONS

High-speed digital computing has made little impact on the modeling process. Scientists, for the most part, continue to follow the same steps taken by their precomputer age predecessors, generally transforming axioms into a differential-integral equation representation. From this representation, numerical techniques are used to give pointwise evaluations of a function. These, in turn, can be used to estimate the parameters which characterize the system. If these steps become too complex (and generally they do), the investigator can throw up his or her hands and use an ad hoc regression model.

In this chapter we have shown how simulation can be used to proceed rapidly from the axioms to the estimation of the characterizing parameters. This concept is, on the one hand, a drastic departure from precomputer age methodology. On the other hand, it simply extends the power of Karl Pearson's concept of goodness of fit. SIMEST enables the estimation of parameters in models far more complex than those tractable in Pearson's day.

We believe that we are fast approaching the time when the potential of high-speed computing to change, fundamentally, the modeling process will be realized. SIMEST is hopefully a step in this direction.

ACKNOWLEDGMENTS

This work was supported in part by the United States Army Research Office (Durham) under DAAG-29-85-K-012, the National Cancer Institute under CA11430, the office of Naval Research under N00014-85-K-0100, and Cray Research, Inc. The authors acknowledge with gratitude the expert word processing of Ms. Betty Schwarz, who created the original of this paper in the TEX language.

REFERENCES

1. Graunt, John, *Natural and Political Observations on the Bills of Mortality* (1662).
2. Poisson, Simeon Denis, *Recherches sur la Probabilité des Jugements* (1837).

3. Atkinson, E. Neely, Bartoszyński, Robert, Brown, Barry W., and Thompson, James R., Simulation techniques for parameter estimation in tumor related stochastic processes, in *Proceedings of the 1983 Computer Simulation Conference,* North-Holland, New York, pp. 754–757 (1983).

4. Atkinson, E. Neely, Bartoszyński, Robert, Brown, Barry W., and Thompson, James R., Maximum likelihood techniques, in *Proceedings of the 44th Meeting of the International Statistical Institute,* Contributed Papers, 2, pp. 494–497 (1983).

5. Diggle, P. J. and Gratton, R. J., Monte Carlo methods of inference for implicit statistical models. *J. R. Statist. Soc. B,* 46:193–227 (1984).

6. Pearson, Karl. Contributions to the mathematical theory of evolution. II. Skew variation in homogeneous material. *Phil. Trans. Roy. Soc. London, Ser. H.,* 186:343–414 (1895).

7. Bayes, Thomas, *Facsimiles of Two Papers by Bayes,* Hafner, New York (1983).

8. Fisher, Ronald, A. *Statistical Methods for Research Workers,* Oliver and Boyd, Edinburgh, p. 21 (1958).

9. Bartoszyński, Robert, Brown, Barry W., McBride, Charles, and Thompson, James R., Some nonparametric techniques for estimating the intensity function of a cancer related nonstationary Poisson process. *Ann. Stat.* 9:1050–1060 (1981).

10. Bartoszyński, Robert, Brown, Barry W., and Thompson, James R., Metastatic and systemic factors in neoplastic progression, in *Probability Models and Cancer* (LeCam and Neyman, eds.), North-Holland, New York, pp. 253–264 (1982).

11. Chandler, J. P., STEPIT, *Behavioral Science, 14*:81 (1969).

12. Nelder, J. A., and Mead, R. A simplex method for function minimization. *Comput. J.,* 7:308–313 (1965).

13. Gay, D. M., Algorithm 611—subroutines for unconstrained minimization using a model/trust region approach. *ACM Trans. Math. Software,* 9:160–169 (1983).

Index